Microsurgical Carotid Endarterectomy

Microsurgical Carotid Endarterectomy

Editors

Julian E. Bailes, M.D.
Department of Neurological Surgery
Allegheny General Hospital
Pittsburgh, Pennsylvania

Robert F. Spetzler, M.D.
Division of Neurological Surgery
Barrow Neurological Institute
Phoenix, Arizona

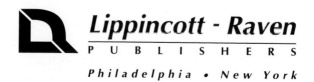

Lippincott - Raven
PUBLISHERS

Philadelphia • New York

Lippincott - Raven Publishers, 227 East Washington Square, Philadelphia, Pennsylvania 19106

Printed in Hong Kong

Library of Congress Cataloging-in-Publication Data

Microsurgical carotid endarterectomy / editors, Julian E. Bailes,
   Robert F. Spetzler.
      p. cm.
   Includes bibliographical references and index.
   ISBN 0-7817-0149-X
   1. Carotid artery—Surgery. 2. Endarterectomy. 3. Microsurgery.
 I. Bailes, Julian E. II. Spetzler, Robert F. (Robert Friedrich),
1944—   .
   [DNLM: 1. Endarterectomy, Carotid. WG 595.5.C2 M626 1995]
 RD598.65.M53 1995
 617.4'13—dc20
 DNLM/DLC
 for Library of Congress   95-7242

9 8 7 6 5 4 3 2 1

Contents

Contributors

Arvind Ahuja, M.D., *Department of Neurological Surgery, Allegheny General Hospital, 320 East North Avenue, Pittsburgh, Pennsylvania 15212*

John A. Anson, M.D., *Assistant Professor, Division of Neurosurgery, University of New Mexico, 2211 Lomas Boulevard, NE, Albuquerque, New Mexico 87131*

Paul J. Apostilides, M.D., *Division of Neurological Surgery, Barrow Neurological Institute, 350 West Thomas Road, Phoenix, Arizona 85013*

Julian E. Bailes, M.D., *Department of Neurological Surgery, Allegheny General Hospital, 320 East North Avenue, Pittsburgh, Pennsylvania 15212*

Jon Brillman, M.D., *Department of Neurology, Medical College of Pennsylvania and Hahnemann University, Allegheny General Hospital, Suite 206, 420 East North Avenue, Pittsburgh, Pennsylvania 15212*

Edwin D. Cacayorin, M.D., *Department of Radiology, Medical College of Pennsylvania and Hahnemann University, Allegheny General Hospital, 320 East North Avenue, Pittsburgh, Pennsylvania 15212*

Donalee A. Davis, C.N.R.N., *Department of Neurovascular Diagnostic Ultrasound, Allegheny General Hospital, 320 East North Avenue, Pittsburgh, Pennsylvania 15212*

Christopher N. Faber, M.D., *Department of Medicine, Allegheny General Hospital, Suite 210, 490 East North Avenue, Pittsburgh, Pennsylvania 15212*

James K. Lanz, M.D., *Department of Medicine, Allegheny General Hospital, Suite 210, 490 East North Avenue, Pittsburgh, Pennsylvania 15212*

Paul LoBaugh, M.D., *Department of Neuroanesthesia, Allegheny General Hospital, Pittsburgh, Pennsylvania 15212-9986*

Patrick W. McCormick, M.D., *The Toledo Hospital; Suite 311, 2213 Cherry Street, Toledo, Ohio 43608*

John R. Robinson, Jr., *Division of Neurological Surgery, Barrow Neurological Institute, 350 West Thomas Road, Phoenix, Arizona 85013-4496*

William E. Rothfus, M.D., *Department of Radiology, Medical College of Pennsylvania and Hahnemann University, Allegheny General Hospital, 320 East North Avenue, Pittsburgh, Pennsylvania 15212*

Thomas F. Scott, M.D., *Medical College of Pennsylvania and Hahnemann University, East Wing Office Building, Suite 206, 420 East North Avenue, Allegheny General Hospital, Pittsburgh, Pennsylvania 15212*

Robert F. Spetzler, M.D., *Division of Neurological Surgery, Barrow Neurological Institute, 350 West Thomas Road, Phoenix, Arizona 85013*

Edward Teeple, Jr., M.D., M.B.A., *Department of Neuroanesthesia, Medical College of Pennsylvania and Hahnemann University, Allegheny General Hospital, 320 East North Avenue, Pittsburgh, Pennsylvania 15212*

Antonios Zikos, M.D., *Department of Medicine, Allegheny General Hospital, Suite 210, 490 East North Avenue, Pittsburgh, Pennsylvania 15212*

Preface

The medical and surgical treatment of cerebrovascular accidents continue to challenge physicians. Our quest for detection and successful treatment of strokes is heightened by our ever-aging population. Although it has been 40 years since carotid endarterectomy was first performed, we are still debating its efficacy and indications in certain situations. The recent publication of several multicenter trials demonstrating the beneficial effects of the operation, especially in symptomatic patients with significant carotid stenosis, has focused this debate.

The procedure of carotid endarterectomy has often been considered as merely a method of increasing ipsilateral cerebral blood flow and of removing angiographically visualized stenoses. Our current knowledge has progressed to allow us to analyze in detail the entire cerebral vascular supply, beginning at the aortic arch and continuing through to the cerebral microcirculation. In conjunction with the neuroradiological investigation, we are able to individualize treatment according to the clinical manifestations of each patient's embolic or hemodynamic phenomena. The past few years have seen tremendous advances in areas such as magnetic resonance angiography, transcranial Doppler ultrasound, critical care medicine, cardiology, anesthesiology, and other areas. These have greatly added to our ability to successfully accomplish carotid endarterectomy in order to improve the natural history of the untreated disease.

Progress is often based on the simplest concepts. Frontiers are pushed forward as much by the application of the familiar to unfamiliar context by the development of sophisticated new technologies. Incorporating the simple concept of magnification into the operative suite has rendered surgery safer and easier. It is astonishing to recall how few years have passed since the use of the operating microscope has become standard in neurosurgery.

The application of the operating microscope has evolved naturally from its use in procedures such as lumbar microdiscectomy and extracranial–intracranial bypasses to its use during carotid endarterectomies for the treatment of carotid atherosclerosis. Clinical series have shown that the technique is effective and reduces the technical difficulties associated with the procedure, thereby leading to fewer postoperative complications. When used appropriately, microsurgical endarterectomy holds great promise for appropriate patients and should become part of the standard vascular armamentarium. This book was designed to make the technique accessible by comprehensively considering the course and treatment of carotid artery disease.

First, we review the epidemiology, natural history, and controversies of carotid stenosis. Once the reader understands these issues, the principles underlying diagnosis with the appropriate imaging modalities—both conventional carotid angiography and the newer noninvasive techniques for imaging the carotid artery, such as magnetic resonance imaging and MR angiography—are discussed. Likewise, the preoperative evaluation of the surgical candidate is reviewed. Current indications are included for selection based on the results of recent and ongoing clinical trials.

Our experience with and technical recommendations for carotid thromboendarterectomy are discussed. Intraoperative techniques intended to improve outcome, such as the use of barbiturates for cerebral protection, electrophysiological monitoring, and transcranial Doppler sonography, are detailed. Anesthetic management is reviewed. The surgical approach for microsurgical endarterectomy is presented step–by–step with ample illustrations. Finally, the patient's postoperative care and optimal medical treatment are addressed. By collecting the entire spectrum of care associated with microsurgical carotid endarterectomy into one reference volume, those unfamiliar with the procedure will be able to explore its utility as a treatment option.

Julian E. Bailes, M.D.
Robert F. Spetzler, M.D.

Acknowledgments

We extend our gratitude to our colleagues who stole time from their already overburdened schedules to share their expertise by contributing discussions on selected topics. Our good-natured and ever-patient editor at Raven Press, Elizabeth Greenspan, must be thanked for shepherding this project from its inception to its completion with alacrity and speed. We also appreciate the constructive criticism offered by Shelley A. Kick, Ph.D., Senior Editor, Barrow Neurological Institute. The outstanding artwork of Randy McKenzie accurately depicts many anatomical features and operative techniques that are essential to successful carotid endarterectomy. Thanks also go to Barbara Berry and Kim Butler who worked behind the scenes to ensure that we met our deadlines.

Microsurgical Carotid Endarterectomy

1

Epidemiology, Natural History, and Controversies in the Treatment of Carotid Stenosis

John R. Robinson, Jr. and
Julian E. Bailes

The ultimate test of a medical treatment is to compare the proposed intervention (and its attendant morbidity and mortality) with the natural history of that particular disease. In the clinical setting, however, treatments are sometimes proposed and utilized well before the natural history of a disease is completely understood. Until the recent publication of several large multicenter randomized clinical trials, many questions about carotid atherosclerosis and its best treatment were unanswered. These studies have elucidated the natural history, effective medical therapies, and the benefits and effectiveness of carotid endarterectomy. This chapter summarizes the development of carotid endarterectomy, the epidemiology of the underlying atherosclerotic disease process, the natural history of carotid stenosis, and controversies regarding its surgical treatment.

EVOLUTION OF CAROTID SURGERY

As a clinical entity, stroke was first recognized thousands of years ago. Hippocrates and perhaps earlier writers described stroke syndromes. Hip-

J. R. Robinson, Jr.: Division of Neurological Surgery, Barrow Neurological Institute, Phoenix, Arizona 85013-4496.
J. E. Bailes: Department of Neurological Surgery, Allegheny General Hospital, Pittsburgh, Pennsylvania 15212.

pocrates used the term apoplexy, meaning "to strike down by an external force," and described strokes, stroke prodromes, and transient ischemic attacks (36). Although Hippocrates's accurate descriptions placed medicine on a more scientific foundation, centuries elapsed before the management of stroke advanced.

Wepfer, Willis, Harvey, Hunter, and others pioneered our knowledge of the cerebral blood supply and our understanding of the collateral flow to the brain. In an 1856 case report, Savoury proposed a link between the pathogenesis of occlusion of the carotid artery and the appearance of stroke (36). In 1914, Hunt elucidated the importance of cervical carotid artery disease in producing the symptoms of amaurosis fugax, hemiplegia, and post-mortem brain softening (36). This work focused the medical community's efforts on the treatment of carotid stenosis.

In 1927, Egas Moniz introduced cerebral angiography, which permitted the preoperative assessment of arterial narrowing (11,36). He described patients with symptoms of internal carotid occlusion and proposed that the diagnosis could be made accurately with angiography.

During the 1940s, it was realized that carotid distribution ischemic symptoms could be caused by narrowing or stenosis of the artery, in addition to embolism and complete occlusion. Fisher later studied several patients suffering embolic ischemic phenomena and could not find thrombus in any of the usual sources of systemic emboli, such as the left heart, ascending aorta, or pulmonary veins. The discovery of these embolic strokes of the middle cerebral artery helped to establish the cervical carotid bifurcation as a common embolic source (Fig. 1). (43). The earliest surgical procedure performed on the carotid artery was ligation for the repair of penetrating injuries and cervical carotid aneurysms. Ligation became standard treatment for many intracranial aneurysms. During the 1940s, cervical carotid excisional ligation and sympathectomy were utilized in attempts to prevent thromboembolism and to abolish symptoms believed to be causative of vasospasm (36). In 1951, C.M. Fisher (42) described the role of carotid bifurcation atheroma and proposed the idea of bypassing carotid stenosis. Following this, surgical efforts then focused on restoring blood flow. Resection and reconstruction of carotid segments followed, performed in 1951 by Carrea, Molins, and Murphy and in 1954 by Eastcott, Pickering, and Rob (32,36).

Endarterectomy, originally developed for the lower extremity, was introduced by Dos Santos in 1946 (36). The technique was adopted and modified for the carotid arteries, leading to the first publication of a successful carotid endarterectomy in 1953 by DeBakey (36). Small series accumulated as did experience with the pitfalls of the technique. Although early studies demonstrated a benefit in certain patients, they also found that some of the best predictors of outcome were patient variables such as hypertension and cardiac disease. Consequently, surgical indications varied widely and the number of procedures performed increased dramatically.

In 1962, the first multicenter cooperative trial began, the Joint Study of Extracranial Arterial Occlusion. Published in 1970, this study enrolled 316 patients in 6 years with a mean follow-up of 42 months (39). The study found that the number of asymptomatic survivors improved; however, it also highlighted a need to refine the surgical indications and to improve the overall morbidity and mortality rates. This study identified cardiac disease as the predominant cause of mortality in all groups studied. Furthermore, it documented that surgical mortality improved significantly between the periods of 1961 to 1965 and 1965 to 1969 (39).

After carotid endarterectomy demonstrated an improved outcome, its use increased from 15,000 cases in 1971 to a peak of about 107,000 cases in 1985 (31,118). By 1982, carotid endarterectomy had become the third most

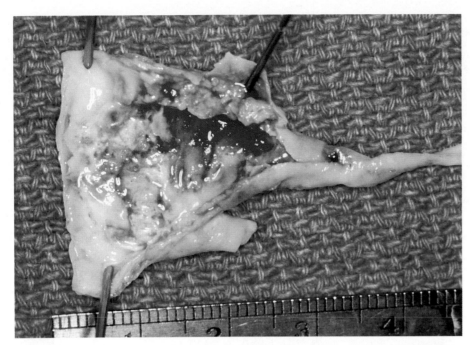

Figure 1. Carotid endarterectomy specimen showing a complex, ulcerated lesion with platelet thrombus formation.

frequently performed surgery in the United States. At this time, serious doubts were raised about the procedure's risk-benefit ratio compared with that of medical therapy using aspirin (9,39,68,113,118). A second large cooperative study to evaluate the benefit of endarterectomy was begun by Shaw et al. (104) in 1965 but was not published until 1984. This study was discontinued after only 41 patients were enrolled because the rates of surgical morbidity and mortality were disproportionately high compared with the patients in the medical control group. Several large, multicenter cooperative trials have recently demonstrated the benefit of carotid endarterectomy and better defined the appropriate indications for its use (35,76,88). These studies have also added to our knowledge of the disease and its ability to progress despite modern medical management. Nonetheless, many controversies about diagnosis, surgical indications, techniques, and patient monitoring still exist. These issues are discussed later in this chapter.

EPIDEMIOLOGY OF STROKE

Stroke has consistently been the third leading cause of death in the United States and the leading cause of morbidity, accounting for 145,340 deaths in 1990 (3). Despite encouraging declines in the number of strokes and in the number of fatalities from stroke during the past 20 years, the number of individuals disabled by stroke is increasing (10,78,102,121,123). The American Heart Association estimates that 3,020,000 people have survived a stroke; many of them require long-term care and have significant disabilities (3). The enormity of the human and economic impact of stroke is obvious and perhaps incalculable. Effective diagnostic methods and prophylactic treatments must be developed.

The term stroke is generic and is not associated with a specific etiology. Infarction is the most common type of stroke and in some studies accounts for 70% of all strokes (3). The frequency of different causes of infarction has been examined in several studies. The Framingham Study, which followed 5,070 patients for 32 years, found that 50% of infarctions were the result of atherosclerotic and thrombotic vessel disease (113). Cardioembolic strokes accounted for 17% to 22% of all strokes. Information from the Stroke Data Bank on 1,273 patients showed that cardioembolic conditions caused 19% of the strokes, whereas large vessel occlusion caused only 14% (80) (Fig. 2). Of these 1,273 strokes, 77% occurred in the territory of penetrating vessels. The origin of 40% was undetermined (23).

Many epidemiologic studies have examined and identified factors that modify a patient's risk (Table 1). These factors, such as age, sex, hypertension, race, cholesterol level, tobacco use, diabetes, and degree of stenosis are important predictors of the severity of the underlying disease (4,20,24,30,65,74,88,119,120,122). Several of the recent cooperative trials examined the importance of risk factors on outcome (35,76,88). The North American

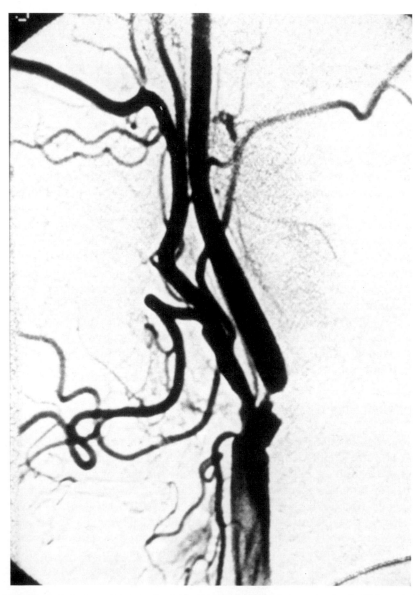

Figure 2. Lateral carotid angiogram in a patient with hemispheric TIAs originating from this 95% ulcerative stenotic lesion.

Table 1. *NASCET risk factors*

Factor	Value
Age	>70 years
Sex	Male
Systolic BP	>160
Diastolic BP	>90
Recent neurologic event	<31 days
Type of neurological event	Stroke
Degree of stenosis	>70%
Angiographic ulceration	Present
History of smoking	Present
Hypertension	Present
Myocardial infarction	Present
Diabetes mellitus	Present
Intermittent claudication	Present
High blood lipids	Present

From Ref. 80.

Symptomatic Carotid Endarterectomy Trial (NASCET) group reported a significant and progressive increase in the risk of stroke for patients with an increasing number of risk factors (88) (Table 2). The NASCET study did not identify the relative contribution of each factor. The prognosis of surgically treated NASCET patients did not vary with the number of risk factors. Numerous other multivariate analyses have demonstrated especially poor outcomes for patients with the risk factors of hypertension, diabetes, or smoking (24,64).

NATURAL HISTORY OF CAROTID ATHEROSCLEROTIC DISEASE

The natural history of carotid artery stenosis is best analyzed by the patients' signs and symptoms at presentation, before the final outcome, infarction, has occurred. The progression of the disease and the contribution of factors that may modify risk (such as plaque ulceration or degree of stenosis) must also be assessed. Carotid occlusion is discussed in Chapter 8. Here we examine the different clinical variables and latest outcome data for patients treated with medical therapy alone.

Bruits

The most common manifestation of extracranial carotid artery disease is a cervical bruit. A bruit is an audible sign that most physicians can readily detect on routine physical examination. Such a finding should initiate an evaluation to determine its cause and significance (82). The differential diagnosis of a carotid bruit is extensive (6,22,49,52–54,57,62,68,98,114,119) (Table 3). A detailed history combined with a thorough physical examination can be used to reduce the list of possibilities.

Table 2. *Number of risk factors and risk of stroke in medically treated patients*

Level of risk	No. of risk factors	% Ipsilateral stroke
Minimal	0–5	17
Moderate	6	23
High	7	39

From Ref. 89.

Table 3. *Differential diagnosis of cervical bruit*

Source	Pathology	Etiology
Arterial	Carotid stenosis: common, internal, or external	Atherosclerosis
		Thrombus
	Carotid occlusion	Fibromuscular dysplasia
	Carotid tortuosity: carotid flow	Contralateral carotid occlusion
		Paget's disease
		Goiter
		Arteriovenous malformation
		Vascular brain tumor
		Vertebral occlusion
Cardiac	Radiated sound from subclavian vein	Thyroid disease
		Anemia
	Radiated heart murmur	Shock
	Hyperdynamic state	Fever
Venous	Venous hum	

Careful auscultation for the timing, tone, and location of the cervical bruit may also help to ascertain its cause. Unfortunately, the characteristics of a neck bruit are difficult to correlate reliably with the underlying degree of carotid stenosis. Over the years, numerous studies have evaluated the significance of bruits. Few modern studies, however, have specified the proportion of bruits attributed to different causes.

Rennie et al. (98) found that carotid atherosclerosis was the most common cause of a cervical bruit in young adults, hospital controls, and stroke patients. Cardiac etiology ranked second, accounting for a significant proportion of bruits in all three groups. Anemia was responsible for 12% to 14% of the bruits.

Bruits related to carotid stenosis are audible vibrations of the carotid wall caused by turbulent flow distal to the stenosis. Although estimates vary, the degree of stenosis necessary to produce a bruit may be as low as 25% (62). The presence of a bruit in a patient with carotid stenosis has been found to indicate a significant level (>50%) of stenosis on angiography in 70% or more of the cases. False-positive rates of 10% to 40% and false-negative rates of 30% to 70% have been reported for cervical bruits.

The overall incidence of an asymptomatic cervical bruit in the general population has been estimated at 440 to 460/100,000 persons, based on data from the Framingham and Evans County, Georgia studies (57,119). These studies have also demonstrated that the number of bruits increases markedly with age, hypertension, and diabetes, and in women (57,119,120).

Numerous studies during the past 20 years have documented the increased risk of neurologic symptoms in patients with bruits who were previously asymptomatic, but the true clinical significance of this finding has been the subject of much debate (17,52,53,57,68,84,91,108,117,120). The Framingham Study found that the risk of stroke and transient ischemic attacks (TIAs) in patients with bruits was two to three times the risk for patients without bruits (120). Furthermore, these patients were 2.5 times more likely to have a myocardial infarction and 1.9 times more likely to die during the period of study. These results were similar to those found by Heyman et al. (56) in the Evans County, Georgia study, which demonstrated over a threefold increase in the risk of a new stroke for patients with bruits. When analyzed more closely, the increased risk of ipsilateral neurologic symptoms is substantially less than it appears to be from these impressive statistics. Thus bruits have been interpreted as general markers of atherosclerosis and as such are worthy of further investigation. They do not, however, necessarily herald a stroke (19,21). Further evaluation by noninvasive studies or angiography is required to discern their importance and the extent of the atherosclerosis and to aid in selecting a treatment.

This sentiment was echoed in the classic study by Chambers and Norris (22) in which 500 patients with asymptomatic bruits were followed for a mean of 23.2 months. These investigators found a 6% annual rate of cerebral ischemia and an actual stroke rate of 1.7% at 12 months. However, only 42% of the strokes were ipsilateral to the carotid bruit. This study also found a 7% annual rate of cardiac ischemic events and a 4% mortality rate for patients with bruits, principally the result of cardiac events.

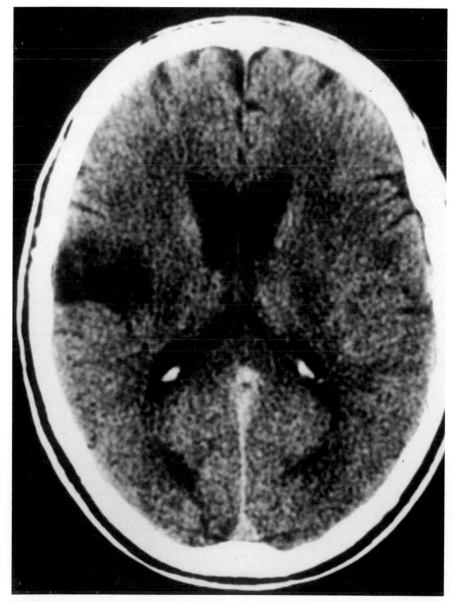

Figure 3. CT scan of a patient presenting with a right hemispheric deficit consistent with this right-sided infarct.

Transient Ischemic Attacks

Another common presentation for carotid artery stenosis is the occurrence of transient neurologic symptoms. This type of presentation may include symptoms caused by retinal ischemia, cerebral ischemia, or both. In 1958, the Committee on Cerebrovascular Nomenclature defined a TIA as a temporary neurologic deficit with an upper limit duration of 1 hour. As knowledge increased, this duration was revised to less than 30 minutes (41). Then in 1990, TIA was redefined as a focal loss of brain function, including loss of vision, lasting less than 24 hours (41,115). The definition was based on clinical conventions despite the ability of neuroimaging modalities such as magnetic resonance imaging (MRI) and computerized tomography (CT) to detect small areas of infarction associated with deficits of 24 hours' duration (41) (Fig. 3). Furthermore, the decision to lump both hemispheric and retinal transient events together cannot be substantiated by the literature. The latest data on this issue were presented at a 1994 meeting in a side analysis of the NASCET study (88). This study found an increase of over twofold in the occurrence of stroke at 2 years for those patients with hemispheric TIAs when compared with patients who had retinal TIAs.

TIAs are characterized by the rapid onset of neurologic symptoms that are usually maximal within 2 minutes but sometimes evolve over 5 minutes (1,41,43,56,92,93,110). Reports indicate that 75% of TIAs resolve within 5 minutes and many last 1 minute or less (41,56,116). TIAs may occasionally persist up to the 24-hour definition. They resolve fully and are typically characterized by a symptom profile associated with the particular vascular distribution (e.g., carotid or vertebrobasilar) in which they occur. The variations in the definition of TIA and how it is distinguished from stroke have created confusion in interpreting studies on this topic. Furthermore, comparison of results across studies, especially those in different decades, must be done with caution.

The rate of occurrence of TIAs in the general population has received little attention during the past three decades. The prevalence of TIAs was examined in two large surveys published in the early 1970s. The Evans County, Georgia survey studied 2,455 people during the 1960s for evidence of stroke. This study contained 551 patients who were 65 years of age and older. The prevalence rate of TIAs in this age group was 18.1/1,000 (56,57). The Cook County Survey, a similar study performed in an urban setting, consisted of 2,772 patients between 65 and 74 years of age. The prevalence rate of TIAs was 63/1,000 (56,92). Numerous explanations concerning the socioeconomic status of the two populations have been developed over the years to account for the differences between the two studies, but none have ever been proved. Despite the population differences, both studies found that risk increased with age and was higher for women (57,93).

The incidence of TIAs in certain populations was examined in the Rochester, Minnesota survey that included 39,012 people, 9,369 of whom were between 45 and 74 years old. The annual incidence in this age group was 93/100,000, and the overall incidence was 31/100,000 (56,115). A similar figure of 110/100,000 was found in the Seal Beach, California study, which covered 10,500 people aged 52 years or older (46,56).

Epidemiologic investigations of TIAs have also found a strong association with other vascular risk factors. In 1978, Toole et al. (109,110) examined the association of risk factors in 225 patients with TIAs: 60% had ischemic cardiac disease, 30% had peripheral vascular disease, 30% had hypertension, and 20% had diabetes mellitus. The Framingham Study followed 171 patients for a mean of 4 years. Four (2.4%) patients had TIAs and 6 (3.5%) patients experienced strokes. The incidence of myocardial infarction was doubled in patients who had bruits (120). The mechanism underlying the occurrence of TIAs and stroke associated with carotid stenosis has been the subject of much speculation. The first mechanism proposed was a relative hypoperfusion state distal to a tight carotid stenosis. Another proposed mechanism was the occurrence of artery-to-artery thromboemboli. Other suggestions included cardiac emboli, arrhythmic perfusion deficits, migraines, and a host of more obscure events (41).

The evidence supports both the hypoperfusion and the thromboembolic theories as likely explanations for TIAs. Early substantiation of the embolic theory was derived from funduscopic observations made by C.M. Fisher (41) during an episode of amaurosis fugax in one of his patients. Angiographic studies, such as that by Pessin et al. (93), have offered further angiographic support for the concept of thromboembolism in 66% of patients with TIAs or strokes. However, the remaining 34% of patients in this study had no evidence of a thromboembolic source. Instead, these patients had significant stenosis with hemodynamic compromise, thus providing support for the hemodynamic theory as well (93).

A 1979 angiographic study found structural lesions that were severe enough to account for strokes in 28 of 40 patients with TIAs localized to the carotid distribution. However, the angiograms of 12 patients lacked structural lesions, thus implicating emboli as the cause of their strokes (112). Similarly, Fields and Lemak (37) found accountable lesions in only 73% of their patients. These findings strongly suggest the possibility of artery-to-artery emboli in patients who lack angiographic evidence of hemodynamically significant lesions to account for their symptoms.

It seems likely that both mechanisms may cause TIAs; therefore the remaining question is how to distinguish them. Studies have revealed that TIAs presumed to be due to emboli (60% of emboli are not associated with TIAs) appear to persist for several hours compared with hemodynamic TIAs, which tend to resolve in minutes (1,41,56,92). Reviewing the records of the Massachusetts General Hospital, Fisher (41) found that when a patient had two or more TIAs or had a TIA and an episode of amaurosis on the same side, the most likely cause was a tight carotid stenosis. In 88.5% of cases with multiple TIAs, the second TIA occurred within 7 days of the first event. When two TIAs occurred on the same day, occlusion was imminent. Further support for the hemodynamic hypothesis came from the pathologic studies of carotid artery plaques by Fisher (41). He found a strong association between residual carotid lumens with a cross-sectional area of 1 mm or less and the occurrence of TIAs (98% of cases) and amaurosis (90%).

The clinical significance of TIAs with regard to the risk of subsequent stroke has been studied extensively for 30 years. Numerous series have cited a subsequent stroke risk of between 2% and 62% in TIA patients (1,3,17, 23,43,47,56,86,92,93,105,110). The consensus figure used by the American Heart Association is that 36% of patients who suffer one or more TIAs will eventually experience a stroke; a large proportion of the remainder become asymptomatic. The data indicate that TIA patients are 9.5 times more likely than those without TIAs to experience a stroke (3). Consequently, TIA is considered an urgent warning sign in need of prompt evaluation.

Plaque Ulceration

In the case of carotid stenosis, as with any clinical problem, certain factors modify a patient's risk. During the early angiographic evaluation of this disease, investigators noted that peculiar features correlated with a higher incidence of stroke and other ischemic symptoms (59). One such feature was the presence of plaque ulceration. Ulceration of the carotid artery has been described and categorized into three groups: small ulcers (type A), large ulcers (type B), and complex, excavated ulcers (type C). Both experimental and clinical experience has shown a higher incidence of stroke as ulceration becomes more complex, with up to seven times more strokes for type C ulcers (Fig. 4).

Despite the apparent increased risk of stroke associated with plaque ulceration, most studies confirm that the risk factor of overwhelming importance is still the degree of stenosis of the ipsilateral vessel (43). In the last 30 years, many studies have documented the progressive risk of ischemia as the level of stenosis increases. This relationship has also been illustrated in the NASCET patients with symptomatic severe stenosis and ulceration. The risk of stroke at 2 years for symptomatic 75% stenosis with ulceration was 26.3%, whereas those with 95% stenosis had a 73.2% risk (88). Several fluid-dynamic studies have modeled the mechanisms responsible for such changes. These data reveal that blood flow remains normal if the vessel diameter decreases by less than 60% (90% narrowing of cross-sectional area) (90). Blood flow decreases rapidly (by 40%) if the luminal diameter is diminished by 75%. If the luminal diameter is decreased by 84%, representing a 96% compromise of the cross-sectional area, blood flow decreases dramatically to 64% of normal (79).

A logical extension of this work implies an even greater increase in the risk of stroke with increasing stenosis in the setting of a contralateral occlusion. An analysis of NASCET data reveals a marked increase in the ipsilateral 2-year stroke rate (56.3%) for the patient with symptomatic severe stenosis and impressive but lower rates for the minimal and moderate stenosis groups at 22.5% and 22.4%, respectively (88).

Although carotid atherosclerotic disease undoubtedly progresses, it is rarely asymptomatic. When the degree of stenosis is critical, it may lead to a recommendation for prophylactic carotid endarterectomy. Javid et al. (64) reported the only angiographic study on the evolution of carotid atherosclerosis. They studied 135 carotid artery bifurcations for 1 to 9 years. During this

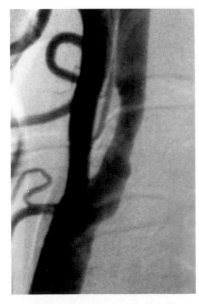 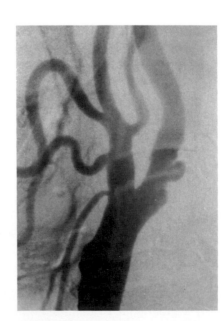 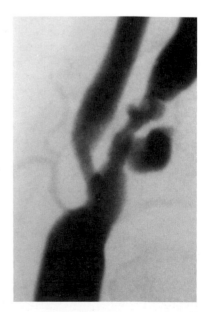

Figure 4. Three categories of carotid artery ulceration. Type A (*left*) is a small shallow ulcer. Type B (*center*) is a simple but deep lesion. Type C (*right*) is both deep and complex.

time, the carotid atherosclerotic lesion progressed in 62% of patients, with 30% having enlargement of the lesions by more than 25% per year. This study suggested that moderate-to-severe atherosclerotic disease is particularly likely to progress to a critical degree of stenosis. In a carotid duplex-scan study, one-third of the carotid arteries progressively narrowed more than 50% (100).

The following factors correlate with plaque progression: plaque size at the time of initial assessment, tobacco use, hypertension, and diabetes mellitus (4,20,24,49,100,102,104,109,112,119,121,122). Patients with known cervical carotid atherosclerotic disease should be followed closely, perhaps more frequently early in their course or if they have any of the other risk factors. Symptomatic patients typically proceed to more aggressive (surgical) treatment. It is believed that control of vasculopathic risk factors may markedly slow the progression of the atherosclerotic process.

Cardiac Disease

In addition to a standard neurologic evaluation, the patient's cardiac status should also be thoroughly evaluated, since the occurrence of TIAs has been strongly associated with ischemic cardiac disease (3,107). Indeed, the most frequent cause of death in many of the large studies of TIA patients has been myocardial infarction. For example, Fields et al. (38) and Toole et al. (110) reported mortality rates attributable to myocardial infarction of 58% and 57%, respectively. Equally important is the percent of patients who have a stroke without warning. In the Rochester, Minnesota survey, Whisnant and his colleagues (116) found that only 10% of the patients reported TIA symptoms before their stroke. Other series, such as that of Pessin et al. (94) in 1979, have found that 54% of patients report TIAs before stroke. Strokes of embolic origin, however, were less likely to be preceded by TIAs (40% of cases). These findings emphasize the need to develop rational surgical guidelines for patients without neurologic symptoms. In summary, the occurrence of a TIA markedly increases the risk of stroke and the risk of death due to ischemic heart disease and thus merits immediate thorough diagnostic evaluation.

CONTROVERSIES IN CAROTID ENDARTERECTOMY

During the last several years, the publication of data from several large multicenter trials has altered much of the controversy regarding carotid endarterectomy. These recent trials have demonstrated the ability of carotid endarterectomy to reduce the risk of stroke in symptomatic and asymptomatic patients with severe ($\geq$70%) stenosis (35,58,76,87,88,111). The current question is how to minimize the risks of the operation. As with any operation, surgeons must constantly reevaluate the indications, methods, and results of carotid endarterectomy, as the literature amply demonstrates.

In the last 30 years, advances in anesthetic procedures, cardiac monitoring, critical care, and operative techniques (e.g., Swan-Ganz catheter measurements) have made carotid endarterectomy a safe and effective therapy against stroke. The reduction in the overall morbidity and mortality rate from about 20% in 1963 to less than 5% has made the procedure a favored therapeutic option. Nonetheless, surgeons continue to debate and investigate ways to improve outcome and to reduce risk.

As with any major surgery, the risks of carotid endarterectomy include infection, neurologic disability, medical complications, and death. The two most common serious complications after an endarterectomy are myocardial infarction and stroke (44). Although myocardial infarction is the most common cause of mortality in the endarterectomy population, it is rarely directly related to the technical aspects of the surgery itself. Instead, careful preoperative evaluation, pulmonary artery pressure monitoring, perioperative nitrates, strict blood pressure control, and other prophylactic measures can be used to decrease the risk of anesthesia and the stress of surgery. The most dreaded neurologic complication associated with carotid endarterectomy is a stroke, be it from bland infarction or hemorrhage.

The risk of stroke in the immediate perioperative period is unlikely to equal that of similar patients who do not undergo the operation. Nonetheless, any intervention or technical improvement that can reduce the risk of stroke significantly should be considered. If the perioperative risk of stroke can be minimized, the usefulness of the procedure may be extended to other groups of patients (e.g., those with moderate stenosis or those with asymptomatic, severe stenosis).

The remainder of this chapter focuses on several of the long-standing surgical and anesthetic controversies surrounding endarterectomy. Issues such as monitoring, cerebral protection, shunting, patching, and anticoagulation are reviewed. Patient selection, radiologic assessment, and cardiac risk are discussed elsewhere in the text. Some of these issues are covered further in Chapter 7.

Anesthetic Technique

The selection of anesthetic technique and agents for carotid endarterectomy has long been controversial. The controversy surrounds the benefit of having a patient under regional anesthetic who is awake and can be assessed neurologically versus the cerebral protection afforded by a general anesthetic. Data on the number of endarterectomies performed under local anesthesia are scarce. However, an informal survey of five major teaching institutions conducted by the authors in 1994 revealed that general anesthesia was used in an overwhelming majority of the procedures.

General anesthesia confers some benefits of cerebral protection including that from barbiturate induction. The use of inhalational agents such as halothane can increase cerebral blood flow (CBF). Another major advantage is the ability to optimize oxygen saturation and to control CBF with P_{CO_2} fluctuations to prevent a reverse steal phenomenon from developing. Finally,

Table 4. *Comparison of regional vs. general anesthetic technique for variables crucial to cerebral ischemia*

	Regional	General
Neurologic assessment	Possible but limited by anxiety	Electrophysiologic
Anxiety	Titratable (but other variables)[a]	Eliminated
Arterial		
P_{O_2}	Limited control[a]	Fully controlled
P_{CO_2}	Limited control[a]	Fully controlled
CBF	Limited control[a]	Increased
Cerebral protection	Limited control	Increased
Arterial BP	Limited control[a]	Fully controlled

[a] Variable may influence other parameters in an awake patient.

general anesthesia avoids the interaction of patient anxiety with other variables such as arterial blood pressure and respiratory parameters that intuitively would seem to influence the probability of a stroke (Table 4).

Nonetheless, several authors have made an eloquent case for regional anesthetic. Some believe that regional anesthesia offers a theoretical increase in the sensitivity of detection of cerebral ischemia at the time of cross-clamping and the ability to distinguish embolic changes from hemodynamic changes. Lee et al. (70) reported their extensive experience with regional anesthesia in 337 carotid endarterectomies. They had two (0.66%) patients with perioperative TIAs, two (0.66%) with perioperative cerebral infarction, and two (0.66%) perioperative deaths. No perioperative (within 30 days) myocardial infarctions occurred. They believed that regional anesthesia was advantageous because it allowed more sensitive monitoring of neurologic function, thus minimizing the need for shunt placement along with its attendant complications, especially embolic phenomena. They also believed that postoperative hypertension and myocardial ischemia occurred less often with regional than with general anesthesia. Most surgeons believe that electrophysiologic monitoring, physiologic measurements of back pressure, and selective shunting based on these assessments provide sufficient information for successful general anesthesia (18).

The argument for an increased sensitivity in detection of ischemia using regional anesthesia is further undermined by the large areas of clinically silent cortex, especially over the right hemisphere. The ability to detect the mechanism of a neurologic deterioration is related to an inference based on the timing of deterioration relative to carotid cross-clamping. This inference is notoriously inaccurate and increasingly so with increased time from the moment of cross-clamping. In any event, the same inference can be made with a higher degree of accuracy (in view of silent cortex) using electrophysiologic means, thereby negating any supposed benefit of regional anesthesia. However, the argument can and has been made that a high rate of false-positive changes is associated with electrophysiologic monitoring during general anesthesia. This important issue is discussed in greater detail in Chapter 5.

Another anesthetic technique that deserves mention is the combination of a regional block (temporary sympathectomy) with a general anesthetic. The rationale behind this technique is to provide the benefits of a general anesthetic along with the reduced intraoperative and postoperative blood pressure fluctuations found with the block. Although the theory is sound, convincing data from a large-scale study are lacking. Thus, whether this approach is of demonstrable benefit to the patient remains to be seen.

Cerebral Protection

The topic of cerebral protection is intimately linked to the choice of anesthetic agent. Multiple therapeutic agents and strategies, apart from anesthesia, have been developed to minimize ischemic complications. The duration of the procedure and its technical perfection are critically important variables. The concept of cerebral protection has been utilized to support shunting of all patients. Because of its technical difficulties and pitfalls, this strategy is considered separately.

Barbiturates have long been used for cerebral protection. Their effectiveness was demonstrated by the work of several investigators (48,50,60,61,77). The mechanism of cerebral protection is still debated but is thought to reflect the reduction in electrical activity of neurons. This reduction markedly decreases the amount of energy required for pumping ions against a concentration gradient. The decreased metabolic requirements reduce oxygen consumption and therefore the risk of ischemia for a given oxygen delivery. Oxygen delivery is also decreased by barbiturate administration; nonetheless, the relative effect of both of these changes has been shown to protect against ischemic damage.

Induced Hypertension

Another strategy with theoretical merit and some practical success in reducing ischemia is the induction of a moderate degree of hypertension during carotid cross-clamping. This technique takes advantage of the Bayliss effect (50,61). Although this strategy is theoretically not as effective as providing blood flow through a shunt system, it is a useful adjunctive technique that has demonstrated its ability to reverse and prevent electrophysiologic changes immediately after and during carotid cross-clamping. Although it is useful to detect minor electroencephalographic (EEG) changes such as mild slowing over the affected hemisphere, this technique should not be relied on if any profound changes are seen in the EEG or a major compromise is indicated by transcranial Doppler sonography.

The underlying mechanism of this strategy is a straightforward increase in blood flow to the affected hemisphere both through intradural circle of Willis collaterals from the contralateral and vertebrobasilar supply and through leptomeningeal and extradural collaterals. Its theoretical drawback is the increased demand on the patient's heart caused by the pressor agents used to induce the hypertension. Administering perioperative nitrates, managing intravenous fluid, monitoring central pressures with Swan-Ganz catheters, and carefully selecting pressor agents may mitigate problems in patients judged to be at significant risk. Induced hypertension may owe part of its success to the stunned autoregulation in the ischemic cerebral vascular bed and to the intact autoregulation in unaffected regions. The net effect is to increase blood flow selectively in a linear fashion to the areas in need with small increases in systematic blood pressure as a result of dysfunctional autoregulation.

Free Radical Scavengers

The use of free radical scavengers has also been proposed as a mechanism to neutralize the deleterious effects of ischemia. Some evidence even shows that barbiturates also use this mechanism in addition to those already discussed. Agents such as mannitol, nonsteroidal antiinflammatory agents, vitamin E, and others have been suggested as potential scavengers or compounds that could ameliorate the damage free radicals afflict on neuronal cell membranes. Newer agents such as lazaroids offer theoretical advantages over other agents and have reduced infarct volume in preliminary studies (51). Other investigators have demonstrated marked reductions in neocortical loss with γ-aminobutyric acid (GABA) receptor antagonists using transient focal ischemia models. The gold standard of cerebral protection remains the use of hypothermia. Mild changes of as little as 2° to 3°C have markedly reduced the size of infarcts (14,15). Furthermore, the benefits of hypothermia can be realized with intra-ischemic induction or with induction at the time of reperfusion as opposed to most interventions, which require prophylactic use (16).

Temporary Intraluminal Shunting

No carotid endarterectomy topic is more controversial than the use of temporary intraluminal shunting. Numerous inadequately designed studies and large retrospective series have contributed to the confusion. Furthermore, shunting is difficult to discuss without becoming entangled in arguments on monitoring techniques. The utilization of carotid shunts is also discussed in detail in Chapter 7.

The goal of reducing the risk of stroke using endarterectomy can only be realized if the perioperative risk of stroke is maintained at an absolute low level. To achieve this level, the surgeon must be able to assess the adequacy of CBF and be prepared to correct inadequate flow within several minutes or to provide flow routinely after a brief interruption of CBF. Despite the strategies discussed above to reverse minimal deficiencies and to ameliorate ischemic damage, nothing can compensate as well as restoring blood flow to the affected cerebral region or hemisphere. Even the staunchest advocates of no-shunt endarterectomies will admit to instances of infarction caused by a lack of blood flow.

Shunts provide enough blood flow to reverse clinical and electrophysiologic changes and supplement arteries with low back pressure. The adverse effects of shunting, which primarily consist of plaque, air, and platelet embolism, are controversial. The increase in the technical difficulty of the procedure itself is another commonly cited disadvantage of shunting. Thus, routinely shunting all patients may needlessly expose those who do not require a shunt to the additional risks inherent in the procedure. The technical difficulty of working with a shunt will probably decrease with experience. It is unlikely, however, that complications from emboli, which are recognized by transcranial Doppler in one-third of cases, will also improve (63). In addition to the risks of air, platelet or atheromatous emboli, damage to the vessel wall (i.e., scuffing or cracking), and the possibility of wall dissection (intimal flap) raise the risk of stroke when a shunt is utilized (Fig. 5). Thus the surgeon

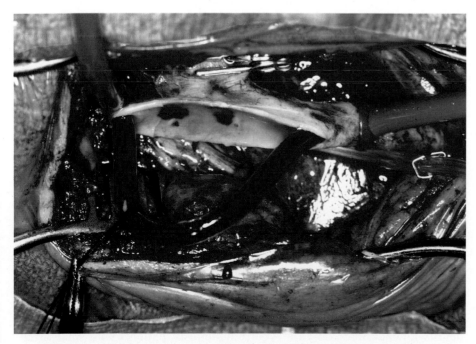

Figure 5. Carotid artery exposed with an indwelling shunt in place.

must assess the risk-benefit ratio of shunting for each patient based on the best available information (i.e., change in neurologic status, EEG, stump pressure, transcranial Doppler, or evoked potentials) at the time of cross-clamping. Selective shunting will minimize the risk to most patients while addressing the special needs of patients who do not tolerate cross-clamping (which has been needed in less than 7% in our series).

Patch Angioplasty

The use of a carotid artery patch during the closure of an endarterectomy has been embroiled in controversy since its inception. Proponents of this technique insist that it enhances blood flow, minimizes early complications, and improves long-term results in an otherwise progressive disease. Although data support some of these claims, the increased risks associated with patch angioplasty, as with shunting, must be balanced against the potential benefits.

Carotid patching has been shown to improve surgical outcome by decreasing the perioperative stroke rate and the risk of early occlusion by 2 to 1 or more (5,55,66,72). The use of a carotid patch may also reduce the rate of early and late restenosis compared with primary closure (7,28,55,66,96). The reduction of symptoms from early restenosis is thought to result from the increased cross-sectional area that provides more flow. The mechanism is a change in the arterial cross-sectional diameter, which in turn reduces shear stress, while small increases in luminal cross section reduce stress on the arterial wall. Evidence suggests that this phenomenon may confer maximal benefit when the vein graft width is 8 mm and that it then reverses itself (40,44). The population of patients who are symptomatic from restenosis is very small and may approach only 1% to 2% a year. Thus it is hard to justify routine patching. Evidence also suggests that an accelerated form of atherosclerosis is associated with venous grafts subjected to arterial pressures.

Patch angioplasty is associated with both real and theoretical increases in risk. In one study, the technique of patching increased the duration of carotid cross-clamping. However, this increase was not associated with a significant change in outcome. A theoretical risk of patching is the increased length of the suture line. In reality, this consideration has not been implicated as a factor in poor neurologic outcomes. In fact, in a recent analysis of catastrophic graft failures, the point of rupture in 16 cases was in the center of the graft and not the suture line (27). The use of a patch graft has also been associated with a slightly higher risk of delayed aneurysm formation than has primary closure (13). Some surgeons now routinely reinforce their endarterectomy patch sites to reduce such physical complications as blow-out and aneurysm formation. This procedure involves either reapproximation of the carotid sheath or placement of a prosthetic mesh graft at the proximal end of the anastomosis. Another risk associated with graft use is persistent bleeding. This complication is normally associated with prosthetic grafts but is occasionally found in conjunction with vein patch angioplasty. This problem is corrected with suture that has a diameter as wide as its needle. Given the risks associated with carotid artery patching and the small number of patients for whom it is actually indicated, it is hard to justify its use in all patients when excellent results can be obtained without primary closure. Intuitively, however, several groups of patients should benefit from this technique: patients with endarterectomy for recurrent stenosis, patients with small arteries, patients who smoke, and patients with hyperlipidemias refractory to treatment.

Advanced microsurgical techniques have made primary vessel closure the best option for most patients. The enhanced illumination, combined with the vastly superior visualization possible with the operating microscope, has allowed primary closures with 6-0 monofilament suture that do not narrow the vessel postoperatively. Postoperative angiographic examination of microsurgical primary closures often reveals postendarterectomy dilation rather than stenosis (106). Furthermore, in head-to-head comparisons in animal models, primary closure was rated superior to closures with wide (10-mm) patches and equal to narrow (5-mm) patch closures in terms of factors related to symptomatic delayed stenosis, shear stress, vascular turbulence, and pressure gradients (40). This topic and the benefits of primary closure are discussed further in Chapter 7, which is devoted to the microsurgical technique of endarterectomy.

Anticoagulation Therapy

The final controversial issue to be examined is the role of postoperative anticoagulation. No disagreement exists on the importance of intraoperative heparin and only minor disagreement on its dosage. No consensus has been reached, however, about whether heparin should be reversed. Questions of if and when to use aspirin postoperatively can further compound the debate (81). Fortunately, as a result of rigorous scientific investigations by Sundt, Ercius and others, the answers to these questions are firmly supported by scientific evidence (29,33,34).

As described by Dirrenberger and Sundt (29) in 1978, the temporal profile of endarterectomy healing reveals a critical period of exposure for the raw endarterectomized vessel during which it is extremely thrombogenic. The thrombogenicity tapers off over the initial 48 postoperative hours. Strong clinical evidence also shows a critical postperfusion period in humans when thromboembolic symptoms are most likely to develop. Together, these two facts strongly support not reversing heparin on a routine basis and waiting a minimum of 10 minutes if reversal must be utilized (95).

Similar evidence supports the use of aspirin pre- and postoperatively. Findings from a canine model support a preoperative dose of 10 mg/kg (101). The rationale for aspirin therapy is similar to that of heparin although a different mechanism inhibits thrombus formation while allowing platelets to adhere to the exposed collagenous surface.

The preoperative use of aspirin and not reversing heparin causes many surgeons concern about intracranial hemorrhages and wound hematomas. These concerns, however, are largely theoretical. To date, no large prospective studies have examined the risk of intracranial hemorrhage from this regimen. However, retrospective reports (exceeding 300 cases) do not indicate any increased risks (106). While a slight increase in the occurrence of wound hematomas has been seen, this can be overcome with techniques designed to achieve meticulous hemostasis.

TANDEM CAROTID LESIONS

Complete assessment of the cerebrovascular circulation begins with angiographic visualization of the aortic arch (45). In such an evaluation it is important to visualize the origins of the carotid and vertebral arteries. Patients with cerebral ischemic symptoms will often have atherosclerotic stenosis, ulcerative lesions, or occlusion of the origin of these great vessels. Full consideration of the cerebral vascular supply and an understanding of the patient's symptomatology is not possible without such a comprehensive evaluation. When tandem lesions exist, they usually involve the cervical carotid bifurcation along with abnormalities in the cavernous portion of the internal carotid artery. However, carotid bifurcation lesions may also exist in tandem with stenosis or occlusion of the origin of the common carotid artery (42).

When atherosclerotic lesions of the origins of the great vessels are believed to be the cause of cerebral ischemic symptoms, several treatment options exist. A direct carotid endarterectomy at the aortic arch carotid origin is possible, as well as reimplantation of the common carotid into adjacent vessels, such as the subclavian, or through another segment of the aortic arch. We have also had experience with a crossover arterial synthetic graft from the aortic arch to the distal common carotid artery. Recently, however, transluminal balloon angioplasty has become a preferred treatment for carotid origin stenotic lesions. Percutaneous carotid angioplasty is possible, and the risk of distal embolization may be prevented by direct open arteriotomy placement into the common carotid in a retrograde fashion (97).

A more common tandem lesion is concomitant cervical carotid bifurcation and carotid siphon stenoses. The carotid siphon is that portion that courses from the carotid's exit from the petrous bone until it enters the dura to become the supraclinoid portion. It has been postulated that the curved shape of the carotid siphon and the associated hemodynamic factors cause greater atherosclerotic formation here than elsewhere in the intracranial internal carotid artery. The siphon also is an area predisposed to calcification, which has been suggested to be relatively protective in avoiding the development of raised atherosclerotic and markedly stenotic lesions in this region (42,99). Roederer et al. (99) analyzed the carotid siphon in 141 patients who underwent carotid angiography. Of 282 carotid arteries examined, carotid siphon disease was present in 84%, with 42% of the lesions manifesting as 20% to 49% of vessel diameter reduction. They found that greater than 50% arterial stenosis was seen in 9% of patients, whereas 10% were occluded. Most carotid siphon lesions in this study were smooth, and no correlation was seen among the degree of cervical carotid bifurcation, atherosclerotic involvement, and siphon atherosclerosis. In 58% of their cases, atherosclerotic plaque had caused significant (greater than half) reduction in carotid bulb diameter. They felt that in 73% of cases the cervical carotid bifurcation lesion was the source of symptomatic cerebral emboli. By contrast, the degree of atherosclerotic disease in the carotid siphon did not appear to correlate with the presence or absence of focal neurologic symptoms. No correlation was found between severity of disease in the siphon and successful performance of carotid endarterectomy or the likelihood of recurrent cerebral ischemic symptoms (99). Other studies have noted an incidence of carotid siphon stenosis in one-third to one-half of patients undergoing carotid endarterectomy (26,103). Keagy et al. (67) found atherosclerotic carotid siphon involvement to be present in 46% of patients in their angiographic study. However, these lesions usually did not have a high degree of stenosis and did not correlate with the amount of cervical carotid bifurcation involvement.

Concerning the natural history of carotid siphon stenosis, studies have shown that it appears to be an important indicator for widespread atherosclerotic disease. Craig et al. (25) found that when the carotid siphon was narrowed by one-third or more, the resultant incidence of stroke was 19%. During their follow-up period, 43% of their 58 patients died; 80% of the deaths were caused by stroke or coronary artery disease. Marzewski et al. (75) reported that with intracranial carotid stenosis of 50% or greater, 27% of patients experienced cerebral ischemic symptoms, 8 (12.1%) had isolated TIAs, and 10 (15.2%) suffered cerebral vascular accidents. This gave an occurrence of stroke 13 times the expected cerebral infarction rate for a normal population. Half of their patients died during the average follow-up of 45 months, and 55% of all deaths were related to cardiac disease. They concluded that intracranial carotid stenosis was a marker of extensive cerebral vascular, systemic atherosclerotic disease and especially coronary artery disease. They also found that patients with tandem extracranial carotid stenosis had a greater risk of stroke than patients with an isolated carotid siphon lesion. Compared with isolated cervical carotid bifurcation atherosclerotic stenosis, the prognosis for ipsilateral stroke with isolated carotid siphon disease may be slightly better (12).

It appears that in patients with tandem carotid bifurcation and carotid siphon lesions, the former are usually responsible for cerebral ischemic symptoms. Cerebral embolization, which is often a middle cerebral artery territory event, is more likely to be of thromboembolic than hemodynamic origin. The characteristics of atheromatous plaques at the internal carotid origin are more likely to provide a substrate for atheromatous debris or thrombotic or platelet aggregate material for embolization than would plaques in the carotid siphon. Therefore removal of an internal carotid origin lesion should eliminate a symptomatic embolic source (83). In addition, studies using oculoplethysmography have shown that cervical carotid bifurcation and carotid siphon stenoses may have an additive affect in hemodynamic terms. In terms of cerebral blood flow, carotid origin lesions have been shown to have a greater detrimental impact than a carotid siphon lesion (67).

Lord et al. (73) have shown that carotid endarterectomy can be successfully performed in patients with coexistent carotid siphon lesions without an apparent increased risk of morbidity and mortality. Day et al. (26) reported two patients with severe preoperative carotid siphon stenosis that resolved following carotid endarterectomy. Their experience emphasizes that tandem lesions are not a contraindication to carotid endarterectomy and that the distal internal carotid artery siphon stenosis may be a reversible phenomenon. Repeat angiography or MRI angiography is indicated to ascertain the status of the carotid siphon lesion. Carotid siphon tandem stenosis can be caused by embolization, reactive arterial spasm, anterograde flow disturbance, or a combination of factors (26). Alcock (2) demonstrated a similar phenomenon with occlusive lesions of the middle cerebral artery. Little et al. (71) had a similar experience in two patients with resolving carotid siphon lesions that they termed *pseudo-tandem stenosis*. They postulated that laminar flow through the poststenotic carotid segment beyond the cervical bifurcation may produce the appearance of marked diminution in arterial caliber, secondary to either a reduced amount of contrast medium or actual slow contrast flow. Collateral flow of a substantial nature through either the anterior cerebral artery or posterior communication artery likewise could displace or dilute a column of contrast medium.

It is generally felt that most patients with tandem carotid lesions are symptomatic from the cervical bifurcation atheromatous plaque. It appears that carotid endarterectomy in such a situation can be safely performed and that no significant increase is seen in incidence of cerebral ischemic symptoms or in the stroke rate following carotid endarterectomy in a patient with tandem carotid lesions (99,103). Due to the potential for an additive effect, carotid endarterectomy can also be recommended (8,15). Carotid siphon stenosis is a predictor of future coronary disease and indicates widespread systemic atherosclerotic changes (67,103).

CONCLUSIONS

Stroke syndromes have been recognized and defined more completely through the years, aided by vast improvements in radiologic imaging techniques. Our ability to diagnose and characterize cerebral ischemic etiology is more sophisticated than ever before. In the last 40 years great interest in surgical treatment of carotid atherosclerotic disease has arisen. Advances in surgical technique, anesthetic management, and postoperative medical and cardiac care have provided much improvement in outcome from carotid endarterectomy. The recent clinical trials have defined the population of symptomatic patients who benefit from this procedure. Despite several technical and management controversies, excellent results are now routinely obtained for symptomatic patients undergoing carotid endarterectomy. These excellent results are most likely to occur in centers with experience and expertise in performing the procedure. We feel that many technical facets of carotid endarterectomy are vital to achieving optimal outcomes, approaching absolute minimal morbidity and mortality rates. These technical issues are discussed in detail in Chapter 7.

With sufficient epidemiologic data to guide us concerning carotid distribution cerebral ischemia and its surgical treatment, we may now make appropriate and accurate recommendations for patient management. Methods of preoperative radiologic assessment leading to patient selection for carotid endarterectomy are detailed in the next chapter.

REFERENCES

1. Adams HP, Putman SF, Corbett JJ et al. Amaurosis fugax: the results of arteriography in 59 patients. *Stroke* 1983;14:742–744.
2. Alcock JM. Occlusion of the middle cerebral artery: serial angiography as a guide to conservative therapy. *J Neurosurg* 1967;27:353–357.
3. American Heart Association. Heart and Stroke Facts Statistics, January 1994.
4. Anderson RJ, Hobson RW, Padberg FT, et al. Carotid endarterectomy for asymptomatic carotid stenosis: a ten-year experience with 120 procedures in a fellowship training program. *Ann Vasc Surg* 1991;5:111–115.
5. Archie JP. Prevention of early restenosis and thrombosis-occlusion after carotid endarterectomy by saphenous vein patch angioplasty. *Stroke* 1986;5:901–905.
6. Arkless HA: Cervical murmurs with normal hearts. *QCIM* 1946;40:114.
7. Awad IA, Little JR. Patch angioplasty in carotid endarterectomy. *Stroke* 1989;20:417–422.
8. Baker WH, Hayes AC, Mahler D. Durability of carotid endarterectomy. *Surgery* 1983;94:112–115.
9. Barnett HJM, Plum F, Walton JN. Carotid endarterectomy—an expression of concern. *Stroke* 1984;15:941–943.
10. Bonita R, Stewart A, Beaglehole R. International trends in stroke mortality: 1970–1985. *Stroke* 1990;21:989–992.
11. Bornstein NM, Chadwick LG, Norris JW. The value of carotid doppler ultrasound in asymptomatic extracranial arterial disease. *Can J Neurol Sci* 1988;15:378–383.
12. Borozan PG, Schuler JJ, LaRosa MP, et al. The natural history of isolated carotid siphon stenosis. *J Vasc Surg* 1984;1:744–749.
13. Branch CL, Davis CH. False aneurysm complicating carotid endarterectomy. *NSG* 1986;19:421–425.
14. Buchan A. Advances in cerebral ischemia: experimental approaches in cerebral ischemia: treatment and prevention. *Neurol Clin* 1992;10:49–61.
15. Busto R, Dietrich WD, Mordecai G et al. Small differences in intraischemic brain temperature critically determines the extent of neuronal injury. *J Cereb Blood Flow Metab* 1987;7:729–738.
16. Busto R, Dietrich WD, Globus MYT et al. Post ischemic moderate hypothermia inhibits CA1 hippocampal ischemic neuronal injury. *Neurosci Lett* 1989;101:299–304.
17. Busuttil RW, Baker JD, Davidson RK. Carotid artery stenosis—hemodynamic significance and clinical course. *JAMA* 1981;245:1438–1441.
18. Callow AD, Matsumoto G, Baker D et al. Protection of the high risk carotid endarterectomy patient by continuous electroencephalography. *J Cardiovasc Surg* 1978;19:55–63.
19. Caplan LR. Carotid artery disease. *N Engl J Med* 1986;315:886–888.
20. CASANOVA Study Group. Carotid surgery versus medical therapy in asymptomatic carotid stenosis. *Stroke* 1991;22:1229–1235.
21. Chambers BR, Norris JW. The case against surgery for asymptomatic carotid stenosis. *Stroke* 1984;15:964–967.
22. Chambers BR, Norris JW. Outcome in patients with asymptomatic neck bruits. *N Engl J Med* 1986;315:860–865.
23. Chimowitz M. Clinical spectrum and natural history of cerebrovascular occlusive disease.

In: Awad, IA, ed. *Cerebrovascular occlusive disease and brain ischemia*. Park Ridge, IL: AANS;1992:59–71.

24. Collins R, Peto R, MacMahon S et al. Epidemiology—blood pressure, stroke, and coronary heart disease. *Lancet* 1990;335:827–838.
25. Craig DR, Meguro K, Watridge C et al. Intracranial internal carotid artery stenosis. *Stroke* 1982;13:825–828.
26. Day AL, Rhoton AL, Quisling RG. Resolving siphon stenosis following endarterectomy. *Stroke* 1980;11:278–281.
27. Day AL, Scott EW, Dolson L et al. Carotid endarterectomy complicated by vein patch rupture. *NSG* 1992;31:373–377.
28. Deriu GP, Ballotta E, Bonavina L et al. The rationale for patch-graft angioplasty after carotid endarterectomy: early and long-term follow-up. *Stroke* 1984;15:972–978.
29. Dirrenberger RA, Sundt TM. Carotid endarterectomy. *J Neurosurg* 1978;48:201–219.
30. Dyken M. Stroke risk factors. In: Norris JW, Hachinski VC, eds. *Prevention of stroke*. New York: Springer-Verlag; 1991:83–101.
31. Dyken ML, Pokras R. The performance of endarterectomy for disease of the extracranial arteries of the head. *Stroke* 1984;15:948–949.
32. Eastcott HHG, Pickering GW, Rob CG. Reconstruction of internal carotid artery. *Lancet* 1954;2:994–996.
33. Ercius MS, Chandler WF, Ford JW et al. Early versus delayed heparin reversal after carotid endarterectomy in the dog. *J Neurosurg* 1983;58:708–713.
34. Ercius MS, Chandler WF, Ford JW et al. Effect of different aspirin doses on arterial thrombosis after canine carotid endarterectomy: a scanning electron microscope and indium-111-labeled platelet study. *Neurosurgery* 1984;14:198–203.
35. European Carotid Surgery Trialists' Collaborative Group. MRC European carotid surgery trial: interim results for symptomatic patients with severe (70–99%) or with mild (0–29%) carotid stenosis. *Lancet* 1991;337:1235–1243.
36. Fein JM. A history of cerebrovascular disease and its surgical management. In: Smith RR, ed. *Stroke and the extracranial vessels*. New York: Raven Press; 1984:1–7.
37. Fields WS, Lemak NA. Joint study of extracranial arterial occlusion. *JAMA* 1976;235:2608–2610.
38. Fields WS, Maslenikov V, Stirling Meyer J et al. Joint study of extracranial arterial occlusion. *JAMA* 1970;211:1993–2003.
39. Fields WS, Lemak NA, Frankowski RF et al. Controlled trial of aspirin in cerebral ischemia. *Stroke* 1977;8:301–315.
40. Fietsam R, Ranval T, Cohn S et al. Hemodynamic effects of primary closure versus patch angioplasty of the carotid artery. *Ann Vasc Surg* 1992;6:443–449.
41. Fisher CM. Concerning transient ischemic attacks. *Clev Clin J Med* 1987;54:3–11.
42. Fisher CM, Gore I, Okabe N, et al. Atherosclerosis of the carotid and vertebral arteries—extracranial and intracranial. *J Neuropathol Exp Neurol* 1965;24:455–476.
43. Flamm ES, Demopoulos HB, Seligman ML et al. Possible molecular mechanisms of barbiturate mediated protection in regional cerebral ischemia. *Acta Neurol Scand* (Suppl) 1977;64:150–151.
44. Fode NC, Sundt TM, Robertson JT et al. Multicenter retrospective review of results and complications of carotid endarterectomy in 1981. *Stroke* 1986;17:370–376.
45. Fox JL. Cerebral arterial revascularization: the value of repeated angiography in selection of patients for operation. *Neurosurgery* 1978;2:205–209.
46. Friedman GD, Wilson WS, Mosier JM et al. Transient ischemic attacks in a community. *JAMA* 1969;210:1428–1434.
47. Gerraty RP, Gatees PC, Doyle JC. Carotid stenosis and perioperative stroke risk in symptomatic and asymptomatic patients undergoing vascular or coronary surgery. *Stroke* 1993;24:1115–1118.
48. Giannotta SL, Dicks RE, Kindt GW. Carotid endarterectomy: technical improvements. *Neurosurgery* 1980;4:309–312.
49. Gilroy J, Meyer JS. Auscultation of the neck in occlusive cerebrovascular disease. *Circulation* 1962;25:300–310.
50. Gross CE, Adams HP, Sokoll MD et al. Use of anticoagulants, electroencephalographic monitoring, and barbiturate cerebral protection in carotid endarterectomy. *Neurosurgery* 1981;9:1–5.
51. Hall ED, Yonkers PA. Attenuation of postischemic cerebral hypoperfusion. *Stroke* 1988;19:340–344.
52. Hammond JH, Eisinger RP. Carotid bruits in 1,000 normal subjects. *Arch Intern Med* 1962;109:563–565.
53. Hennerici M, Hulsbomer HB, Hefter H et al. Natural history of asymptomatic extracranial arterial disease—results of a long-term prospective study. 1987;110:777–791.
54. Hertzer NR, Flanagan RA, O'Hara PJ et al. Surgical versus nonoperative treatment of symptomatic carotid stenosis. *Ann Surg* 1986;2:163–171.
55. Hertzer NR, Beven EG, O'Hara PJ et al. A prospective study of vein patch angioplasty during carotid endarterectomy. *Ann Surg* 1987;628–635.
56. Heyman A, Leviton A, Millikan CH et al. Transient focal cerebral ischemia: epidemiological and clinical aspects. *Stroke* 1974;5:277–283.
57. Heyman A, Wilkinson WE, Heyden S et al. Risk of stroke in asymptomatic persons with cervical arterial bruits. *N Engl J Med* 1986;302:838–841.

58. Hobson RW, Weiss DG, Fields WS et al. Efficacy of carotid endarterectomy for asymptomatic carotid stenosis. *N Engl J Med* 1993;328:221–727.
59. Hunter WJ, Sterpetti AV, Schultz RD et al. Carotid plaque ulceration: its significance in cerebral ischemia. *Stroke* 1989;20:158.
60. Howe JR, Kindt GW. Cerebral protection during carotid endarterectomy. *Stroke* 1974;5:340–343.
61. Imparato AM, Ramirez A, Riles T et al. Cerebral protection in carotid surgery. *Arch Surg* 1982;117:1073–1078.
62. Ingall TJ, Homer D, Whisnant JP et al. Predictive value of carotid bruit for carotid atherosclerosis. *Arch Neurol* 1989;46:418–422.
63. Jansen C, Moll FL, Vermeulen FE et al. Continuous transcranial doppler ultrasonography and electroencephalography during carotid endarterectomy: a multimodal monitoring system to detect intraoperative ischemia. *Ann Vasc Surg* 1993;7:95–101.
64. Javid H, Ostermiller WE, Hengesh JW et al. Natural history of carotid bifurcation atheroma. *Surgery* 1970;67:80–86.
65. Kannel WB, Wolf PA, Verter J. Risk factors for stroke. In: Smith RR, ed. *Stroke and the extracranial vessels*. New York: Raven Press; 1984:47–58.
66. Katz MM, Jones T, Degenhardt J et al. The use of patch angioplasty to alter the incidence of carotid restenosis following thromboendarterectomy. *J Cardiovasc Surg* 1987;28:28–38.
67. Keagy BA, Poole MA, Burnham SJ et al. Frequency, severity, and physiologic importance of carotid siphon lesions. *J Vasc Surg* 1986;3:511–515.
68. Kuller LH, Sutton KC. Carotid artery bruit: is it safe and effective to auscultate the neck? *Stroke* 1984;15:944–947.
69. Kurtzke JF, Barnett HJM, Mohr JP et al. Epidemiology in stroke. In: Barnett HJM, Mohr JP, Stewe BM, et al., eds. *Stroke: pathophysiology, diagnosis, management*. New York: Churchill Livingstone; 1986:3–29.
70. Lee KS, Davis CH Jr, McWhorter JM. Low morbidity and mortality of carotid endarterectomy performed with regional anesthesia. *J Neurosurg* 1988;69:483–487.
71. Little JR, Sawhny B, Weinstein M. Pseudo-tandem stenosis of the internal carotid artery. *Neurosurgery* 1980;7:574–577.
72. Little JR, Bryerton BS, Furlan AJ. Saphenous vein patch grafts in carotid endarterectomy. *J Neurosurg* 1984;61:743–747.
73. Lord RS, Raj TB, Graham AR. Carotid endarterectomy, siphon stenosis, collateral hemispheric pressure, and perioperative cerebral infarction. *J Vasc Surg* 1987;6:391–397.
74. MacMahon S, Peto R, Cutler J. Epidemiology—blood pressure, stroke, and coronary heart disease. *Lancet* 1990;335:765–774.
75. Marjewski DJ, Furhan AJ, St. Louis P, et al. Intracranial internal carotid artery stenosis: long term prognosis. *Stroke* 1982;13:821–824.
76. Mayberg MR, Wilson SE, Yatsu F et al. Carotid endarterectomy and prevention of cerebral ischemia in symptomatic carotid stenosis. *JAMA* 1991;266:3289–3294.
77. Michenfelder JD, Milde JH, Sundt TM. Cerebral protection by barbiturate anesthesia. *Arch Neurol* 1976;33:345–350.
78. Modan B, Wagener DK. Some epidemiological aspects of stroke: mortality/morbidity trends, age, sex, race, socioeconomic status. *Stroke* 1992;23:1230–1236.
79. Mohr JP, Pessin MS. Extracranial carotid artery disease. In Burnett HJM, Mohr JP, Stein BM, Yatsu FM, eds. *Stroke*. New York: Churchill Livingstone; 1986:293–336.
80. Mohr JP, Caplan LR, Melski JW et al. The Harvard Cooperative Stroke Registry: a prospective registry. *Neurology* 1978;28:754–762.
81. Moncada S, Vane JR. Mode of action of aspirin-like drugs. *Adv Int Med* 1979;24:1–20.
82. Moore DJ, Miles RD, Gooley NA et al. Noninvasive assessment of stroke risk in asymptomatic and nonhemispheric patients with suspected carotid disease. *Ann Surg* 1985;202:491–504.
83. Moore WS. Does tandem lesion mean tandem risk in patients with carotid artery disease? *J Vasc Surg* 1988;7:454–455.
84. Moore WS. Extracranial cerebrovascular disease—the carotid artery. 4th edition. New York: W.B. Saunders; 1993:532–575.
85. Moore WS, Boren C, Malone JM et al. Natural history of nonstenotic, asymptomatic ulcerative lesions of the carotid artery. *Arch Surg* 1978;113:1352–1357.
86. Muuronen A. Outcome of surgical treatment of 110 patients with transient ischemic attack. *Stroke* 1984;15:959–963.
87. North American Symptomatic Carotid Endarterectomy Trial (NASCET) Investigators. Clinical alert: benefit of carotid endarterectomy for patients with high-grade stenosis of the internal carotid artery. *Clin Alert* 1991;22:816–817.
88. North American Symptomatic Carotid Endarterectomy Trial (NASCET) Steering Committee. North American symptomatic carotid endarterectomy trial. *Stroke* 1991;22:711–720.
89. North American Symptomatic Carotid Endarterectomy Trial Collaborators. Beneficial effect of carotid endarterectomy in symptomatic patients with high-grade carotid stenosis. *N Engl J Med* 1991;325:445–453.
90. Norris JW, Zhu CZ. Stroke risk and critical carotid stenosis. *J Neurol Neurosurg Psychiatry* 1990;53:235–237.
91. Norris JW, Zhu CZ, Bornstein NM et al. Vascular risks of asymptomatic carotid stenosis. *Stroke* 1991;22:1487–1489.
92. Ostfeld AM, Shekelle RB, Klawans HL. Transient ischemic attacks and risk of stroke in an elderly poor population. *Stroke* 1973;4:980–986.

93. Pessin MS, Duncan GW, Mohr JP et al. Clinical and angiographic features of carotid transient ischemic attacks. *N Engl J Med* 1977;296:358–362.
94. Pessin MS, Hinton RCC, Davis KR et al. Mechanisms of acute carotid stroke. *Ann Neurol* 1979;6:245–255.
95. Piepgras DG, Sundt TM, Sidisheim P. Effect of anticoagulants and inhibitors of platelet aggregation on thrombotic occlusion of endarterectomized cat carotid arteries. *Stroke* 1976;7:249–254.
96. Piepgras DG, Sundt TM, Marsh WR et al. Recurrent carotid stenosis—results and complications of 57 operations. *Am Surg* 1986;203:205–213.
97. Pritz MB, Smolin MF. Treatment of tandem lesions of the extracranial carotid artery. *Neurosurgery* 1984;15:233–236.
98. Rennie L, Ejrup B, McDowell F. Arterial bruits in cerebrovascular disease. *Neurology* 1964;14:751–756.
99. Roederer GO, Langlois YE, Chan ARW, et al. Is siphon disease important in predicting outcome in carotid endarterectomy? *Arch Surg* 1983;118:1177–1181.
100. Roederer GO, Langlois YE, Jager KA et al. The natural history of carotid arterial disease in asymptomatic patients with cervical bruits. *Stroke* 1984;15:605–613.
101. Samuelsson K, Svensson J. Aspirin: optimal dose in stroke prevention. *Stroke* 1993;24:1259–1261.
102. Sarti C, Tuomilehto J, Sivenius J et al. Stroke mortality and case-fatality rates in three geographic areas of Finland from 1983 to 1986. *Stroke* 1993;24:1140–1147.
103. Schuler JJ, Flanigan DP, Lim LT et al. The effect of carotid siphon stenosis on stroke rate, death, and relief of symptoms following elective endarterectomy. *Surgery* 1982;92:1058–1067.
104. Shaw DA, Venables GS, Cartlidge NEF et al. Carotid endarterectomy in patients with transient cerebral ischemia. *J Neurol Sci* 1984;64:45–53.
105. Sorensen S, Marquardsen J, Pedersen H et al. Long-term prognosis of reversible cerebral ischemic attacks. In: *14th International Joint Conference on Stroke and Cerebral Circulation*. San Antonio, Texas 1989.
106. Spetzler RF, Martin N, Hadley MN et al. Microsurgical endarterectomy under barbiturate protection: a prospective study. *J Neurosurg* 1986;65:63–73.
107. Stallones RA. Epidemiology of stroke in relation to the cardiovascular disease complex. *Adv Neurol* 1974;25:117–126.
108. Thompson JE, Patman RD, Talkington CM. Asymptomatic carotid bruit: long-term outcome of patients having endarterectomy compared with unoperated controls. *Ann Surg* 1978;188:308–316.
109. Toole JF. *Cerebrovascular disorders*. 4th edition. New York: Raven Press 1990.
110. Toole JF, Yuson CP, Janeway R et al. Transient ischemic attacks: a prospective study of 225 patients. *Neurology* 1978;28:746–753.
111. Towne JB, Weiss DG, Hobson R. First phase report of cooperative Veterans Administration asymptomatic carotid stenosis study—operative morbidity and mortality. *Vasc Surg* 1990;11:252–259.
112. Ueda K, Toole JF, McHenry LC. Carotid and vertebrobasilar transient ischemic attacks: clinical angiographic correlation. *Neurology* 1979;29:1094–1101.
113. Weksler BB, Lewin M. Anticoagulation in cerebral ischemia. *Stroke* 1983;14:658–663.
114. Welch LK, Crowley WJ. Bruits of the head and neck. *Stroke* 1970;1:245–247.
115. Whisnant JP. Special report from the National Institute of Neurological Disorders and Stroke. Classifications of cerebrovascular diseases III. *Stroke* 1990;21:637–680.
116. Whisnant JP, Matsumoto N, Elveback LR. Transient cerebral ischemic attacks in a community. *Mayo Clin Proc* 1973;48:194–198.
117. Wiebers DO, Whisnant JP, Sandok BA et al. Prospective comparison of a cohort with asymptomatic carotid bruit and a population-based cohort without carotid bruit. *Stroke* 1990;21:984–988.
118. Winslow CM, Solomon DH, Chassin MR et al. The appropriateness of carotid endarterectomy. *N Engl J Med* 1988;318:721–727.
119. Wolf PA. An overview of the epidemiology of stroke. *Stroke* 1990(Suppl. 4–6):21.
120. Wolf PA, Kannel WB, Sorlie P et al. Asymptomatic carotid bruit and risk of stroke. *JAMA* 1981;245:1442–1445.
121. Wolf PA, O'Neill A, D'Agostino RB et al. Declining mortality not declining incidence of stroke. The Framingham Study #101. *Stroke* 1989;20:158.
122. Wolf PA, Belanger AJ, D'Agostino RB. Management of risk factors in cerebral ischemia: treatment and prevention. *Neurol Clin* 1992;177–191.
123. Xue S, Burke GL, Sprafka M et al. Trends in stroke mortality, morbidity, case-fatality and long-term survival from 1970–1985: The Minnesota Heart Survey. In: 17th International Joint Conference on Stroke and Cerebral Circulation, Phoenix, Arizona 1992.
124. Youmans JR, Kindt GW. Efficacy of carbon dioxide in the treatment of cerebral ischemia. *Surg Forum* 1968;19:425–426.

2

Preoperative Evaluation, Risk Assessment, and Patient Selection for Carotid Endarterectomy

Jon Brillman and Thomas F. Scott

The appropriate selection of patients for carotid endarterectomy is, and will always be, the single most important factor in the success or failure of this procedure. Since its inception in the 1950s, carotid endarterectomy has been an extremely popular operation; more than 1 million procedures have been performed (5). Most surgeons now agree that a significant number of these operations were inappropriate (54). Despite the uncertainty of the results of the joint study to evaluate the efficacy of carotid endarterectomy in the late 1960s, the number increased steadily until the mid-1980s, when its indication was subjected to renewed scientific scrutiny (9). The reasons for its early popularity were many. Surgeons were understandably excited about a procedure that promised to prevent the devastation of stroke, and thousands of young physicians were trained in this operation worldwide. The advent of equipment designed to detect the presence and severity of carotid stenosis noninvasively, as well as refinements in angiography, encouraged surgical intervention before adequate data from clinical trials were available to verify the value of the procedure.

During this period, the reported incidence of perioperative complications varied from 3% to more than 21.1%, with an average of about 10% (4,11,

J. Brillman and T. F. Scott: Department of Neurology, Medical College of Pennsylvania and Hahnemann University, Pittsburgh, Pennsylvania 15212.

16,19,21,22,33–36,40,49,54). This discrepancy seemed to depend not only on varying levels of surgical expertise but on the appropriateness of patient selection. It was not sufficient, of course, to define the success of the procedure based on acceptable rates of perioperative morbidity and death; by examining predetermined end points such as stroke, disabling stroke, and vascular mortality, it was imperative to demonstrate that symptomatic patients who underwent surgery had more favorable short- and long-term outcomes than patients on no therapy or on medical therapy alone. The declining incidence of stroke added further urgency to the need to demonstrate the value of surgical treatment (31). Accordingly, several clinical trials were designed in the early 1980s to address the value of surgical intervention for carotid disease.

CLINICAL TRIALS

The joint study in the late 1960s and early 1970s was an early attempt to assess the efficacy of carotid endarterectomy (9,20). Patients were not randomized by degree of stenosis, and the number of patients studied was relatively small. Unfortunately, no firm conclusions could be drawn from the data. A most important well-controlled and well-designed clinical trial to assess the role of surgery in stroke prevention was the Cooperative External Carotid to Internal Carotid Bypass Study completed in the mid-1980s (18). For several years before the inception of this study, many surgeons were trained in this meticulous and painstaking procedure, which attempted to bypass occluded arteries in the neck and intracerebrally. The EC-IC Bypass Study involved 71 centers and randomized 1,377 patients to aspirin therapy and surgery plus aspirin therapy. This study ran for 60 months, and all of the patients were accounted for in follow-up. The patency rate of the bypassed arteries was more than 97%. Although many surgeons had hoped that the study would show the operation to be of value, the results indicated unequivocally that for stroke prevention, it was not (17).

Although the outcome of the EC-IC Bypass Study was discouraging, its study design was adopted for other clinical trials that have proved to be of inestimable value in determining what is and is not successful in stroke prevention. The most widely cited of these is the North American Symptomatic Carotid Endarterectomy Trial (NASCET) study (36,38). Planned in the early 1980s, this trial began to enroll patients in 50 centers in January 1988. Symptomatic, hemispheric, transient ischemic attacks (TIAs), or minor nondisabling stroke patients were randomized into a surgical group and a medical group (on 1,300 mg of aspirin a day) and by degrees of stenosis of the internal carotid artery (30% to 69%; 70% to 99%). The first results from NASCET became available in February 1991, when an independent oversight committee determined that the difference in outcome events in patients with 70% to 99% stenosis was significantly better in the surgically treated patients than in the medical group. The study for patients with high-grade stenosis was therefore terminated. The absolute risk reduction for surgery compared with the best medical therapy at that time was 17%, and the relative risk reduction was 65% for ipsilateral stroke and stroke death. Surgical morbidity was higher only in the first few months. Thereafter, and even until the present time, the difference in stroke outcome has remained consistently better in the surgical group.

Indeed, no matter which subgroup of patients or which end points one studies in NASCET, the surgical patients consistently fare better than medically treated patients (Table 1). Information remains wanting, however, in patients with less than 70% stenosis. The European Carotid Stroke Trial

Table 1. *First adverse events and actuarial failure rates at 2 years of follow-up of patients with severe stenosis in NASCET[a]*

According to the event defining failure[b]	Events (event rate %[c])		Absolute difference ± SE (%)	Relative risk reduction (%)
	Medical patients (n = 331)	Surgical patients (n = 328)		
Any ipsilateral stroke	61 (26.0)	26 (9.0)	17.0 ± 3.5[c]	65
Any stroke	64 (27.6)	34 (12.6)	15.0 ± 3.8[c]	54
Any stroke or death	73 (32.3)	41 (15.8)	16.5 ± 4.2[c]	51
Major or fatal ipsilateral stroke	29 (13.1)	8 (2.5)	10.6 ± 2.6[c]	81
Any major or fatal stroke	29 (13.1)	10 (3.7)	9.4 ± 2.7[c]	72
Any major stroke or death	38 (18.1)	19 (8.0)	10.1 ± 3.5[d]	56

(*From* NASCET Collaborators. *N Engl J Med* 1991;325:445–453, with permission.)

[a] "Death" refers to mortality from all causes. In addition to the events defining treatment failure, each value includes all strokes (any severity and any site) and deaths from any cause: in the surgical patients between randomization and the 30th day after surgery and in the medical patients during the comparable 32-day perirandomization period.

[b] Failure rates were derived from Kaplan-Meier estimates of survival.

[c] $p < 0.001$ for the comparison of the treatment groups.

[d] $p < 0.01$ for the comparison of the treatment groups.

(ECST) demonstrated that patients with less than 30% stenosis fared better with medical therapy (19). Whether the large group of patients in the middle ground (30% to 69% stenosis) benefits from surgical intervention, however, remains unsettled. Indeed, as NASCET continues to enroll patients, some disquieting evidence suggests that physicians may be extrapolating the benefit of surgery from those with higher degrees of stenosis to include those with moderate degrees of stenosis. In a recent article, Barnett et al. (7) have exhorted physicians to randomize their patients objectively.

NASCET not only revealed the value of carotid endarterectomy in certain groups of patients but also enlightened the neurologic community in other areas related to risk assessment. The surgical morbidity and mortality in the first 30 days after carotid endarterectomy was 2.1%. This finding highlighted the fact that centers that perform large numbers of carotid endarterectomy are capable of maintaining a low complication rate. At this writing, some 30 months after the NASCET data became public, the benefit of surgery relative to best medical therapy remains unchanged in terms of absolute risk reduction.

As noted, preliminary evidence suggests that surgery may not be of sufficient value in lower degrees of stenosis to justify its use. Indeed, if one examines the relative advantage of surgery to best medical therapy in the three deciles from 70% to 99%, the benefit for surgical intervention declines with diminishing degrees of stenosis (7). Consequently, patients with less than 70% stenosis may fare as well or better than surgical patients if they are treated medically, particularly if the physician chooses to use newer platelet antiaggregant medication such as ticlopidine, which is superior to aspirin in preventing stroke in symptomatic carotid disease (25).

Some data are available with respect to asymptomatic carotid stenosis. None, however, have clearly determined that surgery is of value in this group of patients. The Veterans Affairs Cooperative Study Group (VACSG) trial published in 1993 showed a benefit for surgery over aspirin in a relatively small series of patients with more than 50% stenosis but only if TIAs were included as end points (27). If one looked at stroke and stroke death alone, surgery was no better than aspirin therapy. The scope of the Asymptomatic Carotid Artery Study (ACAS) is much more extensive having completed randomization favoring surgery over asperin in patients with greater than 50% stenosis. Publication of the results is pending and some discussion by the neurologic community is anticipated (51).

RADIOLOGIC EVALUATION OF CAROTID STENOSIS

Recently, debate regarding the best way to determine the degree of carotid stenosis, thus identifying those patients who may best benefit from surgery, has been vigorous (6). This subject is discussed in more detail in Chapter 4; however, some comment is made here because it is a critical factor in the decision-making process.

The NASCET and ECST studies, both which demonstrated that patients with higher grade carotid stenosis benefit the most from surgery, utilized linear measurements of stenosis identified by angiography (19,36,38). In the NASCET trial, the diameter of the stenotic area was the numerator, and the segment distal to the stenosis was the denominator. The percentage of stenosis was determined by multiplying by 100. The ECST trial utilized the diameter of the carotid bulb. Ultrasonography was not used as a measurement in either trial. Carotid duplex information was available, however, and the correlation with the degree of stenosis as determined by angiography was poor.

Alexandrov et al. (3) have attempted to demonstrate that modern duplex measurements may be more accurate in determining cross-sectional diameter as later determined by analyzing the surgical specimens than are linear measurements or angiography. Nevertheless, the wide variation in instrumentation and radiologic interpretation as well as the need to image the carotid siphon and intracerebral circulation make angiography mandatory. In addition, the simple formula used in NASCET to determine linear stenosis has widespread applicability in the hundreds of centers that currently perform carotid endarterectomy, serving to standardize surgical patients worldwide.

The role of magnetic resonance (MR) angiography, transcranial Doppler, axial MR imaging, and computed tomography (CT) appears to be promising when used as an adjunct to angiography (1,28,41,44). In particular, MRI and transcranial Doppler may provide the vital information required to identify intracerebral stenosis or other lesions that could make carotid endarterectomy imprudent. Based on their evaluation of 24 patients who underwent carotid endarterectomy, Polak et al. (41) concluded that the combined use of Doppler sonography and MRI may be able to replace conventional angiography in as many as 79% of patients. This conclusion was based on "the surgeon's assessment of the appearance and extent of plaque deposition in the internal carotid artery" compared with the results of the noninvasive study. The continued evolution of these techniques suggests that angiography may be unnecessary in the future. However, the well-known difficulty of noninvasive techniques in detecting the difference between high-grade stenosis and occlusion implies that the physician serving this very large group of patients who may benefit from surgery may be subject to planning treatment based on erroneous information gathered during the patient's presurgical evaluation. For the present, therefore, it seems best to encourage the continued use of angiography, which has been established as the standard diagnostic modality in large, accepted clinical trials.

PREOPERATIVE EVALUATION AND PATIENT SELECTION

The preoperative evaluation of the patient for carotid endarterectomy must be designed to ensure that this procedure will not carry a risk that would negate the established benefit of surgery compared with the benefit of medical therapy that has been proved by clinical trials. In addition, the operation must materially benefit the patient in terms of quality of life. Regrettably, this aspect of treatment is often overlooked.

Table 2 identifies the current clinical and radiographic parameters that may suggest the appropriateness of surgical therapy for carotid stenosis. These parameters should serve as a guide only. Various circumstances will force clinicians to use their clinical judgment in deciding the best course for action for an individual patient. A large group of patients, however, still fall into an ''uncertain'' category, and clinical judgment remains the key to mak-

Table 2. *Indications for carotid endarterectomy*

Certain indication
  Symptomatic carotid stenosis, i.e., carotid distribution TIA or minor stroke (recovery up to 80% of premorbid function) in patients with severe (>70%) stenosis ipsilateral to TIA or infarct[a]
Uncertain indication
  (Await results of ongoing clinical trials, retrospective analysis of existing trials or future trials)
  Asymptomatic carotid artery stenosis
  Asymptomatic carotid artery stenosis with progression on successive Doppler studies to >90%
  Symptomatic carotid stenosis of 30–69%
  Patients with severe carotid stenosis who have been asymptomatic for >6 months
  Patients with severe carotid stenosis ipsilateral to symptoms and with contralateral carotid occlusion
  Patients with severe carotid stenosis and ipsilateral amaurosis fugax as the only symptom
  Patients with severe carotid stenosis and completed stroke with significant hemiparesis or aphasia
  Patients with severe carotid stenosis and evolving stroke in the distribution of the carotid lesion
  Patients with severe carotid stenosis, ipsilateral to symptoms and a cardiac embolic source for stroke as determined by echocardiography or the presence of atrial fibrillation
  Patients with severe asymptomatic carotid stenosis prior to coronary revascularization procedures
Surgery not indicated
  Symptomatic carotid stenosis in patients with <30% stenosis ipsilateral to symptoms
  Symptomatic or asymptomatic patients with carotid occlusion, ipsilateral to symptoms
  Nonhemispheric symptoms such as headache, light-headedness, vertigo, syncope, binocular visual blurring, cognitive disturbances even in the presence of severe carotid stenosis
  Vertebrobasilar TIAs
  Severe carotid stenosis with symptoms referable to the opposite hemisphere
  Patients with carotid stenosis and ipsilateral severe stroke with hemiplegia and/or coma
  Patients with severe carotid stenosis and ipsilateral symptoms with serious co-morbid conditions (e.g., metastatic cancer or Alzheimer's disease)

[a] Assumes all other risk factors for stroke, such as age, hypertension, elevated blood lipids, cessation of smoking, and control of diabetes, have been addressed.

ing a wise decision. In all patients, but particularly in this "uncertain" group, it is imperative to consider, and whenever possible, favorably modify risk factors such as hypertension, obesity, smoking, and hyperlipidemia. Certain issues such as age cannot be changed and should be considered as an independent risk factor in terms of surgical risk and comorbid conditions.

Age

Because carotid stenosis is a disease of advanced years, most surgical interventions will be for patients who are 65 years or older. In a random sample of 1,302 patients more than 65 years of age in 1981, Brook et al. (11) found an 11.3% perioperative rate of complications. These patients were controlled for age, race, income, hospital size and type, and physician volume. In addition, they found that if the operating physician was a foreign medical graduate not from a Western European or Canadian medical school, the average complication rate rose from 10.4% to 19.6%. Both of these perioperative morbidity and mortality rates are considered unacceptable today.

In a series from the Mayo Clinic, Meyer et al. (34) examined the records of 479 carotid endarterectomies, 693 of which were performed in patients older than 70 years of age. For this group, the neurologic morbidity was 3.1% and the mortality was 1.3%. Acceptable complication rates therefore occurred in the elderly cohort. In a retrospective analysis of 2,089 patients who had carotid endarterectomy in the mid-1980s, Fisher et al. (21) found that the 30-day perioperative death rate increased for each decile of age, ranging from 1.1% (60–69 years) to 4.7% (over age 80 years). In a large retrospective analysis, McCrory et al. (33) found that an age of more than 75 years doubled the perioperative complication rate of stroke, vascular mortality, and myocardial infarction compared with younger patients.

The perioperative complications, including mortality, therefore increase with a patient's age. However, with careful patient selection, control of other risk factors, and satisfactory surgical expertise, acceptable complication rates can be achieved in older patients.

Carotid Stenosis and Coronary Artery Disease

It is particularly important to assess the status of the coronary circulation preoperatively because the underlying pathology (arteriosclerosis) is similar in stroke and myocardial infarction. It has been known for some time that a significant percentage of patients with TIAs and stroke will die of coronary artery disease. Indeed, the risk of fatal myocardial infarction in symptomatic carotid disease is about 5% a year, exceeding the death rate of recurrent stroke (2). Patients with asymptomatic carotid stenosis are not excluded from this risk (37).

Earlier studies performed at the Cleveland Clinic evaluated candidates for carotid surgery with preoperative coronary arteriography and identified lesions in the coronary arteries in 93% of patients, 86% of whom had no prior indication of coronary artery disease (26). It is unfortunately impractical to perform coronary arteriography on all patients who are appropriate candidates for carotid endarterectomy. Noninvasive cardiac evaluation, however, is widely available in most centers and provides safe, relatively inexpensively obtained information about the status of the coronary circulation. Several studies have demonstrated that myocardial ischemia could be determined in a high percentage (45% to 58%) of patients with symptomatic carotid disease by using exercise stress tests with and without perfusion myocardial scintigraphy (thallium stress test) (15,32,43,46). Further studies have shown that a high percentage of patients who underwent carotid endarterectomy and had identifiable coronary artery lesions on stress testing and perfusional myocardial scintiscans developed ischemic cardiac events (52). Based on the predictive value of these investigations, candidates for carotid endarterectomy can be stratified with respect to their risk of coronary events, and informed decisions regarding the need for coronary arteriography and coronary bypass graft surgery or angioplasty can be made. Further cardiac evaluation of patients with carotid stenosis is discussed in detail in Chapter 4.

Hypertension

The role of hypertension in the pathogenesis of stroke is incontrovertible. Indeed, the declining incidence of stroke over the past three decades can be significantly attributed to the control of hypertension, including the control of mildly elevated blood pressure. What was not fully appreciated until more recently was the importance of controlling isolated systolic hypertension (14,30). Table 3 clearly shows that control of isolated systolic hypertension is associated with a reduced risk of stroke and may be particularly important to the elderly, in whom isolated systolic hypertension often occurs. Although it is beyond the scope of this chapter to discuss the ever increasing number of antihypertensive drugs that are available, angiotensin-converting enzyme inhibitors, beta blockers, and calcium channel blockers are valuable additions to the traditional list of antihypertensives, many of which had unacceptable side effects.

Although it is recommended that patients with hypertension have their blood pressure stabilized slowly with one of these oral agents, individuals who require endarterectomy occasionally need their blood pressure reduced more rapidly. Under these circumstances, parenteral agents such as sodium nitroprusside (8 to 50 μg/min) may be administered by controlled intravenous infusion. Close monitoring to avoid hypertension is required. In these circumstances sublingual or oral nifedipine (5 to 10 mg) may lower the blood pressure within 30 minutes. Close observation is again required to avoid hypotension. Agents that may not require monitoring as close as the rapidly acting drugs in the preoperative period may include intramuscular hydralazine (Apresoline) 5 to 20 mg every 2 to 4 hours or Nitropaste, 1 inch every 4 to 6 hours.

Retrospective analysis has also determined that severe hypertension, de-

Table 3. *Risk of atherothrombotic brain infarction and stroke in the elderly with isolated systolic hypertension (ISH): 36-year follow-up[a]*

	65–74 years old		75–84 years old	
	Men	Women	Men	Women
Atherothrombotic brain infarction				
ISH absent	3.8	3.0	8.2	7.1
ISH present	9.5	7.1	14.5	8.2
Risk ratio	2.5	2.4	1.8	1.2
p value	0.001	0.001	0.12	0.66
Stroke—all types				
ISH absent	8.7	7.3	17.4	15.1
ISH present	17.0	12.6	37.6	20.4
Risk ratio	2.0	1.7	2.2	1.4
p value	0.002	0.002	0.000	0.13

(From Wolf et al. *Neurol Clin* 1992;10:177–191, with permission.)
[a] Average annual incidence per 1,000.

fined as preoperative diastolic blood pressures of more than 110 mmHg, more than doubles the risk of adverse perioperative outcomes. This increased risk is in addition to the continued risk of stroke associated with uncontrolled hypertension, even if carotid endarterectomy is free of complications (33).

RISK OF SURGERY IN ASYMPTOMATIC CAROTID STENOSIS VERSUS SYMPTOMATIC CAROTID STENOSIS

Superficially, it would seem that patients with TIAs and minor stroke treated by carotid endarterectomy would be at a greater risk for complications than patients undergoing a similar procedure in stenotic vessels that have produced no symptoms. The reported incidence of surgical complications in the literature, however, does not always support this commonsense notion. Although complication rates higher than 20% have been reported in many series (both symptomatic and asymptomatic) (16), the NASCET trial reported a remarkably low mortality and morbidity rate of 2.1% (36). The ECST trial had a somewhat higher complication rate of 3.7% (19). The Carotid Artery Stenosis and Narrowing Operation Versus Aspirin (CASANOVA) trial (asymptomatic patients) reported a complication rate of 6.9% (50), and the VACSG trial for asymptomatic carotid stenosis ($\geq$50%) reported a complication rate of 5% (27)—more than twice the rate reported by the NASCET trial, which only included patients with more than 70% stenosis. The ACAS trial, yet to be published, will report a complication rate of 1.9% (J.F. Toole, M.D., personal communication). In their retrospective analysis of 1,160 patients in 12 academic centers, McCrory et al. (33) reported a surgical complication rate of 8.5% in ipsilateral hemispheric TIAs versus 4.5% in asymptomatic patients. Although their data suggested that symptomatic patients have almost twice the risk for complications as asymptomatic patients, this risk factor was considered independently. The many other variables known to alter risk were not taken into account. Indeed, the risk of stroke in asymptomatic patients with more than 75% stenosis approaches that of symptomatic patients (13). Current recommendations are that certain patients with asymptomatic carotid stenosis should undergo surgical intervention. If, however, surgical risk and perioperative morbidity and mortality are not proved to be significantly lower in stenotic arteries in asymptomatic patients, the finding may have negative implications for carotid endarterectomy in patients with less than 70% stenosis whose risk of future stroke may only be marginally improved by surgery.

CORONARY ARTERY BYPASS GRAFT AND ENDARTERECTOMY

A persistent and vexing dilemma continues to face surgeons who plan coronary artery bypass graft procedures in patients with high-grade carotid stenosis. Regrettably, no clinical trials have thus far been performed to define clearly the proper course of action in these circumstances. Experience suggests that a two-stage procedure (carotid endarterectomy and coronary artery bypass graft) poses an unacceptable risk of complications, and that if a decision is made to do a carotid endarterectomy, it should be performed several weeks before the coronary artery bypass graft (10). In a retrospective analysis, Gerraty et al. (23) have recently shown that patients with symptomatic carotid stenosis of more than 50% had a risk of perioperative ipsilateral stroke of 30% in coronary artery bypass graft or vascular surgery. By contrast, the risk in patients with asymptomatic carotid stenosis of more than 50% was not increased. Reed et al. (42) have demonstrated that prior TIAs and congestive heart failure increase the risk of stroke in coronary artery bypass graft surgery. A Cleveland Clinic study examined the clinical outcome of 126 patients with a history of ischemic strokes who underwent open heart surgery (47). Deficits worsened in 17 (13.4%) patients but were moderate to severe in only 4 (3.2%). Extracranial occlusive disease was not a factor. The relatively common discovery of carotid stenosis by preoperative Doppler examination does not warrant surgical intervention if the patient is asymptomatic. Based on all the available studies, it would appear that the most prudent recommendation is that treatment for the patient with symptomatic high-grade (greater than 70%) carotid stenosis who requires coronary artery bypass graft or peripheral vascular surgery should follow the NASCET guidelines, and carotid endarterectomy with the peripheral vascular surgery and coronary artery bypass graft surgery should be postponed for 4 to 6 weeks.

TIMING OF CAROTID ENDARTERECTOMY AFTER STROKE

As mentioned, the NASCET study proved the effectiveness of carotid endarterectomy in selected patients with TIAs or completed minor stroke. Two smaller studies suggest that carotid endarterectomy may be valuable in symptomatic patients regardless of the size of the previous stroke or degree of deficit, although surgery obviously is deferred in some patients with severe neurologic deficits (39,48). In a prospective study, Piotrowsky et al. (39) found low perioperative morbidity and significant long-term risk reduction for recurrent stroke in a group of poststroke patients, most of whom (89/129) were described as moderately or severely disabled.

The traditional acceptable waiting period of 6 weeks between the time of stroke and carotid endarterectomy is substantiated by a single retrospective study and several anecdotal reports (12,24,29,45,56). Giordano et al. (24) reported a high rate of perioperative stroke in patients operated on 3 to 5 weeks after completed stroke. This interval corresponds with a period of intense revascularization of infarcted brain and loss of autoregulation in compromised tissue. The authors recommended a 5-week waiting period before carotid endarterectomy after completed stroke. Two larger studies subsequently failed to confirm Giordano's findings (39,48). One study examined outcomes in patients operated on 2 weeks or longer after stroke; the other included a group of patients operated on between 9 and 21 days after stroke. Neither study revealed an increased stroke risk associated with early versus later intervention. On the basis of these studies and another study of early carotid endarterectomy in patients suffering small strokes, early operation has been recommended as safe in selected patients (53).

An extremely important question concerning the timing of carotid endarterectomy after acute stroke is whether urgent surgery is indicated in patients with tight (>90%) carotid stenosis. Unfortunately, no controlled study has examined the utility of urgent intervention in this setting. It is typically recommended that surgery be deferred until progression of the stroke has ceased. Anticoagulation or antiplatelet therapy with aspirin or ticlopidine is recommended for some patients while they await surgery. Some investigators recommend urgent carotid endarterectomy in patients with very tight stenosis despite the lack of evidence from a controlled study (39). Rosenthal et al. (48) concur with this recommendation but believe that there is some increased (although unproven) risk associated with urgent intervention.

CONCLUSIONS

Table 4 identifies preoperative risk factors associated with poor perioperative outcomes in a recent review (33). Several of these factors may be

Table 4. *Complication rates for potential risk factors*[a]

Factor	Level	Complication rate No./n	Complication rate %	p
Age (years)	<75	19/320	5.9	0.09
	≥75	8/68	11.8	
Symptom status	Ipsilateral hemispheric	23/242	9.5	0.01
	Asymptomatic or other	4/144	2.7	
Severe hypertension	Yes	12/111	11.9	0.02
	No	15/287	5.7	
Preoperative coronary artery bypass graft	Yes	2/5	40.0	<0.01
	No	25/383	6.5	
Angina	Yes	14/141	9.9	0.08
	No	13/247	5.7	
Intraluminal thrombus	Yes	3/12	25.0	0.01
	No	24/376	6.4	
Siphon stenosis	Yes	5/31	16.7	0.04
	No	22/357	6.2	

(From McCrory et al. *Stroke* 1993;24:1285–1291, with permission.)

[a] Complication was defined as any adverse outcome among stroke, death, or myocardial infarction. Results were similar for outcomes of stroke or death. Numerators indicate number of patients with given complication. Denominators indicate total number of patients with given symptom. Univariable probability values for the null hypothesis of no difference among complication rate at variable levels were determined by χ^2 test.

identified by the patient's history and physical examination (e.g., age, symptom status, hypertension, and angina) and angiographic features (e.g., intraluminal thrombosis, siphon stenosis).

With appropriate patient selection, attention to factors such as hypertension, rigid angiographic criteria, and surgeons skilled in microvascular techniques with state-of-the-art intraoperative monitoring, the 30-day mortality rate should certainly be less than the 2% advised by an Ad Hoc Committee on Carotid Surgery Standards of the Stroke Council, American Heart Association (8). Furthermore, the combined 30-day mortality and morbidity rate should not exceed those reported in the most recently published multicenter clinical trials.

REFERENCES

1. Ackerman RH, Candia MR. Assessment of carotid artery stenosis by MR angiography. *AJNR* 1992;13:1005–1008.
2. Adams HP, Kassel NK, Mazuz H. The patient with transient ischemic attack: is this the time for a new therapeutic approach? *Stroke* 1984;15:371–375.
3. Alexandrov AV, Bladin CF, Maggisano R, Norris JW. Measuring carotid stenosis. Time for a reappraisal. *Stroke* 1993;24:1292–1296.
4. Baker WH, Littooy FN, Greisler HP et al. Carotid endarterectomy in private practice by fellowship-trained surgeons. *Stroke* 1987;5:957–958.
5. Barnett HJM. Stroke prevention by surgery for symptomatic disease in the carotid territory. *Neurol Clin* 1992;10:281–292.
6. Barnett HJM, Warlow CP. Carotid endarterectomy and the measurement of stenosis. *Stroke* 1993;24:1281–1284.
7. Barnett HJM, Barnes RW, Clagett GP et al. Symptomatic carotid artery stenosis: a solvable problem. North American Symptomatic Carotid Endarterectomy Trial. *Stroke* 1992;23: 1048–1053.
8. Beebe HG, Clagett GP, DeWeese JA et al. Assessing risk associated with carotid endarterectomy. *Circulation* 1989;79:472–473.
9. Blaisdell WF, Clauss RH, Golbraith JG, Imparato AM, Wylie EJ. Joint study of extracranial arterial occlusion. IV. A review of surgical considerations. *JAMA* 1969;209:1889–1895.
10. Brillman J. Central nervous system complications in coronary artery bypass graft surgery. *Neurol Clin* 1993;11:475–495.

11. Brook RH, Park RE, Chassin NR et al. Carotid endarterectomy for elderly patients: predicting complications. *Ann Intern Med* 1990;113:747–753.
12. Bruetman ME, Fields WS, Crawford ES, DeBakey ME. Cerebral hemorrhage in carotid artery surgery. *Arch Neurol* 1963;9:458–467.
13. Chambers BR, Norris JW. Outcome in patients with asymptomatic neck bruits. *N Engl J Med* 1986;315:860–865.
14. Colandrea MA, Friedman GD, Nichaman MZ et al. Systolic hypertension in the elderly: an epidemiologic assessment. *Circulation* 1970;41:239–245.
15. DiPasquale G, Pinelli G, Grazi P et al. Incidence of silent myocardial ischemia in patients with cerebral ischemia. *Eur Heart J* 1988;9[Suppl. N]:104–107.
16. Easton JD, Sherman DG. Stroke and mortality rate in carotid endarterectomy: 228 consecutive operations. *Stroke* 1977;8:565–568.
17. EC/IC Bypass Study Group: Failure of extracranial-intracranial arterial bypass to reduce the risk of ischemic stroke: results of an international randomized trial. *N Engl J Med* 1985; 331:991–1200.
18. EEC/IC Bypass Study Group: International cooperative study of extracranial/intracranial arterial anastomosis (EC/IC Bypass Study): methodology and entry characteristics. *Stroke* 1985;16:397–405.
19. European Carotid Surgery Trialists' Collaborative Group: MRC European Surgery Trial: interim results for symptomatic patients with severe (70%–99%) or with mild (0%–29%) carotid stenosis. *Lancet* 1991;337:1235–1243.
20. Fields WS, Meslenikov V, Meyer JS et al. Joint study of extracranial arterial occlusion. V. Progress report of prognosis following surgery of nonsurgical treatment of transient ischemic attacks and cervical carotid lesions. *JAMA* 1970;211:1993–2003.
21. Fisher BS, Malenka DJ, Solomon NA, Bubolz TA, Whaley FS, Wennberg JE. Risk of carotid endarterectomy in the elderly. *Am J Public Health* 1989;79:1617–1620.
22. Fode NC, Sundt TM Jr, Robertson JT, Peerless SJ, Shields CB. Multicenter retrospective review of results and complications of carotid endarterectomy in 1981. *Stroke* 1986;17: 370–376.
23. Gerraty RP, Gates PC, Doyle JC. Carotid stenosis and perioperative stroke risk in symptomatic and asymptomatic patients undergoing vascular or coronary surgery. *Stroke* 1993;24: 1115–1118.
24. Giordano JM, Trout HH, Kozloff L, DePalma RG. Timing of carotid artery endarterectomy after stroke. *J Vasc Surg* 1985;2:250–254.
25. Hass WK, Easton JD, Adams HP et al. A randomized trial comparing ticlopidine hydrochloride with aspirin for the prevention of stroke in high risk patients. *N Engl J Med* 1989;321: 501–507.
26. Hertzer NR. The natural history of peripheral vascular disease: implications for its management. *Circulation* 1991;83(Suppl. 1):112–119.
27. Hobson RW II, Weiss DG, Fields WS et al. Efficacy of carotid endarterectomy for asymptomatic carotid stenosis. *N Engl J Med* 1993;4:221–227.
28. Howard G, Sharrett AR, Heiss G et al. Carotid artery intimal-medial thickness distribution in general populations as evaluated by B-mode ultrasound. *Stroke* 1993;24:1297–1304.
29. Hunter JA, Julian OC, Dye WS, Javid H. Emergency operation for acute cerebral ischemia due to carotid artery obstruction. *Ann Surg* 1965;162:901–904.
30. Kannel WB, Wolf PA, McGee DL et al. Systolic blood pressure, arterial rigidity, and risk of stroke: the Framingham Study. *JAMA* 1981;245:1225–1229.
31. Klag MJ, Whelton PK, Seidler AJ. Decline in US stroke mortality: demographic trends and antihypertensive treatment. *Stroke* 1989;20:14–21.
32. Love BB, Grover-McKay M, Biller J, Rezai K, McKay CR. Coronary artery disease and cardiac events with asymptomatic and symptomatic cerebrovascular disease. *Stroke* 1992; 23:939–945.
33. McCrory DC, Goldstein LB, Samsa GP et al. Predicting complications of carotid endarterectomy. *Stroke* 1993;24:1285–1291.
34. Meyer FB, Meissner I, Fode NC, Losasso TJ. Carotid endarterectomy in elderly patients. *Mayo Clin Proc* 1991;66:464–469.
35. Muuronen A. Outcome of surgical treatment of 110 patients with transient ischemic attack. *Stroke* 1984;15:959–964.
36. NASCET Collaborators: Beneficial effect of carotid endarterectomy in symptomatic patients with high-grade carotid stenosis. *N Engl J Med* 1991;325:445–453.
37. Norris JW, Zhu CZ, Borstein NM et al. Vascular risk for asymptomatic carotid stenosis. *Stroke* 1991;22:1485–1490.
38. North American Symptomatic Carotid Endarterectomy Trial (NASCET) Steering Committee. North American Symptomatic Carotid Endarterectomy Trial: methods, patient characteristics, and progress. *Stroke* 1991;22:711–720.
39. Piotrowski JJ, Bernhard VM, Rubin JR et al. Timing of carotid endarterectomy after acute stroke. *J Vasc Surg* 1991;11:45–52.
40. Pokas R, Dyken MS. Dramatic changes in the performance of endarterectomy for diseases of the extracranial arteries of the head. *Stroke* 1988;19:1289–1290.
41. Polak JF, Kalina P, Donaldson MC et al. Carotid endarterectomy: prospective evaluation of combined Doppler sonography and MR angiography. *Neuroradiology* 1993;186:333–338.
42. Reed GL, Singer DE, Picard EH et al. Stroke following coronary-artery bypass surgery: a case control estimate of the risk from carotid bruits. *N Engl J Med* 1988;319:1246–1250.
43. Rihal CS, Gersh BJ, Whisnant JP et al. Influence of coronary artery disease on morbidity

and mortality after carotid endarterectomy: a population-based study in Olmstead County, Minnesota, 1970–1988. *J Am Coll Cardiol* 1992;19:1254–1260.

44. Riles TS, Eidelman EM, Litt AW et al. Comparison of magnetic resonance angiography, conventional angiography and duplex scanning. *Stroke* 1992;23:341–346.

45. Rob CG. Operation for acute completed stroke due to thrombosis of the internal carotid artery. *Surgery* 1969;65:862–865.

46. Rokey R, Rolak LA, Haroti Y et al. Coronary artery disease in patients with cerebrovascular disease: a perspective study. *Ann Neurol* 1984;16:50–53.

47. Rorick MB, Furlan AJ. Risk of cardiac surgery in patients with prior strokes. *Neurology* 1990;40:835–837.

48. Rosenthal D, Borrero E, Clark MD, Lamis PA, Daniel WW. Carotid endarterectomy after reversible ischemic neurologic deficit or stroke: is it of value? *J Vasc Surg* 1988;8:527–534.

49. Sundt TM Jr, Sandok BA, Whisnant JP. Carotid endarterectomy: complications and preoperative assessment of risk. *Mayo Clin Proc* 1975;50:301–306.

50. The CASANOVA Study Group. Carotid surgery versus medical therapy in asymptomatic carotid stenosis. *Stroke* 1991;22:1229–1235.

51. Toole JF, Hobson RW, Howard VJ, Chambers LE. Nearing the finish line? The asymptomatic carotid atherosclerosis study. *Stroke* 1992;23:1054–1055.

52. Urbanati S, DiPasquale G, Andreoli A et al. Frequency and prognostic significance of silent coronary artery disease in patients with cerebral ischemia undergoing carotid endarterectomy. *Am J Cardiol* 1992;69:1166–1170.

53. Whittemore AD, Ruby ST, Couch NP, Mannick JA. Early carotid endarterectomy in patients with small, fixed neurologic deficits. *J Vasc Surg* 1984;1:795–799.

54. Winslow CM, Solomon DH, Chassin MR et al. The appropriateness of carotid endarterectomy. *N Engl J Med* 1988;318:721–727.

55. Wolf PA, Belanger AJ, D'Agostino RB. Management of risk factors. *Neurol Clin* 1992;10:177–191.

56. Wylie EJ, Hein MR, Adams JE. Intracranial hemorrhage following surgical revascularization for treatment of acute strokes. *J Neurosurg* 1964;21:212–215.

3

Carotid Angiography

William E. Rothfus and
Edwin D. Cacayorin

The North American Symptomatic Carotid Endarterectomy Trial (NASCET) collaborators recently concluded that carotid endarterectomy is highly beneficial to symptomatic patients with 70% to 99% carotid stenosis (50). As exemplified by their strong conclusion, precision and accuracy are mandated in the estimation of carotid stenosis.

Duplex and color Doppler sonography are accurate in the evaluation of carotid atherosclerotic disease, but they suffer from operator variability, from artifacts related to calcifications, and from misestimation of stenosis or occlusion. Magnetic resonance (MR) angiography is also accurate in the evaluation of the carotid bifurcation and internal carotid artery, but the exact degree of stenosis may be difficult to determine. Turbulence of blood flow or magnetic susceptibility effects may exaggerate the degree of stenosis (42,62). Both Doppler and MR angiography have a limited field of view. Some researchers believe that these modalities are an adequate replacement for conventional or intra-arterial digital subtraction angiography (55). Currently, however, for most purposes they are used as screening tests to triage patients for subsequent catheter angiography.

Carotid angiography accurately delineates luminal compromise and irregularities. Simultaneously the intracranial circulation can be evaluated for stenotic segments higher in the internal carotid artery, and even for incidental intracranial aneurysms (42). Carotid angiography remains the gold standard for diagnostic modalities used in the evaluation of extracranial and intracra-

W.E. Rothfus and E.D. Cacayorin: Department of Radiology, Medical College of Pennsylvania and Hahnemann University, Allegheny General Hospital, Pennsylvania 15212.

nial carotid circulation and provides a reliable method of communication between subspecialties (62).

TECHNIQUE

Before undergoing angiography, patients are screened for allergies to medications and contrast material, coagulopathy, renal failure, and cardiac failure. Selective characterization of the carotid arteries is accomplished most easily and safely through the transfemoral approach. Following the administration of local anesthesia and light intravenous sedation (our protocol includes a combination of small doses of Fentanyl and Versed), the Seldinger technique is used to puncture the femoral artery (14,46). With a leading guidewire, a soft 4- and 5-F catheter is placed into the aortic arch and then into the common carotid artery. Various catheter shapes are useful. Typically, older or more hypertensive patients need catheters with more pronounced reverse curves because the origins of the carotid and innominate arteries from the aorta are more acutely configured (48). The introduction of "slippery" hydrophilic guidewires has facilitated catheter placement into difficult, tortuous carotids.

Some centers have used a transcubital brachial approach routinely (65), but it can be complicated by arterial spasm and ischemia of the arm (68). When iliofemoral or aortic disease precludes transfemoral catheterization, right axillary puncture is commonly undertaken. Both of these techniques use catheters with reverse curves. They have the advantage of easy ipsilateral vertebral artery catheterization, but injection of the contralateral artery is more difficult. Direct puncture of an aortofemoral graft is typically safe (67). Use of a sheath helps to prevent catheter shearing by graft fibers. Direct carotid puncture is rarely needed.

It is usually most efficacious to study the symptomatic carotid artery first (12). Subsequent vessel injection can then be determined to tailor the examination to address other concerns. Severe unilateral carotid stenosis usually requires contralateral carotid injection. Approximately 9% of stenosis patients will have contralateral internal carotid artery occlusion (70). Collateral flow to the affected hemisphere should be determined because inadequate collateral circulation through the circle of Willis may predispose the patient to intraoperative ischemia, prompting the use of intraluminal shunt during endarterectomy (60). Although directional determination of the circle of Willis can now be made using specialized magnetic resonance velocity-phase contrast techniques, these have not been evaluated extensively in the context of carotid stenosis (54).

It is essential to evaluate not only the carotid bifurcation, but also the intracranial internal carotid artery for stenosis. At present, angiography is the most reliable imaging technique available for this purpose. Ultrasound does not evaluate the intracranial internal carotid artery directly. Magnetic resonance angiography may show flow-related or magnetic susceptibility artifacts that mimic stenosis at the skull base (43), or it may not include that area in the field of view (33). Intracranial stenoses of the middle cerebral artery and anterior cerebral artery are best evaluated by angiography (Fig. 1). Even though MR angiography may demonstrate areas of major arterial narrowing, it is doubtful that stenosis of distal branches can be reliably delineated.

The choice of contrast agent for injection is controversial. Patients feel less discomfort with nonionic than ionic contrast. However, the clinical advantage of one versus the other has never been established in terms of toxic or embolic adverse events. Some evidence suggests that nonionic contrast

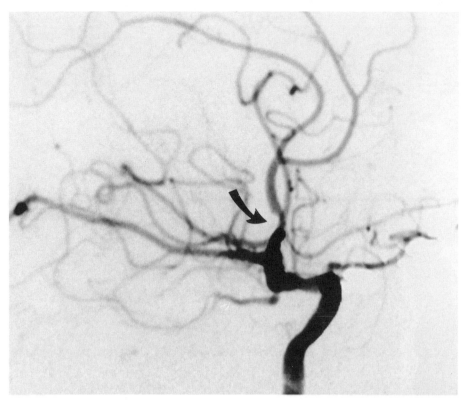

Figure 1. Lateral selective internal carotid artery injection shows focal athero-sclorotic stenosis of the proximal vertical anterior cerebral artery *(arrow)*. Such a stenosis could not be detected with noninvasive imaging.

has less *in vitro* antiplatelet activity than ionic contrast. Whether this characteristic affects complication rates is debatable, especially when the catheter is well flushed with a continuous heparin drip.

At least two image projections are required to evaluate the carotid bifurcation. In most cases, the external carotid artery lies anteromedial to the internal carotid artery. Thus lateral and anteroposterior oblique projections (10°) depict the arteries with less vessel overlap. Since most proximal internal carotid artery ulcers project posterolaterally, these views may best show the niche of the ulcer in silhouette. Considerable anatomic variation does, however, exist. The external carotid artery may be anterolateral to the internal carotid artery in 13% of the cases, and lateral superimposition of the external carotid artery and internal carotid artery occurs in 16% (66). Typically, optimal projections can best be determined during fluoroscopic test injections before filming and instantaneous review of the digital images as obtained. Certainly more than two projections may be needed to assess a complex plaque adequately.

When intra-arterial digital subtraction angiography is used, images should be filmed at a wide gray scale, so that stenosis is not underrepresented (Fig. 2). Calcified plaque may create considerable artifact from misregistration and require standard film-screen imaging or computed tomography (CT) to determine the true luminal size. Nonsubtracted images are essential to determine the exact anatomic level of the bifurcation and its relation to the angle of the mandible, especially in patients with short necks.

The role of aortic arch injection as an adjunct to selective carotid study is controversial (67). Although used commonly, the arch study has a low yield (only about 0.6%) in detecting hemodynamically significant intratho-

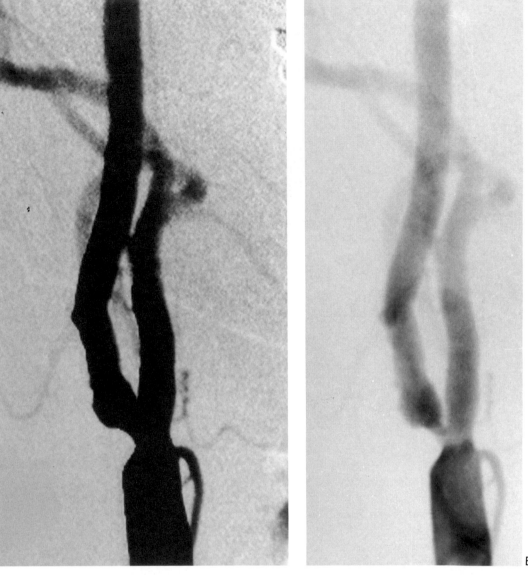

A

B

Figure 2. A: Common carotid injection showing smooth narrowing of the proximal internal carotid artery and bifurcation. At these window settings, luminal narrowing would only approximate 20%. **B:** At wider windows, severe stenosis of about 78% diameter is seen.

racic stenoses and considerably increases the overall dose of contrast (3). It can, however, clarify the diagnosis in patients with multiple vessel stenoses (e.g., subclavian steal) and carotid disease for whom complex surgical or radiologic interventions are contemplated.

ANGIOGRAPHIC RISK

Complications related to carotid angiography have usually been categorized as (a) nonneurologic local, including catheter or puncture-induced hematoma, thrombosis, and pseudoaneurysm; (b) nonneurologic systemic, including hypotension, cardiogenic shock or arrhythmias, allergic reactions, and renal failure; and (c) neurologic, including permanent and reversible deficits. Overall, nonneurologic events occur in 1% to 7% of cases (17,40) and are usually temporary. Permanent risks relate to renal failure (baseline azotemia made worse by contrast), cardiac disease, and limb ischemia. Multiple factors, such as contrast volume, age, hypertension, and difficulty of the procedure correlate with nonneurologic occurrence (19).

The frequency of neurologic complications has been reported to vary from as low as 0% to as high as 28% (17,19,30,40). Hankey et al. (30) reviewed eight prospective and seven retrospective studies of conventional cerebral angiography risk in 17 patients with cerebrovascular disease. As a generalization, they concluded that the risk of any neurologic complication [i.e., transient ischemic attack (TIA) or stroke] was about 4% and that the risk of permanent complication (i.e., major stroke) was about 1%. Complications tended to occur more often in patients with frequent TIAs or stroke-in-evolution, in patients with severe carotid stenosis, and in patients receiving large amounts of contrast material. The tendency was similar in older patients; those in poor health; and those with systemic disease, especially diabetes.

Complications can sometimes be attributed to a known cause, such as catheter-induced arterial dissection (51). In most instances, however, the cause is unclear. Embolic events have been presumed to result from dislodgement of atheromatous debris from catheter and guidewire manipulations and from the formation of microthrombi on catheters or in syringes.

Recently, our group reported transcranial Doppler evidence of microemboli during carotid angiography (16). The emboli occurred most commonly during catheter flushing and contrast injection and were identical to microemboli detected during major cardiovascular surgery. However, they were clinically occult. The source of the emboli was presumed to be otherwise nondetectable gas or small clots formed at the interface of the blood and contrast interface [nonionic contrast may allow red blood cells to aggregate (5)].

Whatever the cause of complications, they are ultimately unavoidable, even in the best of hands. Thus the risks of angiography must be considered carefully and added to the risks of surgery if endarterectomy is contemplated.

STENOSIS

Angiographic methods of determining stenosis vary. Traditionally luminal stenosis has been measured by comparing the diameter of the opacified internal carotid lumen with the imagined original diameter of the carotid bulb (13,24,30) (Fig. 3). This method is fairly reliable, with an interobserver correlation of 0.94 to 0.98. However, differences in determining percent stenosis may vary by more than 9% (13). Reliance on carotid bulb dimensions presumes that the normal variability of bulb dilatation is known and can be estimated exactly, but no such accuracy has been proved. Other methods have been used to quantitate stenosis by comparison with the normal portion of the cervical carotid artery, by subjectively grading the degree of stenosis, and by directly measuring residual luminal diameter (24).

Recent large-scale randomized clinical trials investigating the effect of endarterectomy in carotid stenosis have emphasized the need for precision in determining the degree of stenosis. In the European Carotid Surgery Trial (ECST), angiographic stenosis was calculated using luminal diameter compared with a guesstimate of the diameter of the carotid bulb (Fig. 3). Using this methodology, endarterectomy provided significant risk reduction in patients with severe (70% to 99%) stenosis. After 3 years, the risk was 2.8% for operated patients compared with 16.8% for control patients (23).

A more quantifiable method to determine stenosis was used by NASCET. Luminal diameter was compared with the diameter of the normal carotid

A   B

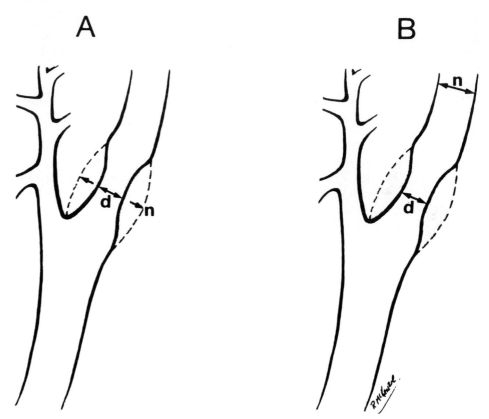

Figure 3. Methods of measuring carotid stenosis. **A:** Method used in European Carotid Surgery Trial requires measurement of residual lumen (d) versus estimation of carotid bulb diameter (n). **B:** Method used in North American Symptomatic Carotid Endarterectomy Trial requires measurement of residual lumen versus measurement of the cervical internal carotid artery well above the stenosis. Luminal narrowing is determined by the formula (1-d/n) × 100.

artery well above the carotid bulb (49) (Fig. 3). Biplane angiography (film-screen or intra-arterial digital subtraction angiography) was required, with stenosis measured in the plane of maximal narrowing. The results showed considerable risk reduction for carotid endarterectomy in symptomatic patients with high-grade stenosis (over 70%); the 2-year stroke risk was 9% for operated patients compared with 26% for controls. Furthermore, the risk reduction depended on degree of stenosis. Patients with 90% to 99% stenosis had 26% reduction; those with 80% to 89% stenosis had 18% reduction; and those with 70% to 79% stenosis had 12% reduction (50). The ongoing trial is investigating patients with moderate (30% to 69%) stenosis to determine the benefit of endarterectomy for lesser degrees of narrowing.

Despite the apparent differences in these two studies (i.e., the denominator is larger in ECST; thus NASCET may underestimate stenosis compared with ECST) (Fig. 4), when ECST measurements are adjusted to NASCET measurements, survival curves from the two studies show considerable correspondence (6). Both methods may underestimate the degree of "true" anatomic stenosis compared with duplex ultrasound (4); however, NASCET found poor overall correlation between angiography and ultrasound.

Overall, NASCET methodology has the strictest criteria for measurement of stenosis. Its proven utility and low interobserver variability recommend its continued use as the standard for further investigations and in everyday clinical decision making (24).

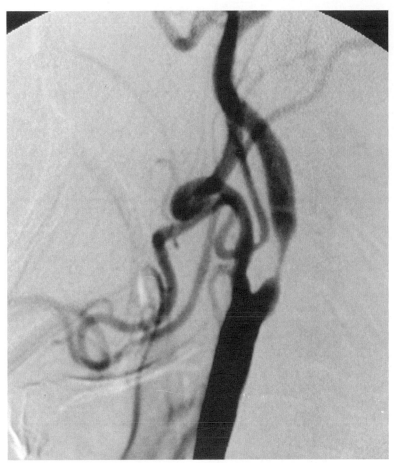

Figure 4. Severe smooth stenosis of proximal internal carotid artery. ECST estimate of luminal narrowing is 90% [(1-1/10) × 100], while NASCET estimate is 83% [(1-1/6) × 100].

PSEUDO-OCCLUSION AND NONTHROMBOSED OCCLUSION

The terms *nearly occluded, pseudo-occlusion, atheromatous pseudo-occlusion,* and *slim-sign* usually indicate that the residual lumen of the proximal internal carotid is extremely small. Because blood flow through a vessel is retarded, the angiographic appearance on cursory examination simulates occlusion (25,56,61,71). However, careful review of delayed subtraction studies shows that a thin stream of contrast progressing cephalad from the severely tapered stenosis finally meets contrast media in the supraclinoid segment of the internal carotid artery, thus proving its patency (Fig. 5). The angiographic appearance of the thin column of contrast presumably relates to a physiologically contracted artery lumen and to dependent layering of contrast (25,61).

Several points are important in recognizing pseudo-occlusion: (a) endarterectomy usually opens the internal carotid artery to normal patency (25,56, 61,71); (b) when coupled with TIAs or acute ipsilateral ischemic deficits, pseudo-occlusion may indicate emergency endarterectomy; (c) pseudo-occlusion occurs in 10% of the cases in which complete occlusion was initially suspected (56); (d) noninvasive ultrasound or MR angiography may fail to detect pseudo-occlusion (1) (Fig. 5); and (e) the somewhat irregular luminal tapering associated with pseudo-occlusion must be distinguished from the smooth, more distal tapering associated with dissection and from the rounded filling defect associated with intraluminal thrombus.

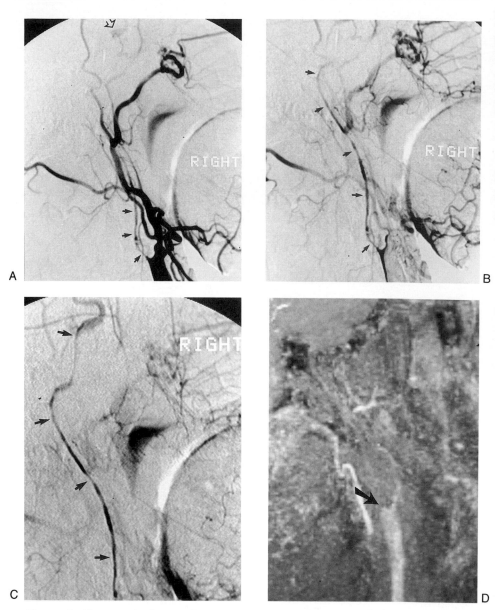

Figure 5. Near occlusion. **A:** Early arterial phase study shows markedly tapered internal carotid artery origin. A very thin stream of contrast is seen progressing superiorly beyond the stenosis *(closed arrows)*. There is faint filling of the supra-clinoid internal carotid artery *(open arrow)*. **B:** Later phase shows filling to the skull base *(arrows)* but still no connection to supraclinoid internal carotid artery. **C:** With more delay, a patent but contracted lumen can be followed throughout the entire course of the internal carotid artery. **D:** Three-dimensional TOF magnetic resonance angiography falsely indicates occlusion at internal carotid artery origin *(arrow)*. Endarterectomy was successful.

Proximal occlusion, but not complete thrombosis, of the internal carotid artery is another important condition to recognize angiographically (2,32,44). In this case, a thin, tapered stream of contrast is present, filling the distal internal carotid artery from external carotid artery collaterals. With delayed filming, the infraophthalmic and then infrapetrosal internal carotid artery segments gradually fill retrogradely. The column of contrast is tapered inferiorly, as opposed to the blunted, convex appearance of complete thrombosis (Fig. 6). Although the etiology of this phenomenon is unclear (it probably

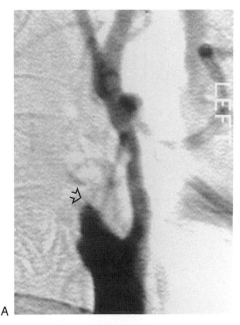

A

Figure 6. **A:** Lateral common carotid injection shows what appears to be complete, although tapered, occlusion of the internal carotid artery *(open arrow).* **B:** Lateral cranial study in early arterial phase demonstrates collateral filing of supraclinoid internal carotid artery *(curved arrow)* via the ophthalmic artery. **C:** Delayed lateral image has more retrograde filling of the petrosal internal carotid artery *(straight arrows).* Note ill-defined lower margin of contrast, indicating layered contrast within the patent lumen, and not thrombus.

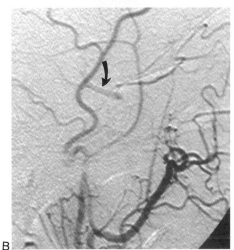

B

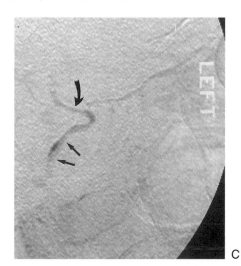

C

represents delayed, minimally turbulent reflux rather than proximal collateralization), its recognition is important. The further the contrast column extends inferiorly, the more likely it is that the endarterectomy will restore patency of the internal carotid artery. Filling to the petrous internal carotid artery indicates a high likelihood of subsequent patency (32).

TANDEM STENOSIS

The NASCET collaborators excluded patients with stenosis of the intracranial carotid artery. This group represented about 2% of the total number of patients studied. Although large cohorts of patients with tandem stenoses have not been examined, some evidence suggests that this group has a higher incidence of ischemic stroke than normal (41). These patients also tend to have a high rate of intraoperative and perioperative complications (45,59). Thus full visualization of the internal carotid artery, both extracranially and intracranially, seems to be warranted in planning an endarterectomy (Fig. 7). Angiographically tandem stenosis must be distinguished from flow artifact

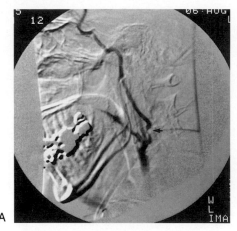
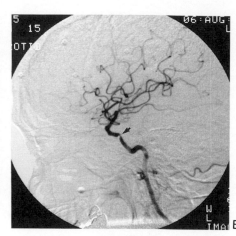

Figure 7. Tandem stenosis. Focal severe atherosclerotic narrowing constricts the lumen of the proximal internal carotid artery **(A)** and precavernous internal carotid artery **(B)** *(arrows)*.

caused by near occlusion (37). In true stenosis, the contrast column has consistent, well-defined edges; in pseudotandem stenosis, the column changes with time (progressive reflux into the internal carotid artery lumen), and the nondependent edge is commonly ill defined (dependent layering of contrast).

RESTENOSIS

The incidence of recurrent stenosis of the carotid artery after endarterectomy varies from less than 1% to more than 14%. Early restenosis (<2 years) is often attributed to neointimal fibromuscular hyperplasia, whereas later restenosis is attributed to atherosclerosis (52). Angiographically neointimal fibromuscular hyperplasia is manifest by smooth, ring-like areas of narrowing usually 2 or more mm long. Restenosis is most commonly diagnosed by ultrasound, but angiography is necessary if surgery or percutaneous transluminal angioplasty is considered.

ULCERATION

Ulceration of a carotid artery plaque has long been considered an important contributor to the pathophysiology of ipsilateral ischemic events (34,47). Presumably, the ulcer represents a site that harbors cholesterol or fibrin-platelet thrombi that later embolize to distal cerebral circulations. However, the exact correlation between ulceration and ischemic symptoms has never been delineated, and its importance is controversial (26,69).

Angiographic criteria for ulceration have neither been rigid nor uniform. Although ulcers are widely accepted to represent a projection of contrast beyond the confines of the opacified lumen, descriptions vary from luminal irregularities (20) to penetrating cavities (8). Blaisdell et al. (8) defined radiologic criteria for ulceration as penetrating niche, irregularity of the luminal silhouette, delayed contrast washout within stenosis (due to slow flow or contrast layering), and double density of the *en face* niche. Of these, the penetrating niche was the most reliable sign of proven ulceration. Overall angiographic accuracy was 86%.

In other series (15,20,22), the correlation between angiographic diagnosis of ulceration and pathologic examination of specimens has been more disappointing, with accuracy rates of 50% to 67%. Irregularities of the lumen, mistaken as ulceration, occur on the surface of smooth, flat plaques. By contrast, thrombogenic ulcers may be so small that they are beyond the resolution of angiography (20,31). The appearance of ulceration can be simulated by the presence of intraplaque hematoma, which push walls of intima inward and leave a central depression. Angiograms usually show fairly smooth, sharply marginated luminal narrowing, surrounding the luminal outpouching (Fig. 8) (20). Although frank ulcerations can be associated with subintimal hematomas, they are usually over the protruding surface of a hematoma rather than in the niche (38).

Interobserver agreement is quite variable in the determination of ulceration. Observers disagree 12.5% to 25% of the time (15). Sometimes it may be possible to distinguish true ulceration (intimal disruption) from intraplaque hematoma. Hypothetically, an ulcer niche that passes beyond the (expected) luminal confines of the carotid bulb has passed through the intima (Fig. 9). Similarly, if the intima is undercut by plaque excavation, true ulceration should be present (Fig. 10). Multiple projections from a luminal outpouching would also suggest true ulceration (Fig. 11).

Stricter criteria are needed before ulceration can be used as a reliable prognostic marker of ipsilateral ischemic disease and then as an indicator for or against surgical intervention.

INTRALUMINAL THROMBUS

Intraluminal thrombus is angiographically identified as a well-defined, elongated, or rounded filling deficit outlined by contrast (Fig. 12). It may

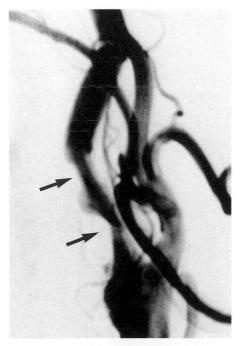

Figure 8. Subintimal hematoma simulating ulceration. Areas of plaque hemorrhage displace the intima upward *(arrows)*, leaving less constricted lumen between them, an appearance similar to an ulcer niche.

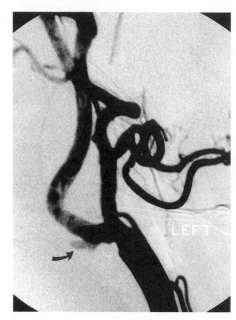

Figure 9. Ulceration. The ulcer niche *(arrow)* projects posteriorly and superiorly well beyond the expected boundary of the carotid bulb.

be small or quite long. It is usually associated with severe atherosclerosis considered by some to indicate a need for emergency endarterectomy. Others have found thrombus to represent a complicating factor (45). In some cases (53), systemic anticoagulant therapy has been effective in clot resolution. No large series of intra-arterial thrombolysis yet exist to determine its effectiveness.

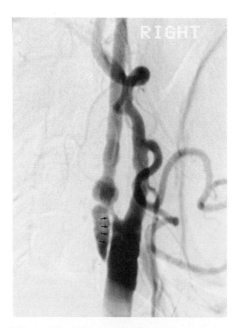

Figure 10. Ulceration. Severely stenotic proximal internal carotid artery plaque is complicated by a large ulcer, which undercuts intact intima *(small arrows).*

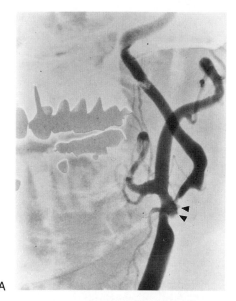

Figure 11. Hemorrhagic plaque. **A:** The oblique anteroposterior view of the left common carotid arteriogram shows an expansile atheromatous plaque that is narrowing (relative by 60% to the lower normal common carotid lumen) the distal common carotid artery and an estimated 80% stenosis of the origin of internal carotid artery (degree of stenosis relative to the higher normal internal carotid lumen). An irregular ulceration of the left common carotid bifurcation is also shown *(arrowheads)*. **B:** Gross endarterectomy specimen. The discolored external appearance of posterolateral aspect of the common carotid bifurcation and proximal internal carotid artery can be appreciated. **C:** Gross dissection of the atheromatous plaque reveals the grossly hemorrhagic subintimal compartment of the carotid bifurcation and proximal internal carotid artery *(arrowheads)*. The endothelial surface also shows multiple focal linear and irregular crevices.

A

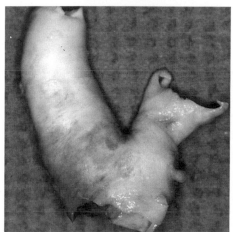

B

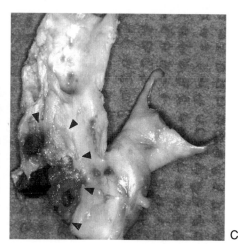

C

INTRAOPERATIVE CAROTID ANGIOGRAPHY

Intraoperative carotid angiography can be performed with ease, speed, and safety at the completion of carotid endarterectomy. The procedure requires the use of a surgical table with a movable radiolucent top, a conventional C-arm imaging unit, and a portable digital subtraction angiography unit. High-resolution digital subtraction angiography (512^2 and $1,024^2$ matrix) imaging units would provide superior quality and detailed images of the carotid lumen.

The intra-arterial digital subtraction angiography is performed through a 21-gauge butterfly needle that is inserted into the common carotid artery below the site of the carotid endarterectomy site (10). Images are acquired in at least two different planes (anteroposterior and lateral) for accurate depiction of the postoperative carotid lumen. Nonionic contrast medium at full angiographic concentration is used. Images are generated at least 3 frames/sec to minimize the influence of carotid pulsation on the image quality.

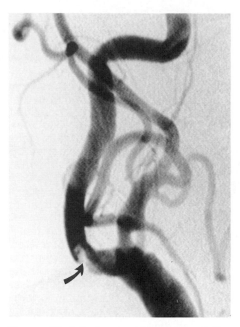

Figure 12. Intraluminal thrombus. A finger-like filling defect projects from a mildly irregular plaque into the lumen *(curved arrow).*

Intraoperative digital subtraction angiography permits recognition of operative complications within the period of reversibility. Most of the complications of carotid endarterectomy relate to anatomic defects at the endarterectomy sites (63). Bradenberg et al. (10) observed instances of tight suture defects, intimal flaps, small platelet aggregates, and thrombi that appeared as luminal irregularities, defects, and narrowings on intraoperative digital subtraction angiography images (Fig. 13). These findings were confirmed on reexploration of the arteriotomies, which were all satisfactory in external appearance and associated with good pulsation distally. Comparing intraoperative digital subtraction angiography studies with preoperative examinations can readily ascertain if the surgical excision of atheromatous plaque was adequate.

In their series of 692 carotid artery reconstructions, Roon and Hoogerwerf (57) found that their combined neurologic morbidity and mortality rate was reduced significantly from 4.5% without intraoperative angiography to 1.3% with intraoperative angiography. Intraoperative angiography demonstrated unsuspected stenosis, occlusions, intimal flaps, and kinks.

PERCUTANEOUS TRANSLUMINAL ANGIOPLASTY

In 1964, Dotter and Judkins originally described percutaneous transluminal angioplasty with a coaxial catheter system (18). A decade later, Gruntzig and Hopff (28) introduced the double-lumen balloon catheter. This advance paved the way toward widespread acceptance of percutaneous transluminal angioplasty and its broad application to coronary, visceral, and limbic atherosclerotic as well as to nonatherosclerotic arterial stenosis (9,27,36,58). The complexities of intrathoracic surgery, coupled with its 23% rate of complications, makes angioplasty an attractive and justifiable alternative for correcting stenosis of the brachiocephalic arteries (7). A success rate of 95.2%, a morbidity rate of 0.5%, and no mortality were attained by Kachel et al. (35),

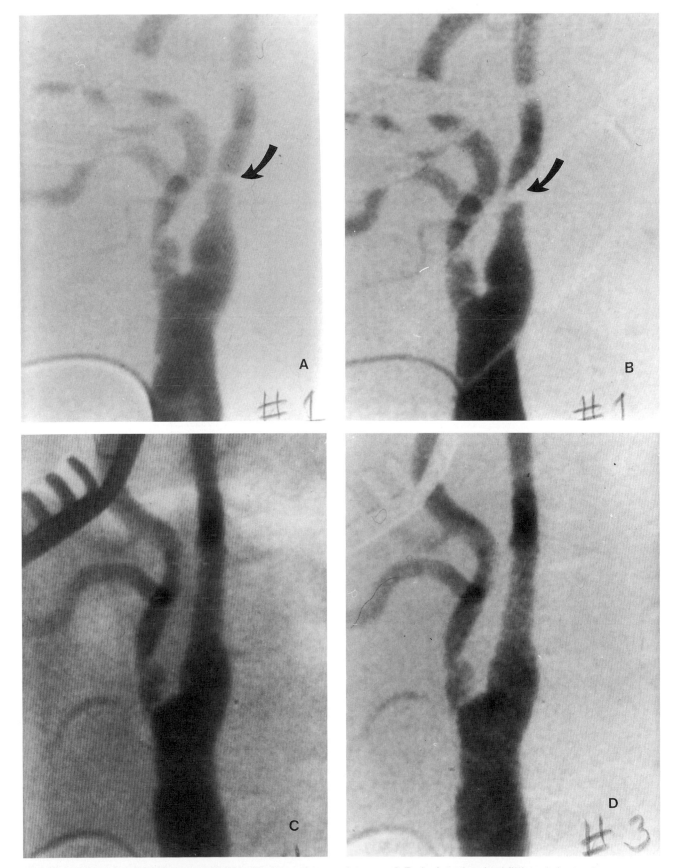

Figure 13. Intraoperative intraarterial digital subtraction angiogram. **A,B:** An intraluminal filling defect enlarges progressively *(right-to-left image)* at the upper end of the endarterectomy site *(curved arrow)*. **C,D:** Postcarotid arteriography revision digital subtraction angiography shows region of smooth internal carotid luminal opacification after removal of the rapidly accumulating platelet aggregates.

who treated 112 stenosed or occluded supra-aortic arteries with percutaneous transluminal angioplasty. A stenotic vertebral artery origin is considered highly amenable to percutaneous transluminal angioplasty; the atherosclerotic plaque is usually smooth-walled and free of ulceration (35).

Angioplasty for a symptomatic stenotic internal carotid artery is controversial. Theron et al. (64) successfully performed carotid angioplasty in 13 patients (10 of whom had TIAs or stroke) using a triple coaxial catheter system. The technique allowed temporary arrest of carotid blood flow and intraluminal flushing, thus minimizing the incidence of cerebroembolic complication. Nevertheless, Lusby et al. (39) and Cacayorin et al. (11) observed a high incidence of subintimal or intraplaque hemorrhage in symptomatic focal internal carotid stenosis. This pathologic observation, along with the high incidence of ulceration that is often difficult to recognize angiographically, mandates that angioplasty be reconsidered for patients with recent embolic manifestations. However, the considerable endothelial, subintimal, and even medial wall-shearing injuries that are inherently sustained in a successful balloon angioplasty must also be considered.

CONCLUSIONS

Catheter angiography is broadly considered to be the gold standard in evaluation of carotid artery atherosclerosis. Unfortunately, surprisingly little uniformity exists in interpreting the significance of angiographic findings. How should stenosis be measured? How important is intracranial stenosis? What is the relevance of ulceration? These and other questions remain, despite years of angiography experience and thousands of carotid surgeries.

Clearly, the answers to these questions require diagnostic accuracy. The use of NASCET methodology illustrates how integral angiographic precision is in determining surgical decisions. As noninvasive imaging (especially MR angiography) evolves, it approaches this angiographic precision, but until potentially dangerous false negatives and false positives (i.e., the risks of noninvasive imaging) become less than the risks of angiography, it will not supplant angiography as the preoperative standard.

REFERENCES

1. Ackerman RH, Candia MR. Assessment of carotid artery stenosis by MR angiography. *AJNR* 1992;13:1005–1008.
2. Ahn HS, Rosenbaum AE, Allen GS et al. Occluded but nonthrombosed internal carotid artery: an indication for endarterectomy. *AJNR* 1983;4:286–288.
3. Akers DL, Markowitz IA, Kerstein MD. The value of aortic arch study in evaluation of cerebrovascular insufficiency. *Am J Surg* 1987;154:230–232.
4. Alexandrov AV, Bladin CF, Maggisano R, Norris JW. Measuring carotid stenosis: time for a reappraisal. *Stroke* 1993;24:1292–1296.
5. Aspelin P. Does nonionic contrast media increase red cell aggregation and clot formation? *Invest Radiol* 1990;1:S119–S120.
6. Barnett HJM, Warlow CP. Carotid endarterectomy and the measurement of stenosis. *Stroke* 1993;24:1281–1284.
7. Beebe HG, Stark R, Johnson ML, Jolly PC, Hill LD. Choices of operation for subclavian-vertebral artery disease. *Am J Surg* 1980;139:616–623.
8. Blaisdell FW, Glickman M, Trunkey DD. Ulcerated atheroma of the carotid artery. *Arch Surg* 1974;108:491–496.
9. Block PC. Percutaneous transluminal coronary angioplasty. *AJR* 1980;135:955–959.
10. Bradenberg CE, Iannettoni M, Rosenbloom M et al. Operative angiography by intraarterial digital subtraction angiography: a new technique for quality control of carotid endarterectomy. *J Vasc Surg* 1989;9:530–534.
11. Cacayorin ED, Hochhauser L, Hodge CJ et al. Comprehensive experience on intraplaque hemorrhage of the carotid artery. *Neuroradiology* 1991;33[Suppl]:75–78.
12. Caplan LR, Wolpert SM. Angiography in patients with occlusive cerebrovascular disease: views of a stroke neurologist and neuroradiologist. *AJNR* 1991;12:593–601.

13. Chikos PM, Fisher LD, Hirsch JH, Harley JD, Thiele BL, Strandness DE Jr. Observer variability in evaluating extracranial carotid artery stenosis. *Stroke* 1983;14:885–892.
14. Conrad MR. Excellent anxiolytic effect achieved with low doses of Versed. *Radiology* 1989;170:579.
15. Croft RJ, Ellam LD, Harrison MJG. Accuracy of carotid angiography in the assessment of atheroma of the internal carotid artery. *Lancet* 1980;1:997–1000.
16. Dagirmanjian A, Davis DA, Rothfus WE, Deeb ZL, Goldberg AL. Silent cerebral microemboli occurring during carotid angiography: frequency as determined with Doppler sonography. *AJR* 1993;161:1037–1040.
17. Dion JE, Gates PC, Fox AJ, Barnett HJM, Blom RJ. Clinical events following neuroangiography: a prospective study. *Stroke* 1987;18:997–1004.
18. Dotter CT, Judkins KP. Transluminal treatment of arteriosclerotic obstruction: description of new technique and preliminary report of its application. *Circulation* 1964;30:654–670.
19. Earnest F IV, Forbes G, Sandok BA et al. Complications of cerebral angiography: prospective assessment of risk. *AJNR* 1983;4:1191–1197.
20. Edwards JH, Kricheff II, Gorstein F, Riles T, Imparato A. Atherosclerotic subintimal hematoma of the carotid artery. *Radiology* 1979;133:123–129.
21. Edwards JH, Kricheff II, Riles T, Imparato A. Angiographically undetected ulceration of the carotid bifurcation as a cause of embolic stroke. *Radiology* 1979;132:369–373.
22. Eikebloom BC, Riles TR, Mintzer R et al. Inaccuracy of angiography in the diagnosis of carotid ulceration. *Stroke* 1983;14:882–885.
23. European Carotid Surgery Trialists' Collaborative Group. MCR European Carotid Surgery Trial: interim results for symptomatic patients with severe (70–99%) or with mild (0–29%) carotid stenosis. *Lancet* 1991;337:1235–1243.
24. Fox AJ. How to measure carotid stenosis. *Radiology* 1993;186:316–318.
25. Gabrielsen TO, Seeger JF, Knake JE, Burke DP, Stilwill EW. The nearly occluded internal carotid artery: a diagnostic trap. *Radiology* 1981;138:611–618.
26. Gomez CR. Carotid plaque morphology and risk for stroke. *Stroke* 1989;24:26–29.
27. Greenfield AJ. Femoral, popliteal, and tibial arteries: percutaneous transluminal angioplasty. *AJR* 1980;135:927–935.
28. Gruntzig A, Hopff H. PerKutane Rekanalisation chronischer arteriellar verschlusse mit einem neuen dilatationskatheter modifikation der Dotter technik. *Dtsch Med Wochenschr* 1974;99:2502–2505.
29. Hankey GJ, Warlow CP. Symptomatic carotid ischemic events: safest and most cost-effective way of selecting patients for angiography, before carotid endarterectomy. *Br Med J* 1990;300:1485–1491.
30. Hankey GJ, Warlow CPW, Sellar RJ. Cerebral angiographic risk in mild cerebrovascular disease. *Stroke* 1990;21:209–222.
31. Hertzer NR, Beven EG, Benjamin SP. Ultramicroscopic ulcerations and thrombi of the carotid bifurcation. *Arch Surg* 1977;112:1394–1402.
32. Hugenholtz H, Elgie RG. Carotid thromboendarterectomy: a reappraisal. *J Neurosurg* 1980;53:776–783.
33. Huston J III, Lewis BD, Wiebers DO, Meyer FB, Riederer SJ, Weaver AL. Carotid artery: prospective blinded comparison of two-dimensional time-of-flight MR angiography with conventional angiography and duplex US. *Radiology* 1993;186:339–344.
34. Julian OC, Dye WS, Javid H et al. Ulcerative lesions of the carotid artery bifurcation. *Arch Surg* 1963;86:803–809.
35. Kachel R, Basche ST, Heerklotz I, Grossmann K, Endler S. Percutaneous transluminal angioplasty (PTA) of supra-aortic arteries especially the internal carotid artery. *Neuroradiology* 1991;33:191–194.
36. Katzen BT, Chang J. Percutaneous transluminal angioplasty with the Gruntzig balloon catheter. *Radiology* 1979;130:623–626.
37. Little JR, Sawhny B, Weinstein M. Pseudo-tandem stenosis of the internal carotid artery. *Neurosurgery* 1980;7:574–577.
38. Lusby RJ, Ferrell LD, Ehrenfeld WK, Stoney RJ, Wylie EJ. Carotid plaque hemorrhage. *Arch Surg* 1982;117:1479–1488.
39. Lusby RJ, Ferrell LD, Ehrenfeld WK, Stoney RJ, Wylie EJ. Carotid plaque hemorrhage: its role in production of cerebral ischemia. *Arch Surg* 1982;117:1479–1488.
40. Mani RL, Eisenberg RL, McDonald EJ Jr, Pollock JA, Mani JR. Complications of catheter cerebral arteriography: analysis of 5,000 procedures. I. criteria and incidence. *AJR* 1978;861–865.
41. Marzewski DJ, Fulan AJ, St. Louis P, Little JR, Modic MT, Williams G. Intracranial internal carotid artery stenosis: long-term prognosis. *Stroke* 1982;13:821–824.
42. Masaryk TJ, Obuchowski NA. Noninvasive carotid imaging: caveat emptor. *Radiology* 1993;186:325–331.
43. Masaryk TJ, Modic MT, Ross JS et al. Intracranial circulation: preliminary clinical results with three-dimensional (volume) MR angiography. *Radiology* 1989;171:793–799.
44. McCormick PW, Spetzler RF, Bailes JE, Zabramski JM, Frey JL. Thromboendarterectomy of the symptomatic occluded internal carotid artery. *J Neurosurg* 1992;76:752–758.
45. McCrory DC, Goldstein LB, Samsa GP et al. Predicting complications of carotid endarterectomy. *Stroke* 1993;24:1285–1291.
46. Miller DL, Wall RT. Fentanyl and diazepam for analgesia and sedation during radiologic special procedures. *Radiology* 1987;162:195–198.
47. Moore WS, Hall AD. Ulcerated atheroma of the carotid artery. *Am J Surg* 1968;116:237–242.

48. Newton TH, Kerber CW. Techniques of catheter cerebral angiography. In: Newton TH, Potts DG, eds. *Radiology of the skull and brain*. Vol. 2, Book 1. St. Louis: CV Mosby; 1974:920–938.

49. North American Symptomatic Carotid Endarterectomy Trial (NASCET) Steering Committee. North American Symptomatic Carotid Endarterectomy Trial: Methods, patient characteristics, and progress. *Stroke* 1991;22:711–720.

50. North American Symptomatic Carotid Endarterectomy Trial Collaborators. Beneficial effect of carotid endarterectomy in symptomatic patients with high grade carotid stenosis. *N Engl J Med* 1991;325:445–453.

51. O'Reilly GV, Naheedy MH, Colucci VM, Hammerschlag SB. The 5-F catheter in cerebral angiography. *Radiology* 1981;141:411–414.

52. Palmaz JC, Hunter G, Carson SN, French SW. Postoperative carotid restenosis due to neointimal fibromuscular hyperplasia: clinical, angiographic and pathological findings. *Radiology* 1983;148:699–702.

53. Pelz DM, Buchan A, Fox AJ, Barnett HJM, Vinuela F. Intraluminal thrombus of the internal carotid arteries: angiographic demonstration of resolution with anticoagulant therapy alone. *Radiology* 1986;160:369–373.

54. Pernicone JR, Siebert JE, Laird TA, Rosenbaum TL, Potchen EJ. Determination of blood flow direction using velocity-phase image display with 3-D phase-contrast MR angiography. *AJNR* 1992;13:1435–1438.

55. Polak JF, Kalina P, Donaldson MC, O'Leary DH, Whittemore AD, Mannick JA. Carotid endarterectomy: preoperative evaluation of candidates with combined Doppler sonography and MR angiography. Work in progress. *Radiology* 1993;186:333–338.

56. Ringelstein EB, Berg-Dammer E, Zeumer H. The so-called atheromatous pseudoocclusion of the internal carotid artery. *Neuroradiology* 1983;25:147–155.

57. Roon AJ, Hoogerwerf D. Intraoperative arteriography and carotid surgery. *J Vasc Surg* 1992;16:239–243.

58. Saddekni S, Sniderman KW, Hilton S, Sos TA. Percutaneous transluminal angioplasty of nonatherosclerotic lesions. *AJR* 1980;135:976–982.

59. Schuler JJ, Flanigan DP, Lim LT, Keifer T, Williams LR, Behrend AJ. The effect of carotid siphon stenosis on stroke rate, death, and relief of symptoms following elective carotid endarterectomy. *Surgery* 1982;92:1058–1065.

60. Schwartz RB, Jones KM, LeClercq GT et al. The value of cerebral angiography in predicting cerebral ischemia during carotid endarterectomy. *AJR* 1992;159:1057–1061.

61. Sekhar LN, Heros RC, Lotz PR, Rosenbaum AE. Atheromatous pseudo-occlusion of the internal carotid artery. *J Neurosurg* 1980;52:782–789.

62. Sitzer M, Furst G, Fischer H et al. Between-method correlation in quantifying internal carotid stenosis. *Stroke* 1993;24:1513–1518.

63. Stead DL, Peitzman AB, Grundy BL, Webster RW. Causes of stroke in carotid endarterectomy. *Surgery* 1982;92:634–641.

64. Theron J, Courtheoux P, Alachkar F, Bovard G, Maiza D. New triple coaxial catheter system for carotid angioplasty with cerebral protection. *AJNR* 1990;11:869–874.

65. Tomac B, Hebrang A. Selective catheterization and digital subtraction angiography of supraaortic arteries via the transcubital approach: a technical note. *AJNR* 1991;12:843–844.

66. Trigaux JP, Delchambre F, Van Beers B. Anatomical variations of the carotid bifurcation: implications for digital subtraction angiography and ultrasonography. *Br J Radiol* 1990;63:181–185.

67. Wade GL, Smith DC, Mohr LL. Follow-up of 50 consecutive angiograms obtained utilizing puncture of prosthetic vascular grafts. *Radiology* 1983;146:663–664.

68. Watkinson AF, Hartnell GG. Complications of direct brachial artery puncture for arteriography: a comparison of techniques. *Clin Radiol* 1991;44:189–191.

69. Weschler LR. Ulceration and carotid artery disease. *Stroke* 1987;22:19–23.

70. Whittemore AD, Kauffman JL, Kahler TR, Mannick JA. Routine electroencephalographic (EEG) monitoring during carotid endarterectomy. *Ann Surg* 1983;197:707–713.

71. Yonas H, Meyer J. Extreme pseudo-occlusion of the internal carotid artery. *Neurosurgery* 1982;11:681–686.

4

Noninvasive Carotid Imaging: Magnetic Resonance Imaging and Magnetic Resonance Angiography

John A. Anson

The availability and efficacy of medical and surgical treatment for atherosclerotic cerebrovascular disease make the accurate detection and depiction of carotid artery stenotic lesions on radiologic studies increasingly important. The advent and continued development of magnetic resonance (MR) angiography permits accurate, noninvasive depiction of the extracranial carotid arteries. Magnetic resonance imaging (MRI) fast is becoming the radiologic study of choice in patients with suspected ischemic neurologic symptoms, and its ability to evaluate the cerebral vasculature directly is particularly appealing.

The results of the North American Symptomatic Carotid Endarterectomy Trial (NASCET) documented the efficacy of carotid endarterectomy for patients with symptomatic stenoses greater than 70% (33). Superiority of surgical treatment, however, is predicated on an acceptably low morbidity of carotid endarterectomy. Although conventional selective carotid angiography has always been considered the gold standard for diagnosis of carotid artery disease, it carries a small but significant risk (40). The risk of minor neurologic events from cerebral angiography has been estimated to range from 1.2% to 4.5%, and the risk of permanent deficit or stroke has been estimated to range from 0.6% to 1.3% (7,15,16,37). These risks must be added to the surgical risk for a true assessment of morbidity if angiography is routinely performed before carotid endarterectomy.

J. A. Anson: Division of Neurosurgery, University of New Mexico Hospital, Albuquerque, New Mexico 87131.

To avoid the risk of angiography, accurate noninvasive methods for diagnosing surgically significant stenoses of the cervical carotid artery have been sought; the most widely described are Doppler ultrasound studies. Although carotid endarterectomy has been performed on the basis of ultrasound blood flow studies alone (14), these studies convey a limited amount of information and may be inaccurate (3,17,19,30). They also include no information about the intracranial vasculature such as tandem stenoses or incidental aneurysms. The angiograms performed in the NASCET study disclosed incidental aneurysms in 2.6% of patients (3).

Magnetic resonance angiography is also noninvasive, but it can visualize the entire length of the carotid and vertebral arteries in a conventional angiographic display. By contrast, ultrasound is more limited to the bifurcation. At the conclusion of a cerebral MRI study, MR angiography is readily performed. In addition to the cervical arteries, additional data concerning the circle of Willis can be obtained by performing an intracranial MR angiogram. Unlike ultrasound studies, whose quality depends on the technician performing the test, MR studies are reader dependent and allow review and independent confirmation of findings by radiologists and clinicians.

PRINCIPLES

Magnetic resonance angiography techniques are based on contrast between moving blood and stationary tissues. The demonstration of blood on MR images is related to the pulse sequence used in the imaging process, incorporating variables such as repetition time, flip angle, and slice orientation. These are also known as *time-of-flight* effects and can be manipulated to increase or decrease vascular signals. The familiar appearance of *flow void* is an example of a time-of-flight effect that decreases vascular signal. As blood moves through the selected imaging slice, the protons (spins) do not remain long enough to be acted upon by both the 90° and 180° radiofrequency (rf) pulses used in conventional spin-echo imaging. Both pulses must be received for the spins to be included in the image. Consequently, spins that receive the first pulse but flow out of the imaging slice before the second pulse, as well as those that flow in after the first pulse and receive only the second pulse, give no signal and appear black in the MR image.

Conversely, time-of-flight effects can be used to increase vascular signal in a process known as *flow-related enhancement*. Normally, signal is detected in MR images when the 90° rf pulse flips the vector of magnetization perpendicular to the main longitudinal magnetic field. Left undisturbed, the transverse magnetization vector gradually returns to the main longitudinal magnetic field. By delivering rapidly repeated 90° rf pulses (short repetition time) before this longitudinal recovery can occur, the protons become partially saturated, and detectable signal is decreased. As signal-rich, unsaturated blood then flows into the imaging slice, it gives increased signal as it is exposed to the rf energy.

Also of importance in maximizing the signal intensity of blood are the signal-localizing gradients (35). These are three orthogonal magnetic fields that are used to localize, or to encode spatially, the voxels in space. These gradients are used to maintain phase coherence of the spins in blood flowing within the imaging plane because loss of coherence results in signal loss. Ross et al. (34) have described this effect as analogous to a tightly collimated searchlight that has much greater intensity than the same light allowed to disperse randomly.

The time-of-flight technique can be implemented with either two- or three-dimensional acquisition techniques (27,34,35). Most centers use two-dimensional time-of-flight for clinical studies of the carotid arteries. Simply put, in two-dimensional imaging, the carotid artery is demonstrated by stacking a series of thin, axial, gradient-echo, two-dimensional images. Postprocessing suppresses the stationary background tissue so that only the blood vessels are demonstrated. To eliminate the venous flow that would otherwise be seen as well, a superior saturation band is used to eliminate signal from the venous blood flowing caudally into the imaging slice.

The major advantage of two-dimensional technique is its excellent flow-related enhancement characteristics, generating high signal intensity of flowing blood for high-resolution images. Its major disadvantage is sensitivity to a patient's movement, which manifests as vessel discontinuity on the stacked axial images.

The current parameters for MR angiography of the carotid bifurcation in use at University of New Mexico Hospital are a two-dimensional time-of-flight technique on a Signa 1.5-Tesla MR imaging system (GE Medical Systems, Milwaukee, WI). Contiguous axial 1.5-mm-thick slices are acquired with a gradient-echo pulse sequence. This sequence, called spoiled gradient-recalled (SPGR) acquisition in the steady state, incorporates either a stepped gradient on the slice-select axis or radiofrequency-phase spoiling to minimize residual signal from stationary tissues. First-order gradient-moment nulling on the slice-select and frequency-encode axes provides constant velocity-flow compensation. A superiorly positioned saturation band is used to suppress caudally directed venous flow.

Usually either 64 or 110 slices are obtained with a repetition time (TR) of 45 ms, an echo time (TE) of 6 ms, and a flip angle of 60°. Matrix size is 256 × 128 with a 20-cm field of view. The resulting axial images are used to construct 19 projected images with a maximum intensity pixel algorithm. The images are projected at 10° increments over a 180° range. An additional collapsed view is constructed demonstrating all the vessels compressed within an axial slab. Imaging time for a study is 12:53 minutes, and the MR angiogram is frequently obtained at the conclusion of a standard cerebral MRI study (Fig. 1).

In three-dimensional time-of-flight technique a thick slab or volume of tissue is excited. The pulse sequence is similar to the two-dimensional technique with an additional phase-encoding gradient for the third dimension. A three-dimensional Fourier transform is used to create the final image. Although three-dimensional technique offers a theoretical increase in the signal-to-noise ratio, current methods are limited to relatively small regions of high flow (35).

An additional technique used for MR angiography is the so-called *black blood* technique, which images uniform signal loss within the vessel compared with *bright blood* techniques, which maximize signal from flowing blood. Although it uses a two-dimensional time-of-flight method, spin dephasing and inferior presaturation below the bifurcation minimize the signal from flowing blood and achieve black vascular contrast that creates an appearance more similar to conventional angiography (9,35). Stenosis is not overestimated with the black blood technique, which therefore may be helpful in cases of severe narrowing of the carotid bifurcation (10).

CORRELATIVE SERIES

A number of reports have demonstrated that MR angiography has a high degree of accuracy compared with that of conventional studies (13,18,21, 24,25,28,39). In a comparative study of 73 carotid arteries at the Barrow Neurological Institute, the correlation of conventional and MR angiography

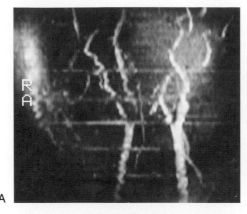

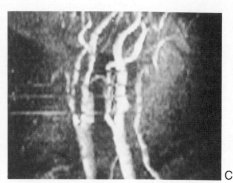

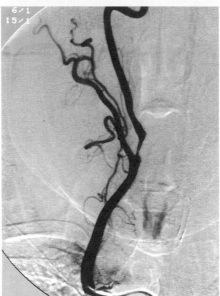

Figure 1. Example of a magnetic resonance (MR) angiogram of the carotid bifurcation in a man aged 64 with a recent mild right hemisphere infarct using two-dimensional, time-of-flight technique with the parameters described in the text. **A:** Preoperative MR angiogram showing the characteristic flow gap in the proximal internal carotid artery suggestive of significant stenosis. Movement artifact is present as horizontal lines across the entire image but does not obscure the pertinent findings. **B:** Conventional angiography confirming the tight stenosis of the proximal internal carotid artery. **C:** Postoperative MR angiogram showing wide patency of the internal carotid artery with good flow.

was strongest when the stenosis was more severe (18). Perfect agreement was found between the two imaging studies for groups with severe stenoses and occlusion. Because symptomatic patients with these lesions are the group that the NASCET study suggests will benefit most from surgical therapy, these results suggest that MR angiography is sensitive enough to identify patients who may benefit from surgical treatment (33). Consequently, we retrospectively compared MR and conventional angiography in 20 patients who underwent carotid endarterectomy (1).

Twenty patients with symptomatic cerebrovascular disease who underwent carotid angiography, MR angiography, and carotid endarterectomy were evaluated retrospectively (1). Seven had minor strokes, eight had amaurosis fugax, and seven had hemispheric transient ischemic attacks (TIAs). Two patients had TIAs associated with minor stroke or transient monocular blindness. The interval between conventional and MR angiography ranged from 1 day to 2 weeks. The patients all underwent carotid endarterectomy based on their cerebrovascular symptoms and on the presence of an occlusion or more than 70% stenosis on conventional angiography.

A two-dimensional, time-of-flight MR angiographic technique, similar to that described above, was performed on a 1.5-Tesla MR imaging system (20). Conventional intra-arterial angiographic studies were performed on all patients with selective common carotid artery injections. Both anteroposterior and lateral images were selected for review. The MR and conventional angiograms were reviewed in a blinded fashion by two experienced neuroradiologists. The angiograms were scored between 0 and 4 according to the narrowing of the diameter of the proximal internal carotid artery. Grades 0 to 4 corresponded respectively to normal (0% to 10% narrowing), mild stenosis (11% to 50%), moderate stenosis (51% to 75%), severe stenosis (76% to 99%), and occlusion. Surgery was performed on 21 carotid arteries.

Results of this series showed 100% correlation between the two readers. The carotid bifurcation had a characteristic appearance on MR angiography in each subgroup. Grade 1 lesions were characterized by mild narrowing of the carotid artery, often along its posterior aspect (Fig. 2). Grade 2 vessels

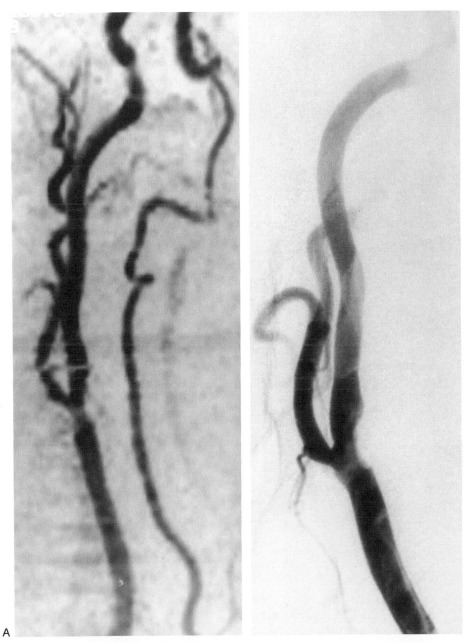

A   B

Figure 2. A: Mild narrowing of the proximal internal carotid artery shown by MR angiography in a 54-year-old man with contralateral transient ischemic attacks. **B:** Conventional angiography confirming mild stenosis.

exhibited moderate narrowing. The MR angiograms usually depicted the morphology of the narrowing accurately, although the length and degree of stenosis can be overestimated. The consistent characteristic appearance of severe stenosis, or grade 3 lesions, on MR angiography was the absence of signal intensity within the internal carotid artery at the level of the stenosis with the reappearance of signal intensity within 2 cm of the bifurcation (Fig. 3). This lack of signal intensity was thought to reflect the loss of laminar flow in the poststenotic portion of the artery. The turbulent flow results in decreased signal intensity, with the length of the signal loss segment roughly

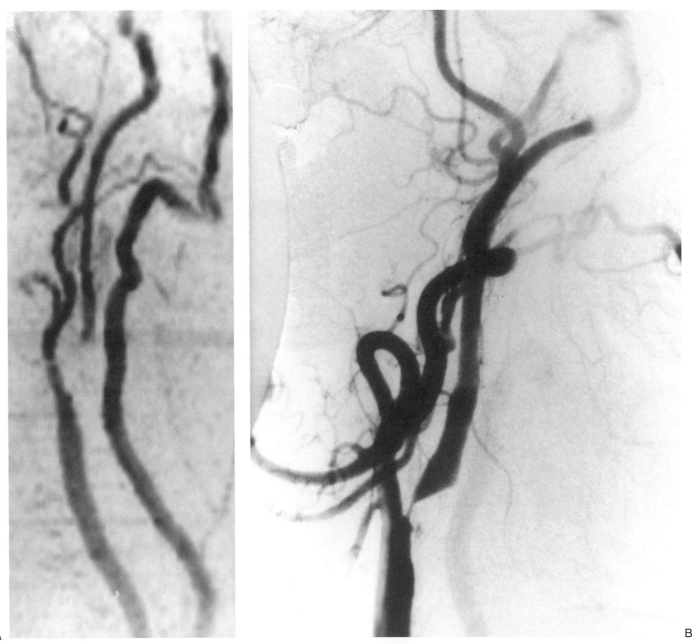

A   B

Figure 3. A: Characteristic findings by MR angiography of signal gap just distal to the bifurcation with distal reappearance indicating severe internal carotid artery stenosis in a 65-year-old man with amaurosis fugax. **B:** Conventional angiography confirming the presence of 95% stenosis of the proximal internal carotid artery. (From *Neurosurgery*)

proportional to the degree of narrowing (11,18). Grade 4 lesions had complete occlusion, as evidenced by absence of the distal reappearance of the signal.

The correlation between MR and conventional angiography in the 21 surgically treated carotid arteries is summarized in Table 1. MR angiography demonstrated severe stenosis in 14 internal carotid arteries. Conventional angiography confirmed the severe stenosis in 12 of these patients. Operative notes reported the presence of severe stenosis in 10 of these vessels. The operative notes did not report the degree of stenosis in the other two cases. Although two vessels were categorized as grade 3 on MR and as grade 2 on conventional angiography, the degree of narrowing was 70%, which qualified these patients for endarterectomy according to the NASCET criteria.

Complete correlation was found between conventional and MR angiography in seven patients with internal carotid artery occlusion. The MR angiogram in these patients showed complete absence of signal intensity distal to the occlusion at the origin of the internal carotid artery, with no distal recovery of signal intensity (Fig. 4). This lack of distal recovery of signal intensity differentiates an occlusion from severe stenosis. At surgery, all seven of these arteries were occluded, confirming both studies. Although four of these vessels had fresh intraluminal thrombus and could be reopened, no characteristic finding identified these cases on MR angiography alone even with a retrospective analysis. Conventional T_1- and T_2-weighted MR images, however, may differentiate between acute and chronic thrombus.

The correlation of MR and conventional angiogram gradings in all 40 carotid arteries (20 patients) is shown in Table 2. One additional case of occlusion was seen on both MR and conventional angiography. Four additional cases were labeled severe stenosis on MR, and three of these correlated with conventional studies; the remaining one was called moderate stenosis on conventional angiography.

Several other series have also documented the accuracy of MR angiography, particularly for high-grade stenoses and occlusions. In a preliminary evaluation of time-of-flight MR angiography, Masaryk et al. (27) reported that it correlated well with conventional angiography in 12 patients. Although one severe stenosis was graded indeterminate on MR angiography, all demonstrations of occlusion were accurate. Edelman et al. (8,9) compared time-of-flight MR angiography and black blood MR angiography in 17 patients. With the time-of-flight technique two false-positive and one false-negative interpretations of occlusion were all correctly interpreted on black blood images.

Litt et al. (25) also found a high degree of correlation between MR and conventional angiography in 94 carotid arteries with severe stenosis. The best correlation was in the severely stenotic category. The poorest correlation was, however, in the occluded category, in which about 25% of the occlusions were graded as severe stenosis. A high rate of accuracy was also reported by Laster et al. (22) in a series of 200 vessels. Using the two-dimensional time-of-flight technique, they detected 100% of the occlusions

Table 1. *MRA (% stenosis)*

	100%	76–99%	51–75%
Conventional angiography			
100%	7	—	—
76–99%	—	12	—
51–75%	—	2	—

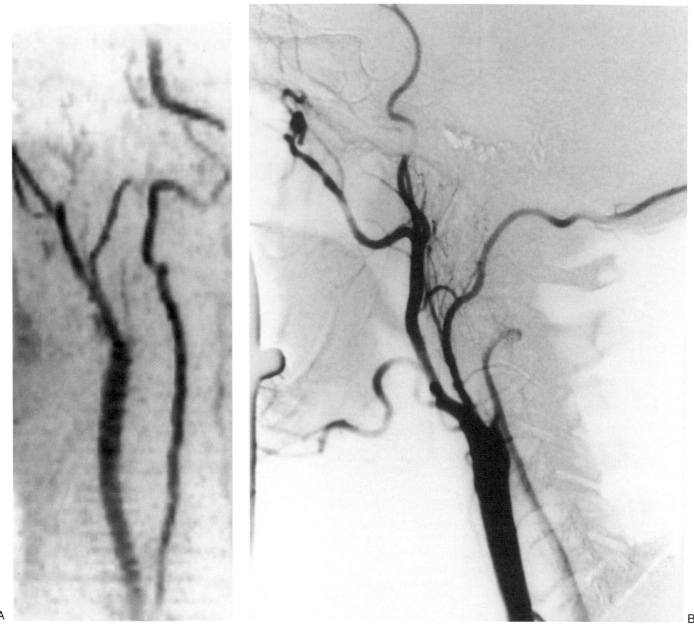

Figure 4. A: Magnetic resonance angiography in a 55-year-old man with left hemisphere transient ischemic attacks demonstrating loss of signal intensity at the bifurcation with no distal reappearance, indicating complete internal carotid artery occlusion. **B:** Conventional angiography confirms complete occlusion of the left internal carotid artery. (From Anson JA et al. *Neurosurgery* 1993;32:335–343, with permission.)

Table 2. *Comparison of MR and conventional angiographic findings of stenosis (%) in 40 carotid arteries in 20 patients*

	MR angiography				
	100	76–99	51–75	11–50	0–10
Conventional angiography					
100	8	—	—	—	—
76–99	—	15	—	—	—
51–75	—	3	4	—	—
11–50	—	—	—	6	1
0–10	—	—	—	1	2

accurately, almost 100% of the normal vessels, and more than 90% of the severely stenotic vessels.

Wesbey et al. (38) compared three-dimensional time-of-flight MR angiography with both contrast angiography and duplex ultrasonography. They reported 75% exact correlation of stenosis grade between MR angiography and duplex examinations, and 86% agreement between MR angiography and conventional angiography. The degree of stenosis seen on MR angiography also agreed with surgical findings in 98% of cases. Mattle et al. (29) also reported that MR angiography was more accurate than duplex ultrasound in a series of 39 carotid arteries studied with duplex, bright blood MR angiography, black blood MR angiography, and conventional angiography. Duplex was inaccurate compared with conventional angiography in six cases: three were overgraded and three were undergraded. Magnetic resonance angiography overgraded the degree of stenosis in three cases. When they evaluated the various methods using a greater-than-70% stenosis as a positive study, the sensitivity of MR angiography was 100% and its specificity was 92%. This result was better than duplex scanning, which had a sensitivity of 86% and specificity of 84%. Cases in which the results of the MR angiography and duplex scanning were in agreement correlated with conventional angiography 100%.

Chiesa et al. (6) also found an excellent correlation between MR and conventional angiography in cases of surgical stenosis in a study of 194 carotid bifurcations. By regression analysis, the sensitivity of MR angiography was 93% and its specificity was 98% with regard to surgically significant stenosis. Their study also demonstrated a shortcoming of MR angiography, namely, its poor sensitivity for detecting ulceration. In their 68 operated cases, Chiesa et al. (6) also reported 100% agreement between postoperative MR angiography and intraoperative angiography performed by direct proximal carotid puncture after completion of the endarterectomy and arteriotomy closure. Intraoperative angiography showed a patent internal carotid artery with satisfactory endarterectomy in all cases. Magnetic resonance angiography performed before hospital discharge also showed a patent internal carotid artery without residual stenosis in all cases. We have also found MR angiography to be the ideal study for routine postoperative evaluation after carotid endarterectomy and now use it routinely without any other intra- or postoperative study (Fig. 1C).

OVERESTIMATION AND ARTIFACT

The most common inaccuracy of MR angiography is a tendency to overestimate the degree of stenosis at the carotid bifurcation (18,27). The maximum intensity pixel projection algorithm used to reconstruct the projection images may artifactually narrow the apparent vessel lumen, producing two effects. One is an overall narrowing of the depicted blood vessels that does not appear to affect interpretation by experienced readers. The other, an accentuation of focal areas of narrowing, is more likely to result in overinterpretation of stenoses.

Normal or mildly stenotic carotid arteries can also be misinterpreted as narrowed because of loss of signal intensity in the region of the posterior aspect of the carotid bulb. This signal loss is produced by local areas of nonlaminar flow. Flow separation, turbulence, and reversal of flow are known to occur at the normal carotid bulb (32). Doppler studies of healthy young volunteers have demonstrated that an average of 33% (range, 8% to 64%) of the area of the carotid bulb is occupied by flow reversal (31). The amount of lost signal intensity attributable to posterior bulb artifact varies and could be confused with focal stenosis. Cases of artifactual signal loss in the posterior bulb are typically characterized by a relative decrease in signal intensity with smooth borders (Fig. 5). Atherosclerotic lesions in this region can usually be differentiated by a more marked loss of signal intensity and less regular borders. Reader experience and technical improvements, such as shorter TE, help to avoid overinterpretation of this pseudonarrowing.

Motion artifact is another common source of interpretive error. Gross motion artifact is usually readily apparent and leads to technically inadequate studies. Local motion artifact from swallowing can also cause apparent ves-

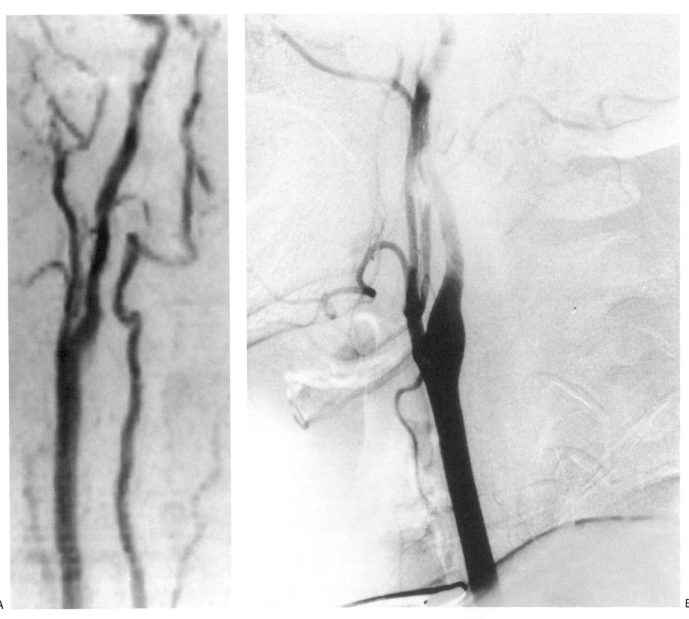

A   B

Figure 5. A: Normal carotid bifurcation by MR angiogram. Posterior carotid bulb produces the appearance of slight focal narrowing, but the location and incomplete loss of signal identify it as artifact. **B:** Angiography confirming that the vessel is normal. (From Anson JA. *Neurosurgery* 1993;32:335–343, with permission.)

sel narrowing, but this error can usually be recognized by the appearance of a band across all the depicted vessels at the same level (18). Susceptibility artifact, caused by bone, is seldom a problem in evaluating the carotid bifurcation, which is not close to any bony structures. Susceptibility artifact should be considered, however, when distal internal carotid artery narrowing is apparently seen. As the carotid artery approaches the skull base, signal loss becomes an unreliable indicator of stenosis and should not necessarily be interpreted as pathologic.

At the carotid bifurcation and proximal internal carotid artery, MR angiography appears to identify reliably severe stenoses that would be considered surgically significant in symptomatic patients. The hallmark finding is a short segment of complete signal loss in the proximal internal carotid artery with reappearance distally along the vessel. In our experience, a vessel that appears constricted on MR angiography but that does not exhibit complete signal loss over a focal segment will have no more than 70% stenosis on conventional contrast angiography. This focal signal loss is thought to represent an area of turbulent nonlaminar flow created by a severe stenosis that results in intravoxel or "spin" dephasing. In other words, the spins (protons) do not rotate coherently because of excessive flow turbulence along the localizing gradient planes, and that loss of coherence results in signal loss (34). The span of the artifactual signal loss is roughly proportional to the degree of stenosis, but this relationship cannot be demonstrated accurately enough to differentiate among different degrees of severe stenosis in clinical situations (18). This inability of MR angiography to differentiate between various degrees of severe stenosis remains a potential limitation to its use as the sole study of symptomatic carotid artery disease. However, shorter TE values can minimize the amount of artifact from turbulent flow and can represent stenosis more accurately. With a TE of 8.7 ms or less, artifact associated with the posterior carotid bulb can be almost eliminated. Acceleration of blood through a stenotic vessel lumen, however, can still be sufficient to lead to spin dephasing and subsequent signal loss.

Biorheologic models of vessel stenosis show that any distortions of blood vessel lumens, even physiologic bendings and bifurcations, produce local flow disturbances (2,4,12). Flow separation and vortices may develop downstream from stenoses, even when flow through the constriction itself is smooth (2). Irregular stenoses can also separate the slower moving, peripheral "boundary layer" from the luminal wall. This separation creates a zone of stasis or stagnation of blood adjacent to the vessel wall, even while high-flow velocities continue on the other side of the boundary layer (12). This phenomenon has also been demonstrated at vessel bifurcations: stagnant areas form on the external wall of the branch vessels or on the side away from the divergence (12). All of these flow anomalies alter the signal intensity of MR angiographic images and must be considered during interpretation (11).

Another potential cause of artifactual signal loss is a loop of carotid artery oriented within and parallel to the imaging slice. This configuration creates in-plane flow that results in apparent signal loss. We have seen a notable example of this phenomenon in a patient whose MR angiogram demonstrated an apparent severe stenosis of the internal carotid artery approximately 3 cm distal to the bifurcation (Fig. 6A). Conventional angiography, however, showed that the lumen of the internal carotid artery was normal but that the vessel looped tortuously at that site (Fig. 6B). The appearance of a stenosis in such an atypical distal location on a preoperative MR angiography should raise suspicion of a loop and prompt the use of conventional angiography for confirmation.

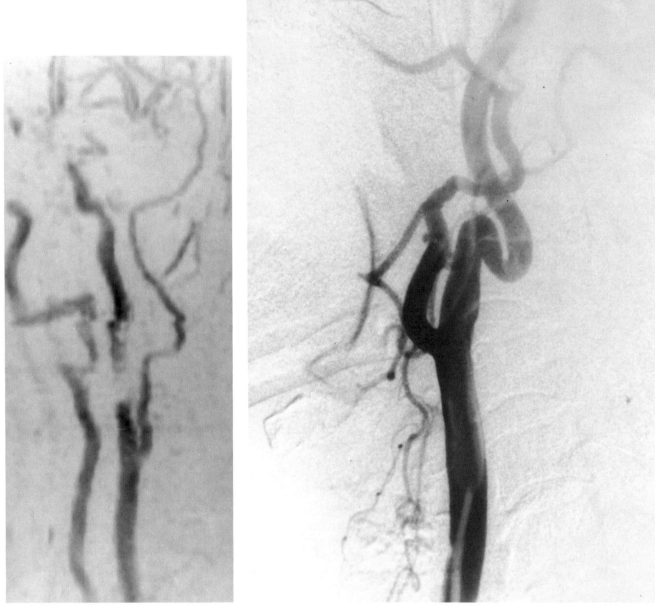

A   B

Figure 6. A: An example of in-plane flow artifact from a vessel loop by MR angiography demonstrating an apparent severe stenosis of the internal carotid artery 3 cm distal to the bifurcation. **B:** Conventional angiography shows a tortuous vessel loop with a normal lumen. The unusual location of this apparent stenosis should suggest the possibility of artifact and indicate the need for conventional angiography. (From Anson JA. *Neurosurgery* 1993;32:335–343, with permission.)

CONCLUSIONS

Magnetic resonance angiography can be an accurate and reliable indicator of surgically significant carotid artery stenosis. Occasional false-positive results may occur, however, particularly if vessels are tortuous or overlap. Careful interpretation for consistency of level and location, including consideration of flow patterns, will minimize these errors. No false-negative studies were seen in our series in symptomatic patients. Experienced readers can differentiate normal or mildly stenotic vessels from severe disease and can distinguish severe stenosis from occlusion.

Because false positives occasionally occur, MR angiography studies of carotid stenosis should still be interpreted cautiously. If, however, a technically adequate MR angiogram demonstrates a flow gap within 2 cm of the carotid bifurcation with distal reappearance of flow at a site consistent with symptoms, it may potentially be considered adequate as the sole preoperative study. Further progress in techniques and interpretation skills will no doubt improve the accuracy of MR angiography and also advance its use as an adequate sole preoperative study for carotid endarterectomy.

With ever-increasing pressure to reduce health care expenditures, the relative costs of preoperative carotid evaluation should be considered as well. At the University of New Mexico Hospital, for example, a conventional anteroposterior and lateral angiogram of both extracranial carotid arteries costs $3,888 (including technical and professional fees plus related hospital costs). An MR angiogram costs only $235 when performed as part of the initial brain MRI examination, which costs $982. In comparison, a duplex study of the carotid arteries costs $393, or 67% more than MR angiography. Eliminating conventional angiography for certain patients offers significant savings in addition to reducing risk (plus the high cost of complications).

MR angiography is less sensitive for the study of atherosclerotic disease in the carotid siphon and intracranial vasculature than it is for evaluation of the carotid bifurcation. Nonetheless, it can provide pertinent information about these areas in preoperative patients that is unavailable by duplex scanning. Recent reports have demonstrated improved visualization of the intracranial vessels that may provide sufficient sensitivity for preoperative evaluation of distal tandem stenoses and collateral circulation as well as of incidental aneurysms (5,8,23,26,36).

Magnetic resonance angiography is accurate, safe, and easy to obtain for the evaluation of patients with cerebrovascular symptoms. It is cheaper and more informative than Doppler studies. At centers that have verified accuracy compared with conventional angiography, MR angiography should be considered potentially suitable as the sole preoperative test in patients with symptomatic atherosclerotic carotid artery disease. It is also an excellent screening test for patients with possible extracranial cerebrovascular pathology and should replace ultrasound screening studies in most cases.

REFERENCES

1. Anson JA, Heiserman JE, Drayer BP, Spetzler RF. Surgical decisions on the basis of magnetic resonance angiography of the carotid arteries. *Neurosurgery* 1993;32:335–343.
2. Azuma T, Fukushima T. Flow patterns in stenotic blood vessel models. *Biorheology* 1976; 13:337–355.
3. Barnett HJM, Barnes RW, Robertson JT. The uncertainties surrounding carotid endarterectomy. *JAMA* 1992;268:3120–3121.
4. Blackshear WM Jr, Phillips DJ, Chikos PM, Harley JD, Thiele BL, Strandness DE Jr. Carotid artery velocity patterns in normal and stenotic vessels. *Stroke* 1980;11:67–71.
5. Blatter DD, Parker DL, Robison RO. Cerebral MR angiography with multiple overlapping thin slab acquisition. Part I. Quantitative analysis of vessel visibility. *Radiology* 1991;179: 805–811.
6. Chiesa R, Melissano G, Castellano R. Three dimensional time-of-flight magnetic resonance angiography in carotid artery surgery: a comparison with digital subtraction angiography. *Eur J Vasc Surg* 1993;7:171–176.
7. Earnest F IV, Forbes G, Sandok BA, et al. Complications of cerebral angiography: prospective assessment of risk. *AJR* 1984;142:247–253.
8. Edelman RR, Mattle HP, O'Reilly GV, Wentz KU, Liu C, Zhao B. Magnetic resonance imaging of flow dynamics in the circle of Willis. *Stroke* 1990;21:56–65.
9. Edelman RR, Mattle HP, Wallner B, et al. Extracranial carotid arteries: evaluation with "black blood" MR angiography. *Radiology* 1990;177:45–50.
10. Edelman RR, Mattle HP, Wallner B, Kleefield J, Atkinson DJ. MR angiography of the extracranial carotid arteries: evaluation of bright and black blood techniques. *Radiology* 1990;177(P):89(abst).

11. Evans AJ, Blinder RA, Herfkens RJ, et al. Effects of turbulence on signal intensity in gradient echo images. *Invest Radiol* 1988;23:512–518.
12. Fox JA, Hugh AE. Static zones in the internal carotid artery: correlation with boundary layer separation and stasis in model flows. *Br J Radiol* 1970;43:370–376.
13. Furuya Y, Isoda H, Hasegawa S, Takahashi M, Kaneko M, Uemura K. Magnetic resonance angiography of extracranial carotid and vertebral arteries, including their origins: comparison with digital subtraction angiography. *Neuroradiology* 1992;35:42–45.
14. Gelebart HA, Moore WS. Carotid endarterectomy without angiography. *Surg Clin North Am* 1990;70:213–223.
15. Hankey GJ, Warlow CP, Molyneux AJ. Complications of cerebral angiography for patients with mild carotid territory ischaemia being considered for carotid endarterectomy. *J Neurol Neurosurg Psychiatry* 1990;53:542–548.
16. Hankey GJ, Warlow CP, Sellar RJ. Cerebral angiographic risk in mild cerebrovascular disease. *Stroke* 1990;21:209–222.
17. Haynes RB, Taylor DW, Sacket DL. Poor performance of Doppler in detecting high-grade carotid stenosis. *Clin Res* 1990;40:184A(abst).
18. Heiserman JE, Drayer BP, Fram EK, et al. Carotid artery stenosis: clinical efficacy of two-dimensional time-of-flight MR angiography. *Radiology* 1992;182:761–768.
19. Howard G, Jones AM, Chambless L, et al. A multicenter validation of Doppler ultrasound versus angiogram: the ACAS experience. *Stroke* 1991;22:147(abst).
20. Keller PJ, Drayer BP, Fram EK, Williams KD. MR angiography with two-dimensional acquisition and three-dimensional display. *Radiology* 1989;173:527–532.
21. Kido DK, Panzer RJ, Szumowski J, et al. Clinical evaluation of stenosis of the carotid bifurcation with magnetic resonance angiographic techniques. *Arch Neurol* 1991;48:484–489.
22. Laster RE, Acker JD, Halford HH, Nauert C. Carotid bifurcation evaluation with vascular MR imaging. *J Magn Reson Imaging* 1991;1:205(abst).
23. Lewin JS, Laub G. Intracranial MR angiography: a direct comparison of three time-of-flight techniques. *AJNR* 1991;12:1133–1139.
24. Link KM, Elster AD, Margosian P, Sattin B. Clinical utility of three-dimensional magnetic resonance angiographic imaging. *Clin Neurosurg* 1989;37:275–288.
25. Litt AW, Eidelman EM, Pinto RS, et al. Diagnosis of carotid artery stenosis: comparison of 2DFT time-of-flight MR angiography with contrast angiography in 50 patients. *AJNR* 1991;12:149–154.
26. Masaryk TJ, Modic MT, Ross JS, et al. Intracranial circulation: Preliminary clinical results with three-dimensional (volume) MR angiography. *Radiology* 1989;171:793–799.
27. Masaryk TJ, Modic MT, Ruggieri PM, et al. Three-dimensional (volume) gradient-echo imaging of the carotid bifurcation: preliminary clinical experience. *Radiology* 1989;171:801–806.
28. Masaryk AM, Ross JS, DiCello MC, Modic MT, Paranandi L, Masaryk TJ. 3DFT MR angiography of the carotid bifurcation: potential and limitations as a screening examination. *Radiology* 1991;179:797–804.
29. Mattle HP, Kent KC, Edelman RR, Atkinson DJ, Skillman JJ. Evaluation of the extracranial carotid arteries: correlation of magnetic resonance angiography, duplex ultrasonography, and conventional angiography. *J Vasc Surg* 1991;13:838–845.
30. Mayberg MR, Wilson SE, Yatsu F. Carotid endarterectomy and prevention of cerebral ischemia in symptomatic carotid stenosis. *JAMA* 1991;266:3289–3294.
31. Middleton WD, Foley WD, Lawson TL. Flow reversal in the normal carotid bifurcation: color Doppler flow imaging analysis. *Radiology* 1988;167:207–210.
32. Motomiya M, Karino T. Flow patterns in the human carotid artery bifurcation. *Stroke* 1984;15:50–56.
33. North American Symptomatic Carotid Endarterectomy Trial Collaborators. Beneficial effect of carotid endarterectomy in symptomatic patients with high-grade carotid stenosis. *N Engl J Med* 1991;325:445–453.
34. Ross JS, Masaryk TJ, Modic MT, Harik SI, Wiznitzer M, Selman WR. Magnetic resonance angiography of the extracranial carotid arteries and intracranial vessels: a review. *Neurology* 1989;39:1369–1376.
35. Ross JS, Masaryk TJ, Ruggieri PM. Magnetic resonance angiography of the carotid bifurcation. *Top Magn Reson Imaging* 1991;3:12–22.
36. Ruggieri PM, Laub GA, Masaryk TJ, Modic MT. Intracranial circulation: pulse-sequence considerations in three-dimensional (volume) MR angiography. *Radiology* 1989;171:785–791.
37. Sundt TM Jr, Houser OW, Fode NC, Whisnant JP. Correlation of postoperative and two-year follow-up angiography with neurological function in 99 carotid endarterectomies in 86 consecutive patients. *Ann Surg* 1986;203:90–100.
38. Wesbey GE, Bergan JJ, Moreland SI, et al. Cerebrovascular magnetic resonance angiography: a critical verification. *J Vasc Surg* 1992;16:619–632.
39. Wilkerson DK, Keller I, Mezrich R, et al. The comparative evaluation of three-dimensional magnetic resonance for carotid artery disease. *J Vasc Surg* 1991;14:803–811.
40. Zabramski JM, Anson JA. Diagnostic evaluation of ischemic cerebrovascular disease. In: Awad I, ed. *Neurological topics series (Book 10). Cerebrovascular occlusive disease and brain ischemia.* Park Ridge IL: AANS; 1992:73–102.

5

Anesthesia and Carotid Endarterectomy

Edward Teeple, Jr. and Paul Lobaugh

Evaluation of outcomes for medical and surgical treatments has recently intensified. Nowhere is this more true than for carotid endarterectomy. This technique is frequently performed, and numerous articles have been written analyzing the impact of the hospital site (community versus tertiary hospital), surgeon, surgical technique, anesthesia, and method of monitoring the patient. The surgeon and the anesthesiologist need to use this information when choosing the method for the procedure. Certain patients' medical conditions may demand certain surgical and anesthetic approaches. Whereas the simpler techniques can be defended on the basis of lucidity, decreased cost, and outcome, they may not be appropriate in all patients. In fact, they may increase incidental complications (perioperative myocardial ischemia, loss of airway during procedure) or be refused by the patient (anxiety, inability to lie still). High-technology approaches may also increase risks (by prolonging the duration of anesthesia or the carotid cross-clamp time). This chapter attempts to elucidate the impact of these variations and the various anesthetic options. With increased understanding, perhaps future outcome studies will report even lower levels of morbidity and mortality for patients undergoing carotid endarterectomy.

INCIDENCE OF STROKE

Preoperative Risk Factors

A number of diseases can have an impact during and after the procedure (Table 1). Hypertension, diabetes, older age, and smoking combined with

E. Teeple, Jr and P. Lobaugh: Department of Neuroanesthesia, Medical College of Pennsylvania and Hahnemann University, Allegheny General Hospital, Pittsburgh, Pennsylvania 15212.

Table 1. *Preoperative disease presentation of carotid endarterectomy patients*

Diseases/symptom	% Patients
Angina	24
Previous myocardial infarction	20
Hypertension	60
Peripheral vascular disease	15
Smoking	
Current	37
Previous	40
Diabetes	19

carotid angiographic abnormalities can increase postoperative cerebral complications (73). Myocardial infarction in the perioperative period is the leading cause of death after carotid endarterectomy (30,46). This speaks for the necessity of a thorough preoperative cardiac work-up and treatment. Also, in patients with diagnosed cardiac dysfunction, rigorous intraoperative and postoperative monitoring and intervention is necessary to prevent subsequent myocardial infarction and death.

Elevated blood sugars intraoperatively have been shown to increase the risk of ischemic brain damage during periods of poor perfusion. Blood glucose levels should be kept below 150 mg/dl if possible (37,99).

Elevated preoperative blood pressures can increase the risks of anesthesia and surgery. Certain authors suggest keeping the blood pressure below 180/100 mmHg preoperatively. Prospective studies of anesthesia and blood pressure suggest an increased risk of complications when the diastolic pressure exceeds 110 mmHg, including postoperative hypertensive crisis, myocardial infarction, wound hematoma, and cerebral hemorrhage (5,41).

Also, a preoperative history of transient ischemic attacks (TIAs) or completed strokes is important to consider. If the stroke or TIA was a flow-related phenomenon, then changes in flow rates may occur during anesthesia induction and during the surgery. If the stroke or TIA was caused by embolization of ulcerated plaque, then surgical manipulation of the field may cause further embolization before the isolation of the carotid artery. Full documentation of the preoperative neurologic status is paramount, since questions may arise as to which symptoms or deficits existed before or after surgery.

Table 2 shows a classification of risk groups for carotid endarterectomy

Table 2. *Risk groups for carotid endarterectomy*

Group	Condition	Morbidity/mortality (%)
1	Neurologically stable No major medical problems Little angiographic risk	1
2	Neurologically stable No major medical problems Significant angiographic risk	2
3	Neurologically stable Major medical problems Significant angiographic risk	7
4	Neurologically unstable Major medical problems Significant angiographic risk	10

(5,71). Risks increase with a more complicated disease presentation. However, lack of significant disease does not imply that less stringent anesthetic and surgical care is permissible or will result in low morbidity and mortality rates, since contemporary rates of morbidity and mortality reflect more aggressive intraoperative and perioperative monitoring and care. A risk exists that less stringent care of more normal patients might allow complication rates to approach the levels of sicker patients. This is not acceptable. All methods of anesthesia and surgery, surgeons, and institutions should be periodically monitored for their effect on outcome to ensure optimum results for patients (27,61). Outcome analysis should be compared with the National Institutes of Health recommendations (morbidity and mortality should be less than 3%) (5,77).

High-risk presentations of carotid arterial disease for carotid endarterectomy include bilateral stenosis (34), contralateral high-grade stenosis (21,22, 60,78), TIA and stenosis (24), contralateral occlusion (64), bilateral occlusion (14), and previous stroke (48). These clinical presentations demand maximum monitoring and careful choice of technique.

Predicting which patients will not have adequate cerebral blood flow (CBF) is unclear at best. Therefore, monitoring the ipsilateral brain's status during cross-clamping is absolutely necessary. Contralateral carotid lesions present a challenge because the operative site will allow little or no blood flow to the ipsilateral brain. Ideally, during cross-clamping, enough blood flow to the ipsilateral brain can be supplied via the contralateral carotid artery in conjunction with adequate collateral flow from the anterior communicating artery (or the posterior circulation to the brain via the circle of Willis). Anatomic variations in the circle of Willis that can compromise collateral flow also exist.

Intraoperative Risk Factors

Induction of anesthesia can be problematic for patients with carotid disease. Coexistent carotid and coronary artery disease is a frequent presentation. Severe disease in either area can compromise a good response to surgical intervention. For instance, a patient with carotid occlusion undergoing coronary artery bypass may have compromised cerebral blood flow due to nonpulsatile flow or decreased mean perfusion pressures. Numerous studies have documented worsened outcomes in patients undergoing bypass without prior carotid endarterectomy (9,30,86) (Table 3). Certain authors recommend performance of simultaneous carotid endarterectomy and coronary bypass. The endarterectomy is done with the bypass apparatus placed intravascularly prior to bypassing the coronary arteries (15,17,27,29,44,51,70,88,91,94). Carotid endarterectomy under local or cervical block immediately followed by bypass (14) or placement of an intra-aortic balloon pump prior to carotid endarterectomy to support cardiac function may be recommended in certain very unstable cardiac patients (68). One author suggests bypass using pro

Table 3. *Operative mortality for simultaneous coronary artery disease (CAD) and carotid disease (CD)*

Procedure	Mortality (%)
CAD and CD	Up to 14
CAD and carotid endarterectomy: simultaneous surgery	5
Coronary artery bypass graft only (CAD and CD)	4–7

found hypothermia with extended circulatory arrest and simultaneous repair (85), although certain discussants of this paper felt that the carotid repair could be performed at normal temperatures with less risk.

Duration of Repair

The initiation of carotid artery occlusion at the start of the surgical repair is usually the critical event that precipitates cerebral ischemia. In cases of contralateral stenosis or carotid occlusion, trial ipsilateral occlusions may be performed to evaluate the need for shunts. Cerebral function and perfusion monitoring is necessary and can be done while the patient is awake or asleep. Monitoring is discussed later in the chapter.

Cerebral ischemia will usually occur within minutes of carotid occlusion, although it does not occur in all cases. Obviously, the shorter the duration of the carotid occlusion the better. Monitoring used to identify ischemia allows for interventions to protect the brain. If extended periods of open carotid dissection are anticipated (more than 5 minutes), careful cerebral perfusion monitoring is mandatory. While some surgeons attempt to minimize carotid occlusion time to avoid ischemia, others feel that diligent surgical dissection and careful repair improve outcome (6,33,42,66,74,79,85,95).

Some authors suggest that certain cerebral protective maneuvers may be indicated, such as placement of a shunt ipsilaterally to maintain CBF. Methods used to determine if shunting is necessary are electroencephalography (EEG) (54,66,74,79,95), somatosensory evoked potentials (SSEP) (32,45), and transcranial Doppler (50) (see Chapter 6). Nevertheless, shunt placement can cause embolization, and it has been shown to have its own morbidity and mortality rate. Some surgeons perform carotid endarterectomy without shunts, only placing one when all other interventions to improve CBF have failed; cerebral monitoring is used to warn the surgeon of pending cerebral perfusion compromise. While this has been our experience in most cases (94%), some surgeons shunt all patients and also monitor cerebral function. Cerebral monitoring is not an infallible way to avoid stroke complications; this may be due to lack of sensitivity following embolic stroke or misdiagnosis (23,54).

Our results indicate that the period of carotid cross-clamping, especially in an anesthetized and pharmacologically protected patient, is perhaps less critical than previously thought. This is especially true when multiple cerebral function monitors are employed. It appears that maintaining adequate collateral flow, including the use of induced moderate blood pressure elevations during carotid cross-clamping, and meticulous surgical dissection technique are more important than the absolute period of temporary inclusion.

CHOICE OF ANESTHESIA

Local and Regional Anesthesia

Local anesthesia plus sedation has been the primary anesthetic technique for carotid endarterectomy since its introduction. Advocates cite the anesthetic's minimal effect on the heart as a benefit. Lower observed changes in blood pressure and lower perioperative myocardial infarction rates are also used to support local anesthesia (18,25,36,40,59,81,89,92). One article recommends the use of droperidol (neurolept sedation) as part of the sedative technique (81). If cerebral monitoring is accomplished via verbal and motor function testing, the anesthesiologist must remember the importance of avoiding deep sedation (10).

Similar methods of sedation are also used with regional anesthesia. Cervical plexus block applied deeply as the nerves exit paravertebrally has been used (8,20,56,64), although a risk exists of temporary vocal cord paralysis or high spinal or hemidiaphragmatic paralysis (13). Cervical plexus block can be accomplished more superficially by blocking the cervical nerve roots as they exit the deep tissues along the posterolateral border of the sternocleidomastoid muscle; this may decrease the complications associated with the deeper cervical plexus blocks.

For superficial cervical plexus block, I have found that injecting along the border all the way to the mastoid process insertion is important. If this is not done, the patient will often complain of severe discomfort when the skin retractors are inserted for the upper cervical dissection. The total volume of Marcaine 0.5% used is approximately 10 to 20 ml. An additional injection must be made under the belly of the sternocleidomastoid to block the nerve supplying the platysma and the skin above it.

Regional anesthesia for carotid surgery using cervical epidural injections has been described (4). However, I would not suggest its use because of the associated high risk of total spinal or spinal cord injury (11).

General Anesthesia

Advocates of local and regional anesthesia cite lower morbidity and mortality rates as evidence of the superiority of their method. However, improved anesthesia techniques and cardiac and cerebral monitoring have significantly decreased complication rates for general anesthesia (2,56,58,64). As discussed in the section on combined coronary and carotid disease, general anesthesia may sometimes be safer than local or regional anesthesia (1,12,19,23,38,47,57,64,67,75,76,80,90).

The type of general anesthetic employed varies. Some authors rely primarily on a nitrous oxide, opioid, amnestic technique to maintain blood pressure and minimize decreases in cerebral perfusion. A few years ago, nitrous oxide was thought to act in a manner deleterious for carotid endarterectomies; however, two recent articles support its use in carotid endarterectomy. Nitrous oxide has not been shown to increase the perioperative myocardial infarction rate (53) and its effect on CBF does not inhibit its use in carotid endarterectomy (28).

Volatile anesthetics have the benefit, however, of better controlling hypertension, which is found in many of these patients. Halothane and isoflurane have not been shown to have any advantage over one another when used for carotid endarterectomy, according to some authors (69,97). Others have suggested that when isoflurane is used, cerebral ischemia occurs at lower CBF values than would normally occur with halothane, nitrous oxide anesthesia (63,65). The use of vasodilators during anesthesia to control hypertension can minimize the effect of the volatile anesthetic on EEG or SSEP monitoring.

Different recommendations have existed as to the optimal level of arterial carbon dioxide during general anesthesia for carotid endarterectomy. It is presently recommended that the arterial carbon dioxide level be kept as close to 40 mmHg as possible to minimize any potential changes in CBF (17,26).

Cerebral Protection

Some surgeons and anesthesiologists consider it very important to use cerebral protection methods during cross-clamping. Theoretically, the advantage of pharmaceutical protection is that it decreases the cerebral metabolic consumption of oxygen. However, others who employ cerebral protection methods have argued that monitoring for cerebral ischemia and placing a shunt if it develops obviate the need for pharmacologic protection. Those who do not favor pharmacologic intervention argue that it effectively blocks only about 20% of oxygen consumption. They also point out that thiopental at doses required for cerebral protection may decrease mean arterial blood pressure and cardiac output, thereby causing decreased effective cerebral perfusion. Drugs used for cerebral protection may leave the patient sedated for a number of hours after the procedure. This may inhibit neurologic evaluation in the immediate postoperative period, which is considered important for picking up cerebral perfusion abnormalities. Surgeons and anesthesiologists who do favor cerebral protection argue that reduced cerebral metabolic consumption may obviate the need to place shunts. Also, one author who uses thiopental in his practice has not noted large decreases in cardiac output or drops in blood pressure (35).

Several points are important when discussing the methodology of a cerebral protective intravenous anesthetic. Thiopental is not the only agent that can decrease cerebral metabolic demand (98). Propofol has been shown to decrease the cerebral metabolic rate of oxygen CMR_{O_2}. Etomidate decreases CMR_{O_2} and is less depressant on the cardiac output and blood pressure (52). Etomidate is used at our institution for cerebral protection in patients with a significant cardiac history. Patients with histories of myocardial infarctions, congestive heart failure, or significant valvular heart disease appear to tolerate higher doses of etomidate than thiopental with more stable fluid, pressure, and cardiac output.

Some authors have suggested the concomitant use of neosynephrine drips at the time of thiopental use for cerebral protection. This is not without risk, since the use of neosynephrine during carotid endarterectomy has been shown to increase the perioperative myocardial infarction rate. Ideally, neosynephrine should never be used prophylactically to maintain blood pressure. It should only be employed in cases of lower blood pressure and documented cerebral ischemia (62). In our institution, it is attempted during cross-clamping to keep the perfusion pressure at 130 to 150 mmHg systolic. If the systolic blood pressure is lower than this, the volatile anesthetic concentration is decreased to 0.4% or less or the anesthetic is changed to a nitrous narcotic technique. If the systolic pressure fails to rise at this point, then a neosynephrine infusion is started to bring the systolic pressure slowly to the desired level.

When cerebral protective drugs are employed, they must be given prior to the carotid cross-clamping, since areas of lowered cerebral perfusion may not get adequate doses of the drug for maximum protection from collateral flow.

Continuous intravenous infusions are better than intermittent infusions for cerebral protection. Intermittent boluses of thiopental give protection for approximately 15 minutes, which is the duration of EEG burst suppression. As the plasma concentration of the drug drops, cerebral metabolism returns toward normal. This means that after the bolus is given and the carotid cross-clamp is applied, the protective effect will be decreasing while the ischemic risk is increasing. Cross-clamping also varies and can last for periods of 15 minutes to 1 hour. This implies that a number of boluses must be given (Fig. 1). Repeated boluses of thiopental may cause prolonged drowsiness after anesthesia. As stated previously, this is undesirable. Another problem with bolus injection of a cerebral protectant is that the high dose required to achieve the desired effect may go too far and cause a flat line on the EEG. This is undesirable because the flat-line effect of the cerebral protectant may mask the onset of ischemic changes on the EEG. Each bolus may create

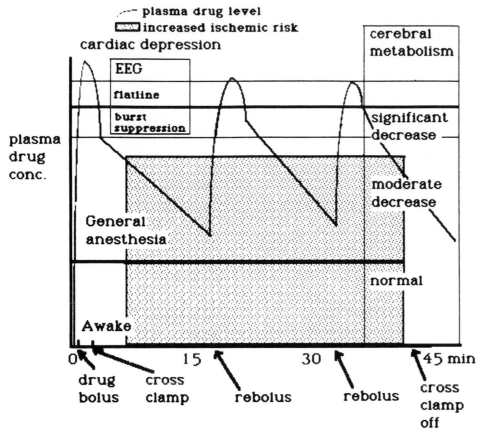

Figure 1. Cerebral protection is attempted during the cross-clamp period by giving bolus injections of a drug that decreases $CMRo_2$. The plasma level of the drug declines and the bolus must be repeated. At the time of the bolus the plasma levels may be high enough to cause cardiac depression and hypotension. The risk of brain ischemia occurs at 4 minutes and continues until the cross-clamp is removed. Periods of low drug level may increase ischemic risk due to increases in $CMRo_2$.

periods of ineffective EEG or SSEP diagnosis, which also is not desirable (83,96).

Continuous infusions of intravenous anesthetics have the benefit of maintaining their cerebroprotective effect over the duration of the carotid occlusion period. Infusions also allow the anesthesiologist to titrate the infusion rate carefully to maintain burst suppression while minimizing the flat-line periods that occur with the bolus technique. Even the initial bolus can be lower, because the pharmacologically effective duration will be maintained by the infusion instead of by the size of the initial bolus (Fig. 2). Figure 3 shows the EEG changes associated with burst suppression. In Figure 4, Tracing A shows the preoperative EEG; Tracing B shows the burst suppression. It is important to understand that the short burst must be maintained to check for adequate neural perfusion. If a flat line exists, one has no idea whether this signifies drug effect or ischemic lack of activity. Tracing C shows the effect of anesthesia with lowered amplitude in the EEG tracing.

Hypothermia of about 34° to 35°C has also been shown to be protective. The problem with the use of hypothermia in a short-duration case like carotid endarterectomy is that it requires time to cool the patient passively externally. This prolongs the anesthesia and increases patient risk. Cooling could

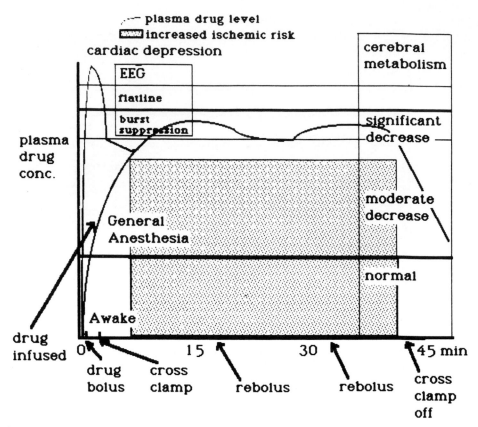

Figure 2. Cerebral protection is attempted during the cross-clamp period using an initial bolus plus a continuous infusion. The infusion is titrated to maintain burst suppression. The plasma level is maintained by adjusting the infusion rate. An attempt is made to avoid increases in CMR_{O_2} during cross-clamp. Avoiding rebolus may decrease potential cardiac depression. Rate is lowered if a flat line occurs.

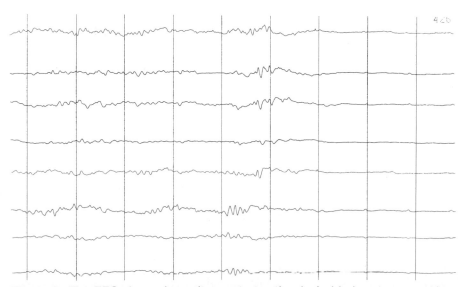

Figure 3. The EEG shown here demonstrates the desirable burst suppression. Burst suppression implies functional brain electrical activity. If a flat line occurs with a bolus injection, the EEG reader is unable to differentiate ischemia from drug effect.

not be considered in awake unparalyzed patients due to shivering. This would also cause acidosis, which may not be beneficial to CBF distribution. Hence hypothermia, although cerebroprotective, is not applicable in most instances of carotid surgery. Hypothermia would be used during cardiac bypass procedures if applicable, usually only after a carotid obstruction has been surgically repaired (84,87).

CHOICE OF MONITORING

Awake Monitoring

The use of local and regional anesthesia with mild sedation for carotid endarterectomy allows effective cerebral monitoring. It is a cost-effective method, and provided the patient does not require heavy sedation because of anxiety, mental status and cerebral function can be followed with repeated oral questions and evaluation of the patient's response. Motor function can also be evaluated on the contralateral side. A clicker, horn, or grip-strength monitor is placed in the patient's hand prior to draping and on request the patient is to click or squeeze the object (10). Both of these methods work but are not perfect, since the onset of neurologic deficit symptoms can lag the cross-clamping by many minutes.

One other problem that can cause difficulty during awake carotid endarterectomy is sudden loss of the airway and/or spontaneous respiration. If the patient develops severe neurologic symptoms or will not lie calmly under the drapes, the patient must be anesthetized and intubated. Intubating under these circumstances may not be ideal. A risk of wound contamination exists. If thiopental is used for the induction, then a risk of hypotension exists, which may further compromise cerebral perfusion. If etomidate is used and the patient is hypertensive, the hypertension may persist or worsen during the induction. The anesthesiologist would do well to call for help during this difficult situation. Once the patient is asleep and the airway is controlled, decisions concerning shunt placement and other means of cerebral monitoring have to be made.

Stump Pressure, Stump Pulsation, and Retrograde Flow

Stump pressure by itself has not been found to be a reliable monitor of cerebral blood flow or perfusion. Stump pressure has been found to correlate with the stump pulse. When the stump pulse is palpable, the stump pressure, measured by inserting a needle into the distal portion of the carotid past the occlusion, is usually greater than 40 mmHg and preferably greater than 50 to 60 mmHg. Stump pressures are considered more important when significant contralateral stenosis or occlusion of the carotid are present. Retrograde flow from the stump has a poor correlation with CBF. However, it is used as a monitor in conjunction with other direct monitors of cerebral function (3,16,21). Stump pressure has also been tested against transcranial Doppler flow measures and found not to correlate closely (82).

Transcranial Doppler

Transcranial Doppler (TCD) monitoring is a recent development in carotid endarterectomy. It allows direct measure of ipsilateral CBF. It is best used by a technician, but the technique can be mastered by the anesthesiologist with some practice and specialized training. The unique quality of TCD is that it can diagnose embolization as it occurs. If embolization occurs during a manipulation, then the manipulation can be stopped and hopefully the embolization will stop as well. Sometimes, though, during a required maneuver the TCD documents a shower of emboli. In this instance the TCD can be worrisome for the surgeon (17,39,43,62).

This technique has been compared with simultaneous EEG; they have been found to correlate loosely. It can be used to measure the effectiveness of shunt placement in improving CBF (31) and may also be used to measure anterior communicating artery collateral flow (59). Finally, TCD is the only method to diagnose whether a patient is having hyperflow in the ipsilateral cerebral arterial system. Hyperflow can cause cerebral edema and neurologic deficits in the patient in the early postoperative period. If hyperflow occurs, careful blood pressure and cardiac output control must be instituted. It can also be used along with duplex scanning in the early postoperative period to diagnose low cerebral perfusion and recurrence of arterial obstruction due to thrombosis or intimal flap obstruction (see Chapter 6).

Electroencephalography and Somatosensory Evoked Potentials

If a patient remains awake during carotid endarterectomy, cerebral function monitoring can be done easily. With general anesthesia, however, the

Figure 4. A: Pre-induction EEG with much high frequency electrical activity.

Figure 4. *Continued.* **B:** After etomidate induction, nitrous oxide, midazolam, and .4% isoflurane are given, the EEG shows a decrease of the high-frequency electrical waves; slower waves are more abundant

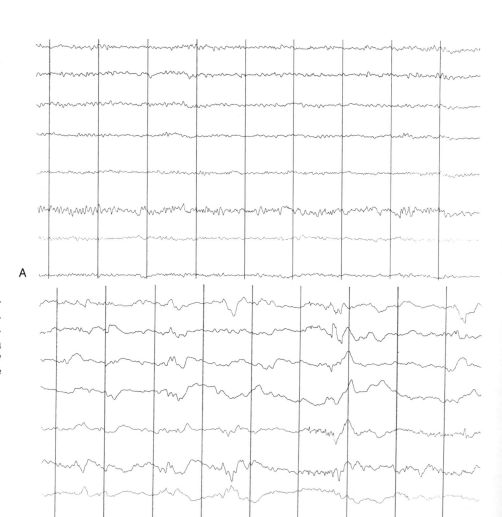

A

B

process of cerebral monitoring becomes more complicated. Various forms of cerebral status monitoring remain possible:

EEG raw (4, 8, 16 channel)
Processed EEG (Lifescan, Spectral Array)
SSEP of the median nerve
Transcranial Doppler
Stump pressure

EEG and other monitoring methods are listed here because many of the reference articles compare EEG monitoring with other methods to elucidate correlations, sensitivity and specificity differences, and incidences of false positives and false negatives.

Electroencephalography has been used to define changes in cerebral electrical activity that can herald the onset of decreased or absent perfusion, anoxia or hypoxia, or embolic activity. During anesthesia EEG changes can vary according to the type of anesthesia used. As the patient enters the anesthetic state, the EEG reflects a slowing of the high-frequency waves and an increase in the number of slower frequency waves. This change should usually be less than 50%. If declines greater than 50% occur with halothane and/or isoflurane at 0.5% to 1.0%, then ischemia should be ruled out.

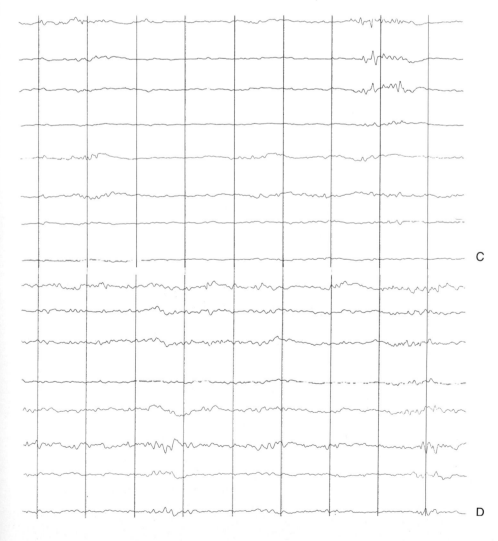

C

D

Figure 4. *Continued.* **C:** Cerebral protection has been started. A bolus of etomidate and a subsequent infusion are given. Burst suppression is induced. Flattened areas are seen between areas of spiked electrical waves.

Figure 4. *Continued.* **D:** After the infusion is stopped. The wave forms return and normal electrical activity is seen bilaterally.

Complete loss of EEG waves in one or both hemispheres usually heralds the onset of severe ischemia and the risk of permanent neurologic deficit (72).

Electroencephalography can be used to diagnose embolic occurrences during surgery. Eight- and 16-channel EEG monitors are required to do this since four-lead EEG monitors are not considered sensitive enough to pick up areas of regional ischemia. Processed EEG machines have been developed to facilitate the EEG interpretation (59). Lifescan has a four-color wave frequency monitor; in real time, with four electrodes it can monitor cerebral function very well. Lifescan's advantage is its ease of interpretation for decreased hemispherical or global EEG changes. However, it would only be able to pick up global or hemispherical ischemia, hypoxia/anoxia, or massive changes from emboli. Another type of processed EEG monitor is the spectral array monitor. This monitor also manipulates the raw EEG into a more readable form (50).

When intravenous anesthetics (thiopental, etomidate, methohexital) are given at high doses, a flat line can occur on the EEG (35). This EEG pattern resembles the flat line of a brain with complete hypoxia or ischemia. If a slightly lower dose of the intravenous drug is used, then the raw EEG wave will show a flat line with intermittent short periods of moderate-frequency activity, usually bilaterally (Fig. 4). This is called a burst suppression. The EEG technician will be much more comfortable monitoring this burst suppression than a pure flat-line EEG, since flat-line EEGs may also mask the onset of severe ischemia or hypoxia. If such a condition occurred while a flat line was induced pharmacologically, the EEG technician would be unable to diagnose the ischemia or anoxia.

Many surgeons will place a shunt when changes indicating potential ischemia are seen on the EEG monitor. Although this is considered safe practice and is recommended by many, certain papers have suggested that shunts may not be needed in all cases. These authors have noted that false-positive and false-negative readings have occurred with the use of EEG monitoring during carotid endarterectomy (9,47,48,79). Recent developments in the use of intraoperative TCD have allowed more effective interpretation of EEG changes. More affirmative interpretations as to the effect of carotid cross-clamping can be made. Also, the response of the cerebral circulation to specific interventions that attempt to improve cerebral circulation can be evaluated. Normal findings for TCD, EEG, and stump pressures in a patient during surgery are correlated with good outcome. However, all monitoring methods even when combined are not perfect (54,55).

Another method of monitoring uses somatosensory evoked potentials to interpret cortical function in the area posterior to the motor strip. The SSEP machine picks up electrical activity in the cortical area and sums it up. As the random impulses cancel each other out, what is left is a wave form that shows a response to a repeated sensory stimulus to a peripheral nerve (see diagram). For each peripheral nerve a particular latency and an amplitude are associated with the SSEP response. For instance, the latency for median nerve will be shorter than for a posterior tibial nerve. This is because the signal takes longer to travel from the leg than the hand. Lam reports that both the EEG and the SSEP suffer a considerable false positive rate. Both EEG and SSEP have similar sensitivity and specificity for monitoring carotid endarterectomy. Amplitude reduction greater than 50% is a better indicator of ischemia than latency increase is in SSEP monitoring. Other articles have also compared EEG and SSEP; one author felt that SSEP was not as good as EEG, since if emboli seeded an area other than the somatosensory area, the SSEP would not detect it (49,51).

COMPLICATIONS

The immediate postoperative period is a time of great risk for the carotid endarterectomy patient. At the end of surgery, the monitoring is removed. The patient is then allowed to awaken from anesthesia. The goal of the anesthesiologist should be to minimize the time from the discontinuance of the anesthetic agent until an effective motor and verbal response can be evaluated. The reason for this is that complications from carotid occlusion or embolization can occur. These complications can be life-threatening and require immediate treatment. The longer the complications remain undiagnosed and untreated, the higher the risk of permanent neurologic deficit. Therefore no patient of this type should be left pharmacologically paralyzed or severely somnolent. Also, if new neurologic deficits are noted when the patient awakens, the surgeon must be immediately notified and a diagnostic work-up performed.

One other potential complication that can change the mental status of the patient is hyperflow in the ipsilateral cerebral hemisphere. If allowed to persist, hyperflow causes cerebral edema, with an altered state of consciousness as the physical sign. The only method of detecting this is TCD; the tracings are compared from before and after the operation. The same technique can also be used to measure the effectiveness of any treatment for the hyperflow. Often the hyperflow phenomenon is accompanied by hypertension. If the systolic blood pressure is controlled below or equal to 130 to 140 mmHg systolic, then the cerebral edema should subside. Hyperflow phenomena should resolve spontaneously over 24 hours, if blood pressure is reasonably controlled.

Labile blood pressure is a serious problem with organs other than the brain. Hypertension as an immediate postoperative problem is very common in carotid endarterectomy patients. The incidence of blood pressure instability is even higher in patients undergoing a second contralateral carotid endarterectomy.

The simplest cause is hypertension associated with anesthetic emergence. This hypertension is usually short lived and resolves spontaneously. Essential hypertension, if it occurs, will continue and not resolve quickly without treatment. Remember that hypertension and high heart rates can cause myocardial ischemia. Perioperative myocardial infarction remains a major cause of severe morbidity and mortality. One of the primary reasons for a decline in morbidity and mortality from carotid endarterectomy has been better monitoring and treatment of blood pressure changes in the perioperative period.

Hypotension or relative hypoperfusion can also be a problem. Autoregulation of brain perfusion can be disturbed. The autoregulatory curves for blood pressure may be shifted to the right in these patients due to long-standing hypertension. Treatment of drops in systolic pressures below 120 mmHg should be treated when they occur. If the systolic pressure is returned to above 120 mmHg and the neurologic deficit persists, then the blood pressure can be carefully titrated upward until the systolic pressure is at 160 mmHg or the neurologic deficit has resolved. Systolic blood pressures above 160 mmHg run the risk of causing a wound hematoma.

A significant wound hematoma can be life threatening. The hematoma can cause significant blood loss or compress vital structures in the neck. If the ipsilateral carotid artery is leaking or compressed, it can impair ipsilateral brain perfusion. If the trachea is compressed it can cause shifts that compromise airflow or even make the intubation more difficult or impossible. Some authors suggest that trying to reintubate under general anesthesia for this group of patients is very risky, and the patients may be difficult to ventilate. If the patient's blood pressure drops during the induction, this may compromise cerebral tissue and cause stroke complications. It is recommended that these patients be intubated with good topicalization.

OTHER INTERVENTIONS

Low-Dose Aspirin Therapy

Since one major postoperative complication is recurrent thrombosis at the carotid arteriotomy site, medical interventions that might decrease this risk have been proposed. One suggested means is to have the patient start mild oral antiplatelet therapy such as aspirin once a day starting 1 day preoperatively (58). This therapy should be avoided in patients with a history of hemorrhage or recent stroke.

Heparin and Protamine Use

Heparin is used at most institutions just before opening the carotid artery and removing the plaque. Usually 5,000 units of heparin are given 3 minutes prior to carotid cross-clamping. No further heparin is given in most cases. Protamine is not usually used because of the concern for rebound hypercoagulability and for a desired prolonged anticoagulant effect. Protamine use may be considered in combined carotid endarterectomy and coronary artery bypass. In these cases, avoidance of hypercoagulability is recommended (93). One other important postoperative measure to prevent rebleeding and wound hematoma is to control and if possible to avoid postoperative hypertension.

ANESTHETIC PRACTICE AT OUR INSTITUTION

For cases involving the neurosurgeons at our institution the following is the usual anesthesia protocol. All patients will have a large-bore intravenous line and a radial arterial line. Electrocardiogram, oxygen saturation, and end-tidal carbon dioxide are also key components. If the patient has significant cardiac disease, then a Swan-Ganz catheter is placed. Vasoactive drips of nitroglycerin and neosynephrine are placed in the intravenous line close to the catheter where it enters the skin. This is to decrease the dead space and time lag for effect when the drug is infused. This avoids large swings in blood pressure during anesthesia when vasoactive agents are infused.

Induction usually involves premedication with midazolam and an opioid drug. Thiopental at the low range of dose 4 to 5 mg/kg is used for induction. If the patient has a significant cardiac history then etomidate, 0.3 to 0.5 mg/kg, is the induction agent. Lidocaine, 0.5 mg/kg, is given to decrease the sympathetic response to induction just before the thiopental or etomidate. Succinylcholine is used for muscle relaxation during intubation. After intubation the patient is given a full loading dose of the opioid and oxygen 40% with nitrous oxide 60%, isoflurane 0.5 to 1% as required to control the systolic blood pressure at 130 to 160 mmHg. If the systolic pressure falls below 130 mmHg systolic, then the isoflurane is turned off. If the systolic blood pressure remains below 130 mmHg at the time of cross-clamping, then low doses of neosynephrine are given to maintain the systolic pressure in the 140- to 150-mmHg range. Pavulon is used for neuromuscular blockade. This much is fairly standard methodology for carotid endarterectomy. However, our practice also has several unique characteristics.

Julian Bailes believes that careful diligent dissection under the microscope is necessary to optimize the outcome, for which increased duration of cross-clamp time is used. In order to minimize the risk of the larger cross-clamp time, aggressive monitoring using a 8-lead EEG is done by a technician. To optimize the oxygen demand and supply balance to the brain further during the cross-clamping period, the systolic pressure is maintained in the 140- to 160-mmHg systolic range. Ideally this is achieved by avoiding isoflurane if necessary and by giving the patient adequate fluids to replace overnight losses. This also helps to maintain adequate perfusion. If these two interventions fail, then neosynephrine is carefully titrated to raise the blood pressure into the desired range.

For the demand side of cerebral oxygen support, the patient is given continuous infusions of cerebral protective agents. Older practices involved giving bolus doses of the cerebral protective agents. This is not optimal, since hypotension is common during the loading and rebolus injections due to the high plasma drug levels that occur as discussed previously in the EEG section. Continuous infusions of cerebral protective agents, on the other hand, have the benefit of a decreased initial loading dose. This decreases the risk of hypotension and decreased perfusion of the brain at the time of cross-clamping. Continuous infusions also tend to maintain the plasma and tissue levels of the protective agents for a longer or continuous period. This avoids the risk during cross-clamping that as the brain becomes more ischemic, the effective plasma level of the protective agent decreases. Intermittent decreases in drug plasma and tissue concentrations occur with bolus dosing (Fig. 1). For patients with minimal history of heart disease (no myocardial infarction, no congestive heart failure, normal activity, and no angina) thiopental is usually used. For patients with a significant cardiac history etomidate is the drug of choice. Etomidate tends to maintain stable blood pressure and cardiac output even at doses that achieve decreased cerebral metabolic demand.

The difficulty with continuous infusions is the calculation of the infusion dose and mixture. The author has developed a standard rate and dose range software (available via A MIXED BAG, Inc., P.O. Box 79182, Pittsburgh, PA) that calculates the correct infusion mixture for thiopental or etomidate. The software provides the recommended dose for the infusion and the recommended loading dose. The loading dose is given 2 minutes before cross-clamping to ensure that the ipsilateral cerebral hemisphere receives the drug. After the loading dose, a continuous infusion is started. The infusion mixture uses a standard range of 10 to 30 ml/hr (Fig. 5). This provides quality control and simplicity of use. The titration is started at 20 ml/hr and titrated to both the patient response and the EEG. The infusion rate is lowered until burst suppression is seen on EEG and is raised if higher frequency brain activity returns. If needed, small boluses of the cerebral protective agent can be given to return to burst suppression. The infusion is given during the whole period of the cross-clamping. As the cross-clamp is removed, the infusion is stopped.

In our experience the longer cross-clamp time (approximately 45 to 60 minutes) has not been associated with a more frequent need for ipsilateral shunting during cross-clamping. Bailes reported that only 6% of his series were shunted.

Failure to use the shunt did not result in a higher incidence of intraoperative cerebral ischemia or postoperative neurologic deficit. We believe this is due to our aggressive balancing of the supply and demand equation. Maintaining the high perfusion pressure supports the supply of oxygen to the brain while the cerebral protective agent decreases the demand for oxygen in the ipsilateral cerebral hemisphere. Although the pharmacologic cerebral protective

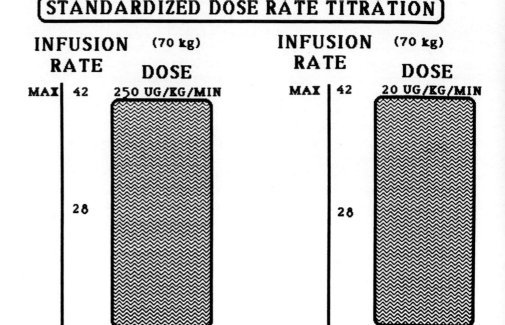

Figure 5. Cerebral protective infusion use: The infusion calculator software from A Mixed Bag, Inc. calculates the correct infusion bag mixture and dose for the cerebral protection. A titration range is shown that allows easy adjustment of the infusion rate. Although 10 to 30 ml/hr is the standard range, the software determined that 42 ml/hr maximum rate of undiluted drug would be required for this application with both drugs for a 70-kg patient. Loading dose recommendations are also provided. The loading dose is given, and the infusion is started in the midtitration range. The EEG output is monitored and the infusion rate is adjusted to maintain burst suppression during the cross-clamp period. (Courtesy of A Mixed Bag, Inc.)

effect is believed to be only 20% of the total cerebral metabolic demand, the decreased metabolic demand and supported perfusion pressure in combination may have adequately supported the brain and avoided damage.

CONCLUSIONS

Carotid endarterectomy remains a challenge for the surgeon and the anesthesiologist. Providing optimal conditions for the brain during cross-clamping remains the biggest challenge. Hopefully this chapter has provided some new insights for the reader to consider in patients having a carotid endarterectomy. Improved understanding of continuous-infusion pharmacokinetics and cerebral protective drugs perhaps will lead to further refinements in outcome.

REFERENCES

1. Allcutt DA, Chakraborty M, Sengupta RP. Neurosurgical experience with carotid endarterectomy: a 12-year study. *Br J Neurosurg* 1991;5:257–264.
2. Allen BT, Anderson CB, Rubin BG, et al. The influence of anesthetic technique on perioperative complications after carotid endarterectomy. *J Vasc Surg* 1994;19:834–843.

3. Ammar AD, Pauls DG. Correlation of carotid artery stump pressure with a palpable carotid artery pulse. *J Cardiovasc Surg* 1992;33:59–61.

4. Asano Y, Hasuo M, Shimosawa S, Nakamura F, Sunohara K. [Carotid endarterectomy under cervical epidural anesthesia.] [Japanese.] *No Shinkei Geka* 1993;21:787–791.

5. Baker AB, Resch JA, Lowenson RB. Hypertension and cerebral atherosclerosis. *Circulation* 1969;39:701.

6. Baker WH, Durner DB, Barnes RW. Carotid endarterectomy: is an indwelling shunt necessary? *Surgery* 1977;82:321.

7. Barash P. In: *Clinical anesthesia*. New York: JB Lippincott; 1979:793–795.

8. Bartoloni A, Savron F, Rigo V, et al. [Effectiveness of regional anesthesia for loco-regional carotid surgery. Retrospective review of 147 interventions.] [Italian.] *Minerva Anestesiol* 1991;57:75–82.

9. Bass A, Krupski WC, Dilley RB, Bernstein EF. Combined carotid endarterectomy and coronary artery revascularization: a sobering review. *Isr J Med Sci* 1992;28:27–32.

10. Benjamin ME, Silva MB Jr, Watt C, et al. Awake patient monitoring to determine the need for shunting during carotid endarterectomy. *Surgery* 1993;114:673–680.

11. Bonnet F, Derosier JP, Pluskwa F, Abhay K, Gaillard A. Cervical epidural anaesthesia for carotid artery surgery. *Can J Anaesth* 1990;37:353–358.

12. Burns RJ, Willoughby JO. South Australian carotid endarterectomy study. *Med J Aust* 1991;154:650–653.

13. Castresana MR, Masters RD, Castresana EJ, Stefansson S, Shaker IJ, Newman WH. Incidence and clinical significance of hemidiaphragmatic paresis in patients undergoing carotid endarterectomy during cervical plexus block anesthesia. *J Neurosurg Anesthesiol* 1994;6:21–23.

14. Castresana MR, Balser JS, Newman WH, Stefansson S. Cervical block for carotid endarterectomy followed immediately by general anesthesia for coronary artery bypass and aortic valve replacement. *Anesth Analg* 1993;77:186–187.

15. Chang BB, Darling RC 3rd, Shah DM, Paty PS, Leather RP. Carotid endarterectomy can be safely performed with acceptable mortality and morbidity in patients requiring coronary artery bypass grafts. *Am J Surg* 1994;168:94–96.

16. Cherry KJ Jr, Roland CF, Hallett JW Jr, et al. Stump pressure, the contralateral carotid artery, and electroencephalographic changes. *Am J Surg* 1991;162:185–189.

17. Chiesa R, Minicucci F, Melissano G, et al. The role of transcranial Doppler in carotid artery surgery. *Eur J Vasc Surg* 1992;6:211–216.

18. Collier PE. Carotid endarterectomy: a safe cost-efficient approach. *J Vasc Surg* 1992;16:926–933.

19. Cristofori G, Bordoni M, Lubatti L, et al. [General anesthesia in carotid endarterectomy.] [Italian.] *Minerva Anestesiol* 1992;58:1121–1122.

20. Davies MJ, Murrell GC, Cronin KD, Meads AC, Dawson A. Carotid endarterectomy under cervical plexus block—a prospective clinical audit. *Anaesth Intensive Care* 1990;18:219–223.

21. DeLaurentis DA, Dougherty MJ, Calligaro KD, Savarese RP, Raviola CA, Bajgier SM. Carotid stump pressure, stump pulse, and retrograde flow. *Am J Surg* 1993;166:152–156.

22. Deriu GP, Franceschi L, Milite D, et al. [Carotid stenosis and obliteration of the contralateral carotid. A prospective study of the risks of a carotid endarterectomy intervention and its long-term results.] [Italian.] *Riv Neurol* 1990;60:51–59.

23. Deruty R, Mottolese C, Pelissou-Guyotat I, Lapras C. [Cervical carotid endarterectomy. Evaluation of a 12 years' experience (260 operations).] [Review] [French.] *Neurochirurgie* 1991;37:241–247.

24. Dippel DW, Vermeulen M, Braakman R, Habbema JD. Transient ischemic attacks, carotid stenosis, and an incidental intracranial aneurysm. A decision analysis. *Neurosurgery* 1994;34:449–458.

25. Donato AT, Hill SL. Carotid arterial surgery using local anesthesia: a private practice retrospective study. *Am Surg* 1992;58:446–450.

26. Donegan JH. Anesthesia for carotid endarterectomy. In: Miller RD, ed. *Anesthesia*. 2nd ed. New York: Churchill Livingstone; 1986.

27. Earnshaw JJ, Hayward JK, Horrocks M, Baird RN. The importance of vascular surgical audit to surgeons, patient and purchasers. *Eur J Vasc Surg* 1992;6:540–544.

28. Eger EI 2d, Lampe GH, Wauk LZ, Whitendale P, Cahalan MK, Donegan JH. Clinical pharmacology of nitrous oxide: an argument for its continued use. *Anesth Analg* 1990;71:575–585.

29. Emery RW, Cohn LH, Whittemore AD. Coexistent carotid and coronary disease. *Arch Surg* 1983;118:1035–1038.

30. Ennix CL, Lawrie GM, Morris GE, et al. Improved results of carotid endarterectomy in patients with symptomatic coronary artery disease: an analysis of 11,546 consecutive carotid operations. *Stroke* 1979;10:122–125.

31. Facco E, Deriu GP, Dona B, et al. EEG monitoring of carotid endarterectomy with routine patch-graft angioplasty: an experience in a large series. *Neurophysiol Clin* 1992;22:437–446.

32. Fava E, Bortolani E, Ducati A, Schieppati M. Role of SEP in identifying patients requiring temporary shunt during carotid endarterectomy. *Electroencephalogr Clin Neurophysiol* 1992;84:426–432.

33. Ferguson GC. Intraoperative monitoring and internal shunts: are they necessary in carotid endarterectomy. *Stroke* 1982;13:287.

34. Fraunhofer S, Kiossis D, Helmberger H, Von Sommoggy S, Maurer PC. Severe bilateral carotid stenosis. *J Mal Vasc* 1993;18:225–228.

35. Frawley JE, Hicks RG, Horton DA, Gray LJ, Niesche JW, Matheson JM. Thiopental sodium cerebral protection during carotid endarterectomy: perioperative disease and death. *J Vasc Surg* 1994;19:732–738.

36. Fried KS, Elias SM, Raggi R. Carotid endarterectomy under local anesthesia. *NJ Med* 1990;87:795–797.

37. Frost EAM. Preanesthetic assessment—the patient for carotid endarterectomy. Lesson 119. *Anesthesiol News* December, 1994;18–25.

38. Gaspar MR. Carotid endarterectomy. *Am J Surg* 1990;159:252–255.

39. Gaunt ME, Ratliff DA, Martin PJ, Smith JL, Bell PR, Naylor AR. On-table diagnosis of incipient carotid artery thrombosis during carotid endarterectomy by transcranial Doppler scanning. *J Vasc Surg* 1994;20:104–107.

40. Gianferrari P, Conforti M, Forlani G, et al. [Loco-regional anesthesia vs general anesthesia in carotid endarterectomy. Response to the surgical stress.] [Italian.] *Minerva Anestesiol* 1992;58:263–267.

41. Goldman L, Coldera DL. Risks of general anesthesia and elective operation in the hypertensive patient. *Anesthesiology* 1979;50:285.

42. Graham AM, Gewertz BL, Zarins CK. Predicting cerebral ischemia during carotid endarterectomy. *Arch* 1986;121:595.

43. Granry JC. [Transcranial Doppler in anesthesia and intensive care.] [Review] [French.] *Ann Fr Anesth Reanim* 1991;10:127–136.

44. Halpin DP, Riggins S, Carmichael JD, et al. Management of coexistent carotid and coronary artery disease. *South Med J* 1994;87:187–189.

45. Halsey JH Jr. Risks and benefits of shunting in carotid endarterectomy. The International Transcranial Doppler Collaborators [see Comments]. *Stroke* 1992;23:1583–1587.

46. Hertzer NR, Beven EG, Young JR, et al. Coronary artery disease in peripheral vascular surgery patients. A classification of 1000 coronary angiograms and the results of surgical management. *Ann Surg* 1984;199:223–233.

47. Iversen T, Vea H, Sorlie D, Joakimsen O. [Carotid endarterectomy. Surgical complications and long-term prognosis.] [Review] [Norwegian.] *Tidsskr Nor Laegeforen* 1991;111:2253–2255.

48. Jorgensen LG, Schroeder TV. Transcranial Doppler for detection of cerebral ischaemia during carotid endarterectomy. *Eur J Vasc Surg* 1992;6:142–147.

49. Kearse LA Jr, Brown EN, McPeck K. Somatosensory evoked potentials sensitivity relative to electroencephalography for cerebral ischemia during carotid endarterectomy. *Stroke* 1992;23:498–505.

50. Kearse LA Jr, Martin D, McPeck K, Lopez-Bresnahan M. Computer-derived density spectral array in detection of mild analog electroencephalographic ischemic pattern changes during carotid endarterectomy. *J Neurosurg* 1993;78:884–890.

51. Klima U, Wimmer-Greinecker G, Harringer W, Mair R, Gross C, Brucke P. [Surgical management of coronary heart disease and simultaneous carotid artery stenosis.] [German.] *Wien Klin Wochenschr* 1993;105:76–78.

52. Kochs E, Hoffman WE, Werner C, Thomas C, Albrecht RF, Schulte am Esch J. The effects of propofol on brain electrical activity, neurologic outcome and neuronal damage following incomplete ischemia in rats. *Anesthesiology* 1992;76:245–252.

53. Kozmary SV, Lampe GH, Benefiel D, et al. No finding of increased myocardial ischemia during or after carotid endarterectomy under anesthesia with nitrous oxide. *Anesth Analg* 1990;71:591–596.

54. Kresowik TF, Worsey MJ, Khoury MD, et al. Limitations of electroencephalographic monitoring in the detection of cerebral ischemia accompanying carotid endarterectomy. *J Vasc Surg* 1991;13:439–443.

55. Lam AM, Manninen PH, Ferguson GG, Nantau W. Monitoring electrophysiologic function during carotid endarterectomy: a comparison of somatosensory evoked potentials and conventional electroencephalogram. *Anesthesiology* 1991;75:15–21.

56. Landesberg G, Erel J, Anner H, et al. Perioperative myocardial ischemia in carotid endarterectomy under cervical plexus block and prophylactic nitroglycerin infusion [see Comments]. *J Cardiothorac Vasc Anesth* 1993;7:259–265.

57. Lehot JJ, Durand PG, Mure PY, et al. [Anesthesia for carotid endarterectomy.] [Review] [French.] *Ann Fr Anesth Reanim* 1994;13:33–48.

58. Lindblad B, Persson NH, Takolander R, Bergqvist D. Does low-dose acetylsalicylic acid prevent stroke after carotid surgery? A double-blind, placebo-controlled randomized trial. *Stroke* 1993;24:1125–1128.

59. Lopez-Bresnahan MV, Kearse LA Jr, Yanez P, Young TI. Anterior communicating artery collateral flow protection against ischemic change during carotid endarterectomy. *J Neurosurg* 1993;79:379–382.

60. Mackey WC, O'Donnell TF Jr, Callow AD. Carotid endarterectomy contralateral to an occluded carotid artery: perioperative risk and late results. *J Vasc Surg* 1990;11:778–785.

61. Mattos MA, Hodgson KJ, Londrey GL, et al. Carotid endarterectomy: operative risks, recurrent stenosis, and long-term stroke rates in a modern series. *J Cardiovasc Surg* 1992;33:387–400.

62. McDowell HA Jr, Gross GM, Halsey JH. Carotid endarterectomy monitored with transcranial Doppler. *Ann Surg* 1992;215:514–519.

63. Messick JM, Casement B, Sharbough FW, et al. Correlation of regional cerebral blood flow (rCBF) with EEG changes during isoflurane anesthesia for carotid endarterectomy: critical rCBF. *Anesthesiology* 1987;69:344–349.

64. Meyer FB, Fode NC, Marsh WR, Piepgras DG. Carotid endarterectomy in patients with contralateral carotid occlusion. *Mayo Clin Proc* 1993;68:337–342.
65. Michenfelder JD, Sundt TM, Fode N, et al. Isoflurane when compared to enflurane and halothane decreases the frequency of cerebral ischemia during carotid endarterectomy. *Anesthesiology* 1987;67:336–340.
66. Modica PA, Tempelhoff R, Rich KM, Grubb RL Jr. Computerized electroencephalographic monitoring and selective shunting: influence on intraoperative administration of phenylephrine and myocardial infarction after general anesthesia for carotid endarterectomy. *Neurosurgery* 1992;30:842–846.
67. Murie JA, John TG, Morris PJ. Carotid endarterectomy in Great Britain and Ireland: practice between 1984 and 1992. *Br J Surg* 1994;81:827–831.
68. Myers SI, Valentine RJ, Estrera A, Clagett GP. The intra-aortic balloon pump, a novel addition to staged repair of combined symptomatic cerebrovascular and coronary artery disease. *Ann Vasc Surg* 1993;7:239–242.
69. Nebbs DG, Todd MM, Spetzler RF, et al. A comparison of the cerebral protective effects of isoflurane and barbiturates during temporary local ischemia in primates. *Anesthesiology* 1987;66:453–454.
70. Nishizawa J, Konishi Y, Matsumoto M, Yuasa S. [Coronary artery bypass grafting in the patients with previous cerebral infarction: the risk of perioperative cerebral complications.] [Japanese.] *Kyobu Geka* 1994;47:187–190.
71. North American Symptomatic Carotid Endarterectomy Trial Steering Committee. North American Symptomatic Carotid Endarterectomy Trial: methods, patient characteristics, and progress. *Stroke* 1991;22:711–720.
72. Nuwer MR. Intraoperative electroencephalography [Review]. *SO J Clin Neurophysiol* 1993;10:437–444.
73. Otis S, Ringelstein E. Findings associated with extracranial occlusive disease. In: Newell D, Aaslid R, eds. *Transcranial Doppler*. New York: Raven Press; 1992:153–160.
74. Redekop G, Ferguson G. Correlation of contralateral stenosis and intraoperative electroencephalogram change with risk of stroke during carotid endarterectomy [see Comments]. *Neurosurgery* 1992;30:191–194.
75. Richardson JV. Contemporary results of carotid endarterectomy [see Comments]. *Ala Med* 1991;61:10–12.
76. Riles TS, Fisher FS, Lamparello PJ, et al. Immediate and long-term results of carotid endarterectomy for asymptomatic high-grade stenosis [Review]. *Ann Vasc Surg* 1994;8:144–149.
77. Roizen MF. Anesthesia for vascular surgery. In: Barash PG, Cullen BF, Stoelting RK, eds. *Clinical anesthesia*. New York: JB Lippincott; 1989:1015–1016.
78. Saccani S, Beghi C, Fragnito C, Barboso G, Fesani F. Carotid endarterectomy under hypothermic extracorporeal circulation: a method of brain protection for special patients. *J Cardiovasc Surg* 1992;33:311–314.
79. Sbarigia E, Speziale F, Colonna M, et al. The selection for shunting in patients with severe bilateral carotid lesions. *Eur J Vasc Surg* 1993;7[Suppl A]:3–7.
80. Shima T, Matsumura S, Okada Y, et al. [Experience of carotid endarterectomy.] [Japanese.] *Neurol Med Chir* 1990;30(11 Spec No):813–819.
81. Slutzki S, Behar M, Negri M, Hod G, Zaidenstein L, Bogokowsky H. Carotid endarterectomy under local anesthesia supplemented with neuroleptic analgesia. *Surg Gynecol Obstet* 1990;170:141–144.
82. Spencer MP, Thomas GI, Moehring MA. Relation between middle cerebral artery blood flow velocity and stump pressure during carotid endarterectomy. *Stroke* 1992;23:1439–1445.
83. Spetzler RF, Hadley MN. Protection against cerebral ischemia: the role of barbiturates [Review]. *Cerebrovasc Brain Metab Rev* 1989;1:212–229.
84. Steen PA, Newberg L, Milde JH, et al. Hypothermia and barbiturates: individual and combined effects on canine cerebral oxygen consumption. *Anesthesiology* 1983;58:527–532.
85. Sundt TM, Sharbrough FW, Piepgrap DG, et al. Correlation of cerebral blood flow and electroencephalographic changes during carotid endarterectomy with the results of surgery and hemodynamics of cerebral ischemia. *Mayo Clinic Proc* 1981;56:533–543.
86. Thompson J, Carver JM, Murphy DA. Concomitant carotid and coronary artery reconstruction. *Am Surg* 1982;195:712–720.
87. Todd MM, Warner DS. A comfortable hypothesis reevaluated: cerebral metabolic depression and brain protection during ischemia [Review]. *Anesthesiology* 1992;76:161–164.
88. Tsujimoto T, Suzuki T, Kinoshita T. [Anesthesia for combined carotid endarterectomy and coronary artery bypass grafting.] [Japanese.] *Nippon Geka Hokan* 1991;60:354–357.
89. Usmanov NU, Gul'muradov TG, Sultanov DD, Lipatsev II, Tursunkulova VG. [Advantages of endarterectomy of the carotid arteries under local anesthesia.] [Russian.] *Grud Serdechnososudistaia Khir* 1991;4:22–25.
90. van Crevel H. [Consensus cerebrovascular accident.] [Review] [Dutch.] *Ned Tijdschr Geneeskd* 1991;135:2280–2288.
91. Vassilidze TV, Cernaianu AC, Gaprindashvili T, Gallucci JG, Cilley JH Jr, DelRossi AJ. Simultaneous coronary artery bypass and carotid endarterectomy. Determinants of outcome. *Tex Heart Inst J* 1994;21:119–124.
92. Viglione GC, Rivetti R, Lavagne F, Costa C. [Role of loco-regional anesthesia in the surgical treatment of atheromatous lesions of the carotid bifurcation.] [Italian.] *Minerva Chir* 1992;47:1135–1137.
93. Wakefield TW, Lindblad B, Stanley TJ, et al. Heparin and protamine use in peripheral

vascular surgery: a comparison between surgeons of the Society for Vascular Surgery and the European Society for Vascular Surgery. *Eur J Vasc Surg* 1994;8:193–198.

94. Weiss SJ, Sutter FP, Shannon TO, Goldman SM. Combined cardiac operation and carotid endarterectomy during aortic cross-clamping [see Comments]. *Ann Thorac Surg* 1992;53: 813–816.

95. West H, Burton R, Roon AJ. Comparative risk of operation and expectant management for carotid artery disease. *Stroke* 1979;10:117–121.

96. Young WL, Prohovnik I, Correll JW, Ostapkovich N, Ornstein E. Thiopental effect on cerebral blood flow during carotid endarterectomy. *J Neurosurg Anesthesiol* 1991;3: 265–269.

97. Young WL, Prohovnik I, Correll JW, Ostapkovich N, Ornstein E, Quest DO. A comparison of cerebral blood flow reactivity to CO_2 during halothane versus isoflurane anesthesia for carotid endarterectomy [Review]. *Anesth Analg* 1991;73:416–421.

98. Young WL, Prohovnik I, Correll JW, et al. Effect of cerebral blood flow during carotid endarterectomy. *J Neurosurg Anesth* 1991;3:265–269.

99. Zornow M, Scheller M. Intraoperative fluid management during craniotomy. In: Cottrell J, Smith D, eds. *Anesthesia and neurosurgery*. St. Louis: CV Mosby; 1994:253–254.

6

Intraoperative Transcranial Doppler Monitoring in Carotid Endarterectomy

Donalee A. Davis

Transcranial Doppler (TCD) is a relatively new application of ultrasound that permits the hemodynamic evaluation of intracranial cerebral arteries and offers the unique potential for continuous real-time evaluation coupled with a physiologic assessment (2,5,13,29). It has emerged as a useful method of measuring the velocity of blood flow through the ipsilateral middle cerebral artery during carotid endarterectomy procedures (10,17). It provides the surgical team with an immediate assessment of distal flow to the ipsilateral cortex during cross-clamping of the internal or common carotid arteries. This technology can detect a number of hazards such as microembolization, inadvertent kinking of the shunt, carotid thrombus *in situ,* and postoperative hyperperfusion syndrome (9).

TRANSCRANIAL DOPPLER TECHNOLOGY

Intracranial Doppler is based on the same physical principles as is extracranial Doppler (28). The Doppler principle describes the relationship between the velocity of objects and transmitted and collected wave frequencies. In the Doppler effect, a reflected wave is shifted to a frequency that is higher or lower than the transmitted frequency if the reflector is in motion. When the reflector moves toward the transducer, the reflected frequency increases; when it moves away, the frequency decreases. The accurate estimation of

D. A. Davis: Neurovascular Diagnostic Ultrasound, Allegheny General Hospital, Pittsburgh, Pennsylvania 15212.

Doppler frequency requires knowledge of the angle of insonation. Current TCD applications assume a 0° angle of insonation. Relatively low transducer frequencies (2 MHz) are used for TCD, due to the high attenuation of signals in bone compounds.

Vessel Identification

This technique allows blood velocities to be recorded from intracranial arteries at selected cranial foramina or thin regions of the skull (3) (Fig. 1). Through the temporal bone, blood flow velocities in the middle cerebral artery, the terminal branch of the internal carotid arteries, and the proximal portions of the anterior and posterior cerebral arteries can be evaluated.

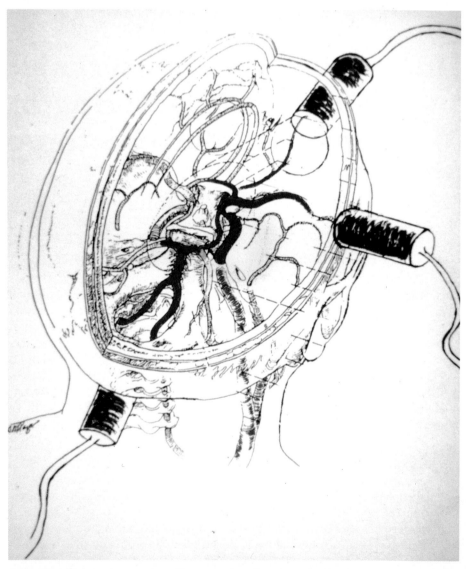

Figure 1. Cranial insonation. Transtemporal approach allows for insonation of the middle cerebral artery, the terminal branch of the internal carotid artery, the anterior cerebral artery, and the posterior cerebral artery. Transforaminal approach allows for insonation of the basilar artery and vertebral arteries. Transorbital approach allows for insonation of the ophthalmic artery and siphon internal carotid artery (parasellar, supraclinoid, genu). (From Nicolet Medical, Inc., Atlanta, GA, with permission.)

Insonation through the foramen magnum permits frequencies to be recorded from intracranial vertebral and basilar arteries. The orbital approach yields information about the siphon portion of the internal carotid arteries and ophthalmic arteries (Fig. 2). Criteria for vessel identification are based on approach, depth of insonation, and blood flow direction. Inability to insonate through the temporal bone is common among elderly women and blacks. Hyperostosis frontalis interna of the temporal bone occurs in 5% to 10% of evaluations.

Data Interpretation

Once a vessel is identified, analysis by fast-Fourier transform permits systolic, diastolic, and mean velocities to be calculated and displayed. Blood flow is measured in centimeters per second (cm/s). Normal reference values for TCD are shown in Table 1. A wide range of variables affects TCD findings. Age, gender, hematocrit, cardiac output, and carbon dioxide levels are a few of the factors that may be reflected in blood flow measurement. Alterations in cerebral blood flow correlate with changes in blood flow velocity. This correlation occurs because the large basal cerebral arteries act as "stiff pipe" noncapacitance vessels. Vascular reactivity occurs in the precapillary arteriole beds (6). Direct middle cerebral artery measurements have revealed that moderate changes in P_{CO_2} and blood pressure cause only slight changes in vessel diameter (10). In addition to flow evaluation, the Gosling

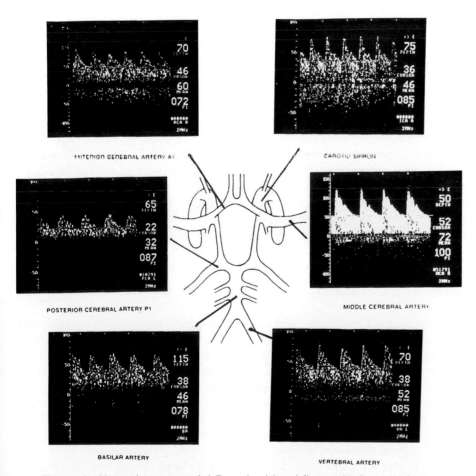

Figure 2. Normal transcranial Doppler blood flow velocity waveforms.

Table 1. *Normal mean reference values for blood velocity as measured by transcranial Doppler sonography (cm/s)*

Age (years)	MCA	ACA	PCA	VA	BA	ICA
<50	46–86	41–76	33–64	27–55	30–57	28–45
>50	34–61	33–55	28–49	27–47	25–39	28–45

MCA, middle cerebral artery; ACA, anterior cerebral artery; PCA, posterior cerebral artery; VA, vertebral artery; BA, basilar artery; ICA, internal carotid artery.

pulsatility index (pulsatility index = systolic-diastolic/mean velocity), which measures vascular resistance distal to the vessel being insonated, can be used (7,12). A normal pulsatility index is 0.80 to 1.20. In the presence of a hemodynamically significant carotid lesion, middle cerebral artery velocities are typically decreased and have a low pulsatility index due to maximal dilatation in the distal arterial circulation and the presence of a "low-flow" state (11,16) (Fig. 3). If middle cerebral artery velocities and pulsatility indices are normal and symmetrical in the presence of carotid disease, the lesion is probably not hemodynamically significant to brain perfusion (15,23).

Emboli Detection

In addition to evaluating cerebral hemodynamic status, TCD is capable of detecting intravascular microembolization (4,19). This capability is based upon the difference in acoustic impedance of embolic material compared with that of surrounding red blood cells. Identifiable differences in the intensity of the spectral display result in characteristic high-amplitude signatures (Fig. 4). All emboli, whether solid or gaseous, demonstrate a high-frequency response with a harmonic quality similar to a chirping or whistling sound. Air emboli produce a particularly intense signal, which, depending on the TCD equipment, extend beyond the Doppler waveform. Signals from some types of solid emboli may remain enveloped within the Doppler waveform (24). The technique is sensitive enough to detect emboli from 30 to 50 μm in diameter (20,21). The composition and size of an embolus, however, cannot be determined accurately based on the Doppler characteristics noted above. Unlike emboli, artifacts produce scratchy, sonorous, nonharmonic sounds and appear bidirectional on spectral display. At this time, the detection of emboli requires auditory as well as visual identification. Intrinsic emboli detector software packages will one day be standard in all TCD equipment.

Intraoperative Monitoring

During carotid endarterectomy, the transtemporal approach is used. To measure flow accurately, it is important that the Ml segment of the middle cerebral artery be correctly identified. Insonation should begin at a depth of 55 mm, and the vessel should be followed to a more superficial depth of 45 mm from the temporal bone surface. Use of these criteria will increase the probability that it is the middle cerebral artery and not the posterior cerebral artery or terminal internal carotid artery that is being insonated. At depths of 55 or 60 mm, part or all of the waveform may be generated from the carotid siphon (terminal internal carotid artery). In such cases, velocities may disappear altogether after cross-clamping, even though middle cerebral artery flow is adequate. The posterior cerebral artery can also be identified

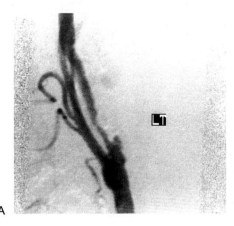

A

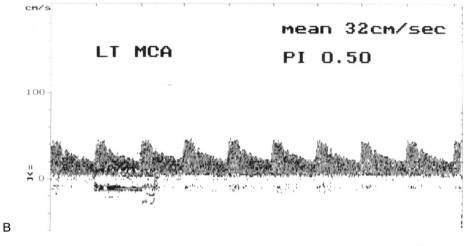

B

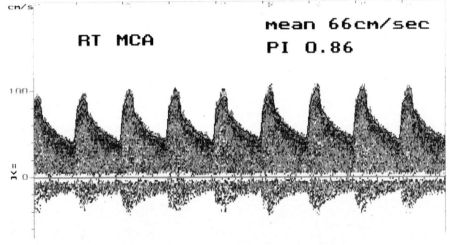

C

Figure 3. Hemodynamically significant lesions. **A**: Cerebral angiogram reveals 99% stenosis of the left internal carotid artery. Mean flow velocities and pulsatility indices in the left middle cerebral artery **(B)** are lower than in the right middle cerebral artery **(C)**.

at depths of 55 or 60 mm. Insonation of this vessel will not reflect a valid index of ischemia except in rare instances when the posterior cerebral artery arises from the internal carotid artery. During vessel dissection, transient decreases in flow velocities, correlated with surgical vessel manipulation, ensure correct middle cerebral artery insonation.

Once the middle cerebral artery has been identified, the skin surface is marked and the operative probe mount is attached with an elastic band around the head (Fig. 5). Insonation must be optimal throughout the procedure because anatomic landmarks are obscured once the signal is lost after

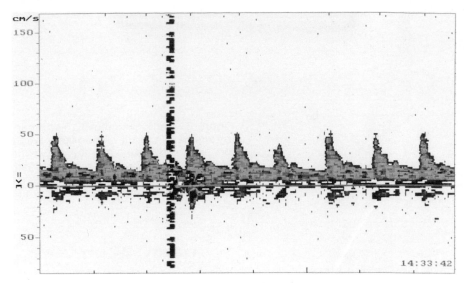

Figure 4. Microembolic events. Microemboli can be detected during any part of the cardiac cycle. The signals produced are of a higher intensity and may appear unidirectional or bidirectional or remain within the spectral envelope.

sterile draping. Insonation can be optimized by placing a small Mayo stand over the patient's head before draping. The stand does not interfere with the surgical procedure, and the anesthetist will find that monitoring the patient is easier. Because it does not interfere with lead placement or signal reception, TCD can be used with alternative methods of monitoring [e.g., electroencephalogram (EEG), life scan]. Velocities are recorded throughout the procedure and stored on computer disc and/or video cassette recorder tape.

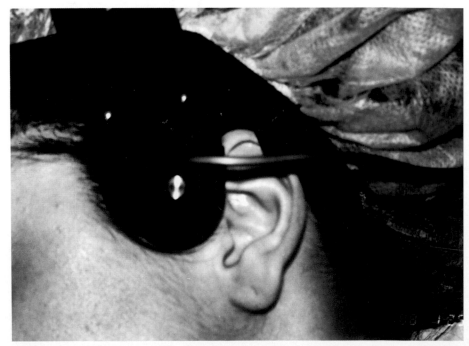

Figure 5. Placement of operative probe and mount over the temporal bone above the zygomatic arch.

Intraoperative Findings

Mean blood flow velocities in the ipsilateral middle cerebral artery can be correlated with surgical events. Velocities in the middle cerebral artery always decrease after cross-clamping of the common carotid artery. The percentage of decrease in flow depends on the individual's cerebrovascular reserve from anterior and posterior collateralization (1,22). In the presence of a competent collateral reserve system, middle cerebral artery velocities may decrease very little after cross-clamping. Figure 6 demonstrates middle cerebral artery response to cross-clamping in a patient who has a competent reserve system. Flow velocities in this case dropped only 30% of the pre-clamp mean. Figure 7 shows a case of the complete absence of middle cerebral artery flow velocity after cross-clamping of the common carotid artery. This finding indicates a lack of a collateral reserve system from communicator pathways or leptomeningeal anastomoses (10,17). Unlike EEG, TCD determines flow from the main trunk of the middle cerebral artery and its immediate distribution in the lenticulostriate territory of the basal ganglia and internal capsule. An EEG evaluates electrical activity in the cerebral convexity, where flows are influenced by cortical collaterals from distal anterior and posterior cerebral artery branches.

Shunt Intervention

The amount of intraoperative cerebral ischemia that follows carotid clamping is influenced by collateral competency. The ischemic tolerance of neural tissue and the need for selective shunting remain controversial (27). Shunt intervention to prevent ischemia during this procedure is typically instituted at the preference of the surgeon.

Early research by Padayachee et al. (17) using TCD monitoring to identify ischemia during carotid endarterectomy expressed the reduction of blood flow velocity after clamping as an absolute value of cm/s. They theorized that the 20-cm/s residual flow velocity in the middle cerebral artery was the

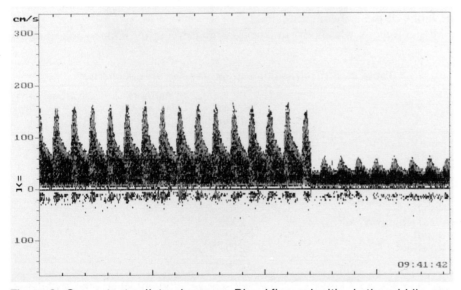

Figure 6. Competent collateral reserve. Blood flow velocities in the middle cerebral artery following clamping of the internal carotid artery indicate competent collateral pathways.

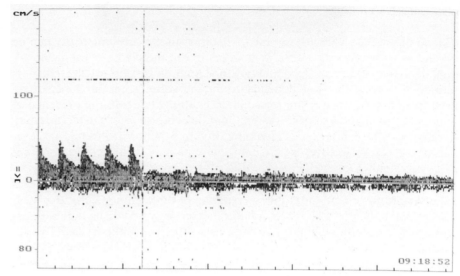

Figure 7. Incompetent collateral reserve. Blood flow velocities in the middle cerebral artery following clamping of the internal carotid artery indicating an exhausted collateral reserve system.

critical ischemic threshold level. However, this finding was disputed when researchers performed carotid endarterectomy with TCD under local cervical anesthesia and observed that patients could tolerate flow velocities below 20 cm/s without neurologic sequelae. Under regional anesthesia, patients could tolerate a 50% to 60% drop in mean flow velocity from the preclamp baseline before a neurologic deficit occurred (unpublished data).

A more accurate assessment of the ischemic threshold would be to evaluate residual flow not as an absolute value but as a percentage of the baseline. Halsey and his colleagues (8,10) used TCD, EEG, and regional cerebral blood flow studies to identify an ischemic threshold following clamping under general anesthesia. Table 2 illustrates findings from Halsey's research identifying stroke that results from intraoperative ischemia in shunted and nonshunted cases. The patient whose mean flow velocity decreased 60% of the baseline preclamp mean or had a 40% residual baseline appeared to be within the limits of the ischemic threshold.

Most surgeons who perform carotid endarterectomy under general anes-

Table 2. *Stroke resulting from intraoperative ischemia[a]*

	No. of patients	Patients with stroke [no. (%)]	Patients with EEG changes [no. (%)]
Severe ischemia (MV 0–15%)[b]	26		17 (65)
Shunt	14	0 (0)	
No shunt	12	4 (33)	
Mild ischemia (MV 16–40%)	37		11 (30)
Shunt	12	0 (0)	
No shunt	25	1 (4)	
No ischemia (MV >40%)	235		0 (0)
Shunt	20	3 (15)	
No shunt	215	4 (1.9)	
Total	298		

[a] The difference between the shunted and nonshunted cases was significant for the severe ischemia ($p < 0.02$) and no ischemia ($p < 0.01$) groups.
[b] MV (mean velocity) expressed as percent of preclamp levels.
(From Halsey, *Transcranial Doppler ultrasonography*, 1992:216–221, with permission.)

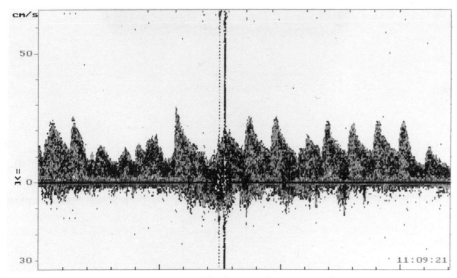

Figure 8. Intraoperative emboli. Middle cerebral artery flow alterations during vessel dissection with proliferation of formed microemboli.

thesia prefer to shunt all patients. TCD monitoring during this phase of the operation provides a surgeon with information about the patency of the temporary intraluminal shunt. Inadvertent kinking of the shunt can be identified immediately and corrected.

Microembolization

Spontaneous microemboli can occur before, during, and after surgical dissection. Preoperatively, emboli are associated with intraluminal platelet thrombi from plaque ulcerations. During vessel dissection, TCD can detect changes in flow velocity and the proliferation of microembolic (Fig. 8) events that occur after shunt intervention and the reinstitution of the carotid blood flow (24) (Fig. 9). Intraoperative air or particulate emboli are frequently associated with shunt intervention, despite careful flushing and venting of

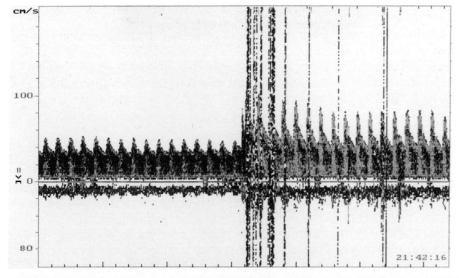

Figure 9. Intraoperative emboli. Microembolic events occurring in the middle cerebral artery following flow restoration of the internal carotid artery.

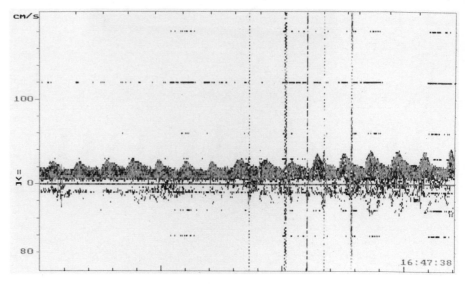

Figure 10. Intraoperative emboli. Emboli occurring in the middle cerebral artery before internal carotid artery clamp release during backflushing into the external carotid artery.

the arterial lumina. Shunt insertion is always associated with the risk of dislodging atheromatous material into the cerebral circulation. Emboli reported at the time of recirculation are probably gaseous rather than particulate. In general, intraoperative emboli have no consequences. However, one researcher reported a large number of emboli correlated with a paroxysmal deterioration of the EEG at the time of recirculation (25). Upon awakening, the patient had a transient hemiparesis that resolved within 1 hour. The quick regression of this neurologic deficit suggests air embolism. Figure 10 demonstrates emboli occurring during backflushing into the external carotid artery before clamp release. In this case, the emboli presumably passed retrogradely through the ophthalmic artery to the middle cerebral artery branches.

DETECTION OF COMPLICATIONS

Controversy exists about the origin of cerebral complications that accompany carotid endarterectomy procedures. Resulting deficits may be a consequence of ischemia that occurs during operative clamping or may be due to perioperative emboli (e.g., intraluminal debris or thrombus formation at the operative site).

In situ Thrombus

Common causes of postoperative thrombus formation *in situ* include intimal flap dissection, vessel kinking, stenotic arterial closure, and hemorrhage into residual intraluminal plaque. Thrombosis of the operative vessel attributable to technical errors is most likely to occur within the first hour after surgery. Blood flow velocities of the middle cerebral artery gradually decrease as the thrombus induces a hemodynamic state that causes the pulsatility index to drop and the waveform to become truncated. Continuous TCD monitoring during skin closure and in the immediate postoperative period can quickly identify and potentially diagnose such critical events. The following case illustrates the value of early detection.

Case 1

A 62-year-old man underwent a carotid endarterectomy performed under cervical anesthesia. Criteria for shunting were based on the patient's level of consciousness and motor function. Following cross-clamping of the internal carotid artery, TCD velocities dropped only 20% of the preclamp mean. The patient tolerated the clamp time well and experienced no neurologic deficit. The endarterectomy was performed without incident until skin closure (Fig. 11A), when the velocities and pulsatility index began to drop, indicating a hemodynamic compromise proximal to the middle cerebral artery (Fig. 11B). Velocities fell from 52 cm/s to 30 cm/s, yet the patient remained neurologically intact. The surgeon was informed of the TCD waveform pattern, and a decision was made to reexplore the vessel (Fig. 11C). Velocities continued to drop despite an increase in arterial pressure. The patient became unconscious when the mean flow velocity fell to 20 cm/s, which was 60% of the preoperative mean. A Javid shunt was placed, and flow was restored within minutes. The patient regained consciousness with full motor and cognitive function. Reexploration of the vessel revealed an intimal flap dissection of the internal carotid artery with thrombus formation. The dissection was repaired and a patch-graft angioplasty performed. Mean flow velocities in the middle cerebral artery, as well as the pulsatility index, returned to normal (Fig. 11D). The patient suffered no postoperative neurologic deficits.

Postcarotid Endarterectomy Hyperemia

Postoperative hyperperfusion syndrome occurs in a subset of patients after carotid endarterectomy (25). An elevated middle cerebral artery mean flow velocity following restoration may exceed 60% of the preoperative mean. This phenomenon has been reported by Steiger et al. (26) and Lindegaard et al. (14), but the exact etiology remains unclear. No consistent correlation has been found between percent stenosis or plaque morphology. Of clinical relevance is the fact that postoperative hyperemia may be a consequence of impaired autoregulation, and uncontrolled hypertension can predispose high-risk patients to cerebral infarctions (18). In patients who display complications postoperatively, TCD may help differentiate hemorrhage from occlusion. The following case illustrates this complication.

Case 2

A 64-year-old man suffered a left hemispheric cerebrovascular accident 4 weeks before surgery. A left carotid endarterectomy was performed under local cervical block. The procedure was unremarkable except for labile arterial blood pressures. After the internal carotid artery was clamped, TCD demonstrated a 40% decrease in middle cerebral artery flow velocities. The patient remained responsive with full motor function. Immediately before cross-clamp release, the patient became hypertensive. Flow restoration produced a hyperemic response (84 cm/s) that was double the preclamp mean of 42 cm/s. Flow velocities remained elevated despite a return to normotension. During skin closure, the patient became extremely restless, right hemiparetic, and aphasic. Intubation was necessary due to a progressive state of obtundation and seizure activity. Figure 12A represents a hyperemic re-

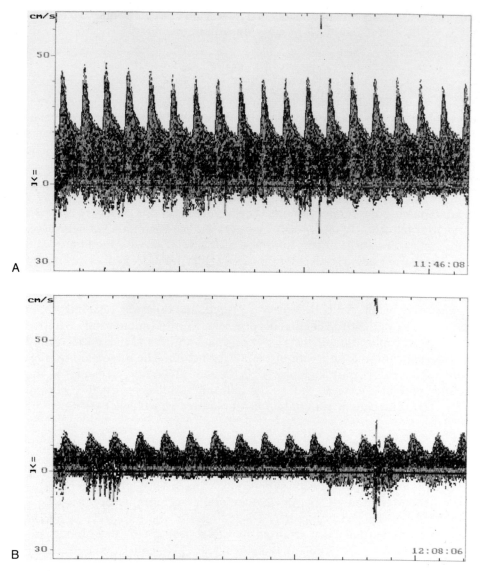

Figure 11. *In situ* thrombus formation. **A:** Middle cerebral artery blood flow velocities following endarterectomy. **B:** Decrease in middle cerebral artery flow with low pulsatility index occurring during skin closure.

sponse following clamp release. The elevated pulsatility indices after the procedure indicate extreme distal resistance in the distribution territory of the middle cerebral artery (Fig. 12B). A computed tomography scan of the brain immediately after surgery revealed a massive hemorrhagic infarction in the left cerebral hemisphere, and the patient died 20 hours after surgery.

TECHNICAL DIFFICULTIES OF INTRAOPERATIVE MONITORING

As previously mentioned, failure to insonate the middle cerebral artery due to hyperostosis occurs in approximately 10% of patients. All patients should be evaluated for hyperostosis before surgery. Once the vessel is identified, the major problem is maintaining optimal position of the transducer after the operative probe mount is attached. Satisfactory protection of the transducer is the key to successful long-term monitoring. Identification of an incorrect vessel is another problem. Using the criteria discussed earlier will help prevent this mishap.

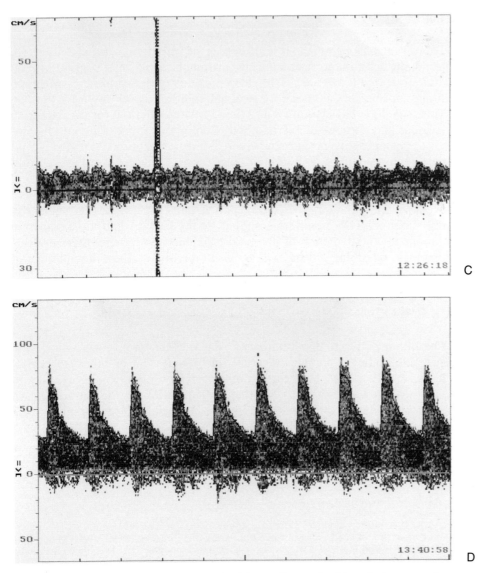

Figure 11. *Continued* **C:** Middle cerebral artery flow velocities during reexploration with embolic event. **D:** Restoration of middle cerebral artery blood flow following thrombectomy.

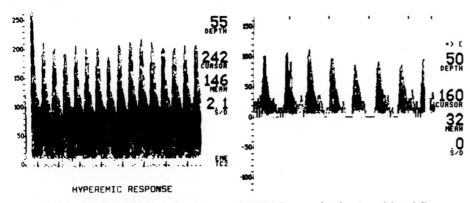

Figure 12. Hyperperfusion syndrome. **A:** Middle cerebral artery blood flow velocities at clamp release. **B:** Middle cerebral artery flow 30 minutes after clamp release. Elevated pulsatility index reflects extreme distal resistance. The patient was obtunded with seizure activity.

CONCLUSIONS

Transcranial Doppler has a high degree of sensitivity and specificity in determining cerebral perfusion during carotid clamping. It is continuous and quantitative, and it can access the deep portions of the cerebral hemisphere that may not be well assessed by regional cerebral blood flow or EEG.

This technique has also proved to be a sensitive method for the detection of gaseous and particulate microemboli. Continuous monitoring into the immediate postoperative period can help to delineate the etiology of postcarotid endarterectomy stroke. Differential diagnoses include hemorrhage, carotid occlusion, or isolated middle cerebral artery occlusion.

Most neurologic complications associated with carotid endarterectomy procedures are secondary to hemodynamic changes. Because it is a hemodynamic monitor, TCD monitoring should be the earliest and most sensitive technique for the detection of potential problems. As more centers use this technology, its ultimate value will be based on how it alters the outcome of the procedure.

ACKNOWLEDGMENTS

The author wishes to thank Barbara C. Good, PhD, for editorial comments, Claire S. Rasimczyk for her assistance in preparation of this manuscript, and Richard E. Clark, MD, for his review. The author would also like to thank the following surgeons for their participation in the intraoperative transcranial Doppler monitoring: J. Bailes, D. Benckart, M. Javan, G. Magovern, Jr., S. Park, and J. Rams.

REFERENCES

1. Aaslid R. Cerebral hemodynamics. In: Newell D, Aaslid R, eds. *Transcranial Doppler*. New York: Raven Press; 1992:49–55.
2. Aaslid RM, Marhwalder TM, Nores H. Non-invasive transcranial Doppler ultrasound recording of flow velocity in basal cerebral arteries. *J Neurosurg* 1982;57:769–774.
3. Arnolds BJ, Von Reutern GM. Transcranial Doppler sonography. Examination technique and normal reference values. *Ultrasound Med Biol* 1986;12:115–123.
4. Berger M, Tegler C. Embolus detection using ultrasonography In: Babikian VL, Wechsler L, eds. *Transcranial Doppler ultrasonography*. New York: Mosby; 1992:232–241.
5. Bishop C, Powell S, Rutt D, Browse N. Transcranial Doppler measurement of middle cerebral artery blood velocity: a validation study. *Stroke* 1986;17:913–920.
6. Giller CA. Diameter changes in cerebral arteries during craniotomy. *J Cardiovasc Technol* 1990;9:51–52.
7. Giller CA, Hodges K, Batjer HH. Transcranial Doppler pulsatility in vasodilatation and stenosis. *J Neurosurg* 1990;72:901–906.
8. Halsey J. Monitoring blood flow velocity in the middle cerebral artery during carotid endarterectomy. In: Babikian VL, Wechsler L, eds. *Transcranial Doppler ultrasonography*. New York: Mosby; 1992:216–221.
9. Halsey J. Risks and benefits of shunting in carotid endarterectomy. *Stroke* 1992;23:1583–1587.
10. Halsey J, McDowell H, Gelman S, Morawetz R. Blood velocity in the middle cerebral and regional cerebral blood flow during carotid endarterectomy. *Stroke* 1989;20:53–58.
11. Kelly R, Namon R, Juang S, Lee S, Chang J. Transcranial Doppler ultrasonography of the middle cerebral artery in the hemodynamic assessment of internal carotid artery stenosis. *Arch Neurol* 1990;47:960–964.
12. Lindegaard KF. Indices of pulsatility. In: Newell D, Aaslid R, eds. *Transcranial Doppler*. New York: Raven Press; 1992:67–82.
13. Lindegaard KF, Bakke SJ, Grolinund P, Aaslid R, Huber P, Nornes H. Assessment of intracranial hemodynamics in carotid artery disease by transcranial Doppler ultrasound. *J Neurosurg* 1985;63:890–898.
14. Lindegaard KF, Lundar T, Wilberg J, et al. Variations in middle cerebral artery blood flow investigated with noninvasive transcranial blood velocity measurements. *Stroke* 1987;18:1025–1030.
15. Norris JW, Krajewski A, Bornstein N. The clinical rate of the cerebral collateral circulation in carotid occlusion. *J Vasc Surg* 1990;12:113–118.

16. Otis S, Ringelstein EB. Findings associated with extracranial occlusive disease. In: Newell D, Aaslid R, eds. *Transcranial Doppler*. New York: Raven Press; 1992:153–160.
17. Padayachee TS, Gosling RG, Bishop CC, Burnard K, Bowser NL. Monitoring middle cerebral artery blood velocity during carotid endarterectomy. *Br J Surg* 1986;73:98–100.
18. Piepgras DB, Morgan M, Sundt T, et al. Intracranial hemorrhage after carotid endarterectomy. *J Neurosurg* 1988;68:532–536.
19. Pugsley W. The use of Doppler ultrasound in the assessment of microemboli during carotid surgery. *Perfusion* 1989;4:115–122.
20. Russell D, Brucher R, Madden KP, Clark WM, Sandset PM, Zivin JA. The intensity of the Doppler signal caused by arterial emboli depends on embolus type and size. *Stroke* 1992;23(I):158(abst).
21. Russell D, Madden K, Clark W, Sandset PM, Zivin J. Detection of arterial emboli using Doppler ultrasound in rabbit. *Stroke* 1991;22:253–258.
22. Schneider PA, Ringelstein EB, Rossman ME, Dilley RB, Otis SM, Berstein EF. Importance of cerebral collateral pathways during carotid endarterectomy. *Stroke* 1988;19:1328–1334.
23. Schneider PA, Rossman ME, Bernstein EF, Torem S, Ringelstein EB, Otis S. Effect of internal carotid artery occlusion on intracranial hemodynamics. Transcranial Doppler evaluation and clinical correlation. *Stroke* 1988;19:589–593.
24. Spencer MP, Thomas GI, Nichalls SC, Sauvage LR. Detection of the middle cerebral artery emboli during carotid endarterectomy using transcranial Doppler ultrasonography. *Stroke* 1990;21:415–423.
25. Steiger HJ. Monitoring for carotid surgery. In: Newell D, Aaslid R, eds. *Transcranial Doppler*. New York: Raven Press; 1992:197–205.
26. Steiger HJ, Schaffler L, Boll J, et al. Results of microsurgical carotid endarterectomy: a prospective study with transcranial Doppler and EEG monitoring and elective shunting. *Acta Neurochir* 1989;100:31–38.
27. Sundt TM. The ischemic tolerance of neural tissue and the need for monitoring and selective shunting during carotid endarterectomy. *Stroke* 1983;14:93–98.
28. Tegler C, Eicke M. Physics and principles of transcranial Doppler ultrasound. In: Babikian VL, Wechsler L, eds. *Transcranial Doppler ultrasonography*. New York: Mosby; 1992: 3–9.
29. Wechsler L, Ropper A, Kistler JP. Transcranial Doppler in cerebrovascular disease. *Stroke* 1986;17:905–912.

7

Rationale and Protocol for Microsurgical Carotid Endarterectomy

Robert F. Spetzler, Julian E. Bailes, and
Paul J. Apostolides

Carotid endarterectomy has undergone an evolution in indications, preoperative patient assessment, intraoperative technique, anesthetic management, and postoperative patient care. In the mid-1950s, the atherosclerotic carotid origin of cerebral symptoms was recognized and successful carotid endarterectomy was performed. Over the ensuing years, refinements in all aspects of this operation took place. Great interest in intraoperative cerebral ischemia and techniques of monitoring intraoperative cerebral function dominated clinical research. While carotid endarterectomy became an accepted prophylactic procedure for cerebral ischemic disease, it has been associated with controversy. Neurosurgeons have participated in the refinements and progress of the procedure. In the current application of endarterectomy, several issues concerning technical variations and surgical methodology are still being debated. We believe that carotid endarterectomy is a safe and effective treatment that is optimized when attention is directed to several considerations.

Technical improvements in carotid endarterectomy have centered around the avoidance of cerebral ischemia. Although earlier reports stressed the

R. F. Spetzler and P. J. Apostolides: Division of Neurological Surgery, Barrow Neurological Institute, Phoenix, Arizona 85013.

J. E. Bailes: Department of Neurological Surgery, Allegheny General Hospital, Pittsburgh, Pennsylvania 15212.

importance of indwelling shunts to supply blood to the brain during the period of carotid artery cross-clamping, recent evidence suggests that a substantial reduction in cerebral blood flow and considerable cerebral ischemia can be tolerated. Although the issue remains controversial, our experience has led us to conclude that the routine use of carotid shunts is unwarranted. Intraluminal shunts and other technical aspects of carotid endarterectomy justify careful consideration, and the implementation of a surgical protocol should be based on obtaining the desired results. Neurosurgeons are most intimately involved in the diagnosis and treatment of disease processes affecting the cerebral blood supply. Our protocol, based on certain modern principles of neurologic surgery such as the use of the operating microscope, intraoperative monitoring of cerebral function, and pharmacologic protection, has yielded favorable outcomes in patients undergoing endarterectomy. This chapter details our rationale for this protocol and presents our results obtained with this method.

SURGICAL ANATOMY AND TECHNIQUE

The patient is placed supine with the head turned slightly to the contralateral side. Rotating the patient's neck places the internal carotid artery in a more lateral and accessible location than its normal position, posterior to the external carotid artery. The degree of rotation required can be assessed from the cervical angiogram. Excessive rotation can cause the internal jugular vein to cover the internal carotid artery and should be avoided. Theoretically, if the turn of the head is exaggerated, the collateral circulation could be compromised by reducing or eliminating blood flow in the ipsilateral vertebral artery. In obese patients or those with thick necks, a towel roll may be placed in the interscapular area to permit cervical extension and to improve deep exposure. Surgical access may also be improved by placing some patients in a modified Trendelenburg position. The occipital area rests on a doughnut foam pad. The skin is carefully prepared with gentle scrubbing, alcohol, and a povidone solution. Using only the latter will minimize the likelihood of mechanical dislodgement of atheromatous or thrombotic debris. If a vein patch angioplasty may be necessary, a lower extremity should be prepared and draped accordingly (Fig. 1).

Surgical Opening

The surgical incision begins about 2 fingerwidths above the clavicle and sternal notch along the anterior border of the sternocleidomastoid muscle and proceeds superiorly until it approaches the angle of the mandible (Fig. 2). Further cephalad exposure is attained by gently curving the incision posteriorly toward the mastoid tip. Directing the incision away from the side of the cheek improves cosmesis and avoids injury to the marginal mandibular branch of the facial nerve. A hemostatic scalpel may assist in attaining the complete hemostasis in those patients who will require full heparinization later in the procedure.

Correct operative planning requires review of the angiogram to ascertain the location of the carotid bifurcation as well as the location and extent of the carotid lesion, which are noted in relation to the cervical vertebral bodies and mandibular angle. When the bifurcation is unusually high or low, the incision may be adjusted accordingly. A submandibular incision 1 cm below and parallel to the lower mandibular margin and a zigzag incision along the anterior border of the sternocleidomastoid muscle are alternatives that can also improve cosmesis. These incisions, however, require developing wide

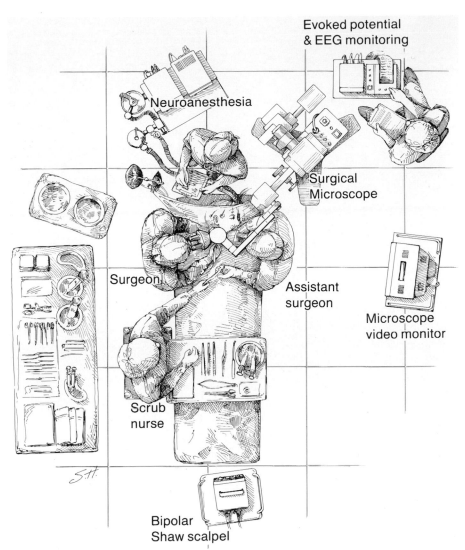

Figure 1. An artist's conceptual drawing of the optimal operating room arrangement for performing carotid microendarterectomy. Reprinted with permission of Barrow Neurological Institute.

skin flaps and do not offer as good an exposure, particularly proximally on the common carotid. The incision along the anterior edge of the sternocleidomastoid is preferred and gives fully acceptable cosmetic results, especially with subcuticular suture closure.

The incision proceeds through the subcutaneous tissues and platysma along the medial border of the sternocleidomastoid muscle. Hemostasis from the skin incision down to the carotid artery must be complete and meticulous since heparinization is not reversed at the end of the procedure. The loose areolar tissue, which attaches the sternocleidomastoid muscle to the strap muscles overlying the trachea, is dissected, and a deep self-retaining retractor is placed to expose the carotid sheath. The common carotid pulse can serve as a guide to proper location during the dissection.

Several nerves are in the vicinity of the exposure, superficial to the sternocleidomastoid muscle. The great auricular nerve crosses obliquely over the sternocleidomastoid toward the posterior auricular region and mandibular angle. The lesser occipital nerve courses across the posterior sternocleidomastoid attachment to the occipital and mastoid regions. The spinal accessory nerve runs on the posterior aspect of the sternocleidomastoid muscle

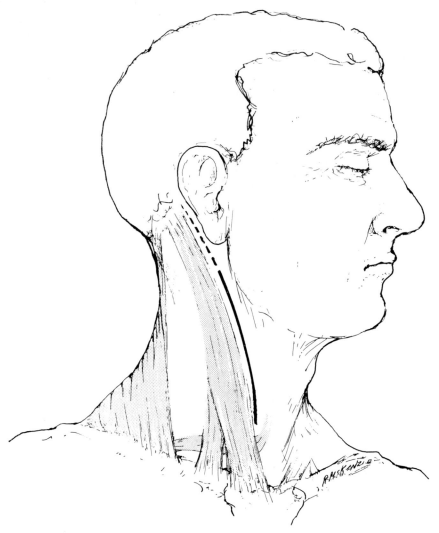

Figure 2. Exposure of the carotid artery is accomplished with an anterocervical longitudinal incision parallel to the medial border of the sternocleidomastoid for lesions that extend distally on the internal carotid artery. The incision is curved posteriorly behind the ear for cosmetic reasons and to avoid the facial nerve branches.

across the posterior triangle to innervate the trapezius muscle. Finally, a cervical branch of the facial nerve runs deep to the platysma. If the dissection is maintained in the correct plane, these nerves will not typically be encountered or injured during the endarterectomy. Often, however, the transverse cervical nerve, which crosses the midbelly of the sternocleidomastoid muscle, is transected. The anterior neck will then be numb. Regeneration typically occurs, and the numbness disappears by 6 months.

As the dissection proceeds posteriorly, lymph nodes, which are best handled by medial dissection and lateral deflection, may be encountered. In the upper end of the incision, the parotid gland may be recognized by its lobulated architecture and pale color compared with subcutaneous adipose tissue.

Once encountered, the carotid sheath is opened with sharp dissection and careful bipolar coagulation of any small vessels within the fibrous sheath. The common carotid artery, located in the proximal region of the dissection posteromedial to the internal jugular vein, is exposed first. Typically, the vagus nerve is dorsal to the vessels within the carotid sheath. The internal

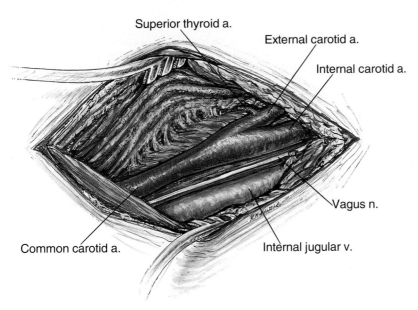

Superior thyroid a.

External carotid a.

Internal carotid a.

Vagus n.

Common carotid a.

Internal jugular v.

Figure 3. The dissection is carried posteriorly and the carotid sheath is opened to isolate the common external and internal carotid arteries. This is best accomplished by always retracting the internal jugular vein laterally. Crossing venous tributaries of the internal jugular are ligated and divided.

jugular vein must be mobilized, which often requires dividing medial venous tributaries, the largest of which is usually the common facial vein located near the carotid bifurcation. Access to the carotid bifurcation and internal carotid artery is best facilitated by reflecting the internal jugular laterally (Fig. 3).

The omohyoid muscle is usually the proximal extent of the exposure. Rarely, this muscle must be divided partially or completely to attain adequate access to the common carotid. The dissection proceeds cephalad. The ansa cervicalis is encountered. It is composed of an inferior division, which originates from the ventral rami of the second and third cervical nerves, and a superior division, which descends from the hypoglossal nerve and connects with the inferior division after the latter courses over the internal jugular vein. Dividing the descending limb of the ansa can afford better access to the carotid artery. This maneuver will also shift the hypoglossal nerve medially and slightly superiorly away from the carotid bifurcation. The carotid bifurcation is most often located at the level of the thyroid cartilage. In about 20% of the cases, however, it bifurcates between the thyroid cartilage and the hyoid bone. Rarely, the bifurcation is below the thyroid cartilage, or the common carotid artery is absent, and the internal and external carotid arteries originate directly from the aortic arch or the innominate artery. These details are discernible on the preoperative angiogram and should be considered during the preoperative planning stage.

The common carotid artery typically possesses no branches, although the superior thyroid artery often may originate within 2 cm proximal to the carotid bifurcation. When the superior thyroid artery is dissected for temporary clipping, its posterior aspect—a location where the superior laryngeal nerve may be injured—should be avoided. The carotid body is ovoid, usually less than 5 mm, and is situated immediately dorsal to the carotid bifurcation. Its chemoreceptor elements form a portion of the visceral afferent system innervated by the vagus nerve.

The routine injection of local anesthetic into the carotid body to avoid reflexive bradycardia and hypotension is often advocated. In our experience, however, a carotid-body injection does not affect the patient's cardiovascular response significantly, and we do not use the technique. If, however, the anesthesiologist notes any hemodynamically significant changes during dissection or handling of this area, the physiologic effects may be blocked temporarily with an injection of 1% lidocaine (2 to 3 ml).

The distal internal carotid artery must be accessed, usually 3 to 5 cm distal to the bifurcation, depending on the extent of the carotid plaque. This distal exposure is readily gained by dissecting laterally and superiorly to the hypoglossal nerve. Leaving the areolar connective tissue attached on the medial side will tend to pull the hypoglossal nerve somewhat medially and superiorly as desired. Occasionally, distal exposure is improved by careful placement of retraction sutures in the medial connective tissue or perineum or by dividing or incising the digastric muscle.

Often an external carotid branch to the sternocleidomastoid muscle, accompanied by a vein, will be encountered and must be divided. Rarely, this structure, together with the 12th nerve, has been the source of carotid compression, the so-called carotid sling. In our experience, more complex maneuvers for distal exposure, such as osteotomy of the mandibular ramus, have been unnecessary. Careful and deliberate dissection along the distal internal carotid artery, working lateral to the hypoglossal nerve, usually provides adequate cephalad exposure. The adventitial layer, which must be included within the arteriotomy closure, should be avoided. Small venous tributaries of the internal jugular vein, which are often encountered in this area, can readily be handled by bipolar coagulation. The external carotid artery is dissected for about 2 cm beyond the bifurcation. Exposure is necessary only to guarantee vascular control and sufficient space for temporary clipping.

Intraoperative Technique

Once the exposure is completed, the carotid artery is inspected for the extent of the plaque (Fig. 4). The plaque is usually tinged yellow compared with the gray walls of a healthy carotid artery. The step-off transition zone

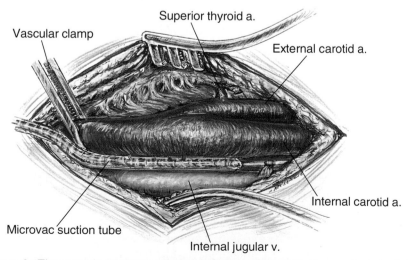

Figure 4. The vessels are then prepared for temporary clipping and an occlusive vascular clamp is positioned on the common carotid artery until needed. An indwelling suction tube is laid parallel with the carotid artery for a constant evacuation of heparinized irrigant, which frees an assistant from performing the task of constant suction.

at the distal end of the lesion can be palpated gently with a moistened gloved finger. This intraoperative judgment is combined with the preoperative angiographic data to confirm plaque location, placement of the arteriotomy, and adequacy of proximal and distal dissection and thus vascular control.

At this junction in the procedure, the patient undergoes full systemic heparinization by an anesthesiologist who administers 100 IU/kg intravenously. Cerebral protection is attained by placing the patient in 15- to 30-s electroencephalographic (EEG) burst suppression, usually with bolus doses of thiopental (150 to 250 mg). Patients with considerable myocardial dysfunction receive an intravenous bolus loading dose of etomidate (0.4 to 0.5 mg/kg) and then 0.1 mg/kg to maintain burst suppression. During infusion of these agents, and particularly during carotid cross-clamping when a moderate degree of hypertension is desired to optimize collateral cerebral blood flow, blood pressure must be controlled carefully. Phenylephrine infusion is occasionally required to maintain systemic blood pressure in the desired range.

Once blood pressure and the EEG have been stabilized, the distal internal carotid artery is occluded with a temporary aneurysm clip. The proximal common carotid artery is immediately occluded with a 45° angled DeBakey vascular clamp, tightened only enough to prevent hemorrhage. The external carotid and superior thyroid arteries are closed using temporary aneurysm clips. For ultimate proximal vascular control, a vascular loop with a rubber tubing occluder (Rummell tourniquet) can be placed proximal to the DeBakey clamp. When encircling tapes are placed for occlusion, the vessel should be dissected from its underlying soft tissue only where the tape is to be passed. Otherwise, troublesome oozing can occur from the relatively inaccessible back wall, especially with heparinization.

Using the angiographic data to judge the proximal extent of the lesion, the common carotid artery is incised, usually about 2 cm proximal to the carotid bifurcation (Fig. 5). The incision must completely penetrate through the plaque and proceed into the carotid lumen, extending about 5 mm in length. Otherwise, the muscularis layer may contract and, together with the adventitial layer, occlude the incision.

An angled Pott's scissors is used to extend the arteriotomy cephalad into the internal carotid artery until the distal extent of the atherosclerotic plaque is passed. The arteriotomy must extend down the center axis of the internal carotid artery. The closure will be more difficult if the arteriotomy veers either medially into the region of the bifurcation or laterally on the vessel. Especially in tightly stenotic carotid arteries, it is important that the lower blade of the scissors should seek and follow the remaining luminal channel.

The endarterectomy is performed using two Penfield #4 dissectors, which are used to find the cleavage plane between the atherosclerotic plaque and the arterial wall (Fig. 6). The characteristics of these lesions vary, however. They usually begin in the distal common carotid artery, are thickest in the anterolateral position of the carotid sinus, and thin distally after considerable involvement at the internal carotid artery origin. Typically, the atherosclerotic plaque is first separated from the tunica media in the common carotid artery using the dissectors to pass along the back or dorsal wall of the artery. The plaque is incised at its proximal end and lifted superiorly as the plaque-media interface is dissected in a distal direction into the internal carotid artery (Fig. 7). The back wall must not be injured nor should the media be dissected through the adventitial layer, which can be identified by its pinkish coloration.

The portion of the plaque extending into the external carotid is recovered by an eversion technique that circumferentially dissects the plaque off the artery. Simultaneously, the external carotid artery is grasped with forceps and pulled away from the atheroma. Removal of this external carotid plaque

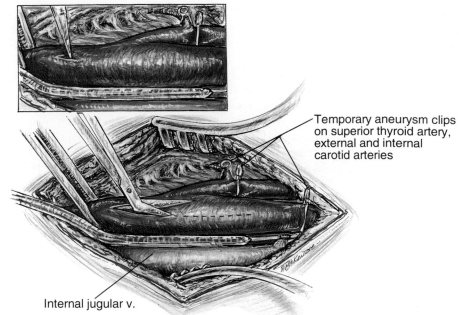

Temporary aneurysm clips
on superior thyroid artery,
external and internal
carotid arteries

Internal jugular v.

Figure 5. Once the common carotid is occluded with the vascular clamp and the thyroid external and internal carotid arteries are occluded with temporary aneurysm clips, the arteriotomy is started by creating a 5-mm incision with a #11 scalpel blade. Using an angled Pott's scissors, the arteriotomy is performed beginning in the common carotid artery proximal to the atherosclerotic lesion and extending distally in the internal carotid artery to a point beyond the lesion. Care must be taken not to extend the arteriotomy too far medial, which will cause it to veer into the bifurcation or region of the origin of the external carotid artery. Likewise, making the arteriotomy too far laterally in the internal carotid artery will cause difficulty with subsequent closure.

can be assisted by briefly opening the temporary clip, allowing the tail of the lesion to be removed.

Technically, the most important portion of the plaque to be removed is that within the distal internal carotid artery. Gentle elevation and traction of the plaque will often cause it to break with an even contour or a feathering effect at the distal internal carotid artery transition zone. This maneuver not only removes the remainder of the hemodynamically offending lesion but also prevents an intimal flap from developing. In some instances, the final cleavage of the plaque can be optimized by combining traction and eversion of the plaque as the back wall of the vessel is pushed away (Fig. 8). Transecting the plaque proximal to the end of the arteriotomy makes closure easier and avoids stenosis of the vessel. When the vessel wall is handled, the layers of the wall should not be separated. Rather, the walls should be held together with little pressure, using only wide-grip vascular forceps. Fine sutures should not be picked up or pinched between the jaws of the forceps because this may cause the suture to crimp and weaken.

At this stage in the procedure, the operating microscope is positioned to allow the surgeon and assistant to have unimpeded binocular vision. The internal surface of the carotid artery is carefully inspected. Remaining atheromatous debris is removed, usually by circumferentially stripping it from the medial surface. Small fragments of plaque filaments are likewise removed. The media is inspected proximally but especially distally, where thrombosis-causing intimal flaps are usually located. Rarely, an abrupt transition zone is seen in the distal internal carotid artery, or if the intima adheres loosely to the media, interrupted 8-0 monofilament tacking sutures should be placed.

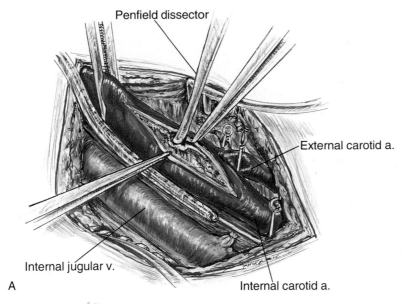

Penfield dissector

External carotid a.

Internal jugular v.

A

Internal carotid a.

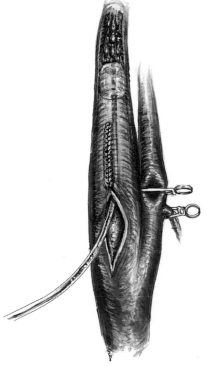

B

Figure 6. A: Following the completion of the arteriotomy and confirming hemostasis, the endarterectomy is begun by finding the correct plane between the arterial wall and the atherosclerotic plaque. This is best accomplished using Penfield #4 instruments, dissecting in a longitudinal direction and circumferentially. **B:** If distal internal carotid artery vascular control is ever lost or is incompletely accessible during the endarterectomy, hemostasis can be achieved with careful insertion of a balloon occlusive catheter.

The luminal surface is inspected in detail using the superior lighting and magnification afforded by the operating microscope (Fig. 9).

Shunting is not performed routinely and is reserved for patients who experience major EEG changes that cannot be reversed by inducing moderate hypertension (vide infra). Both internal (e.g., Sundt) and external (e.g., Javid) shunts have been used successfully. Our recent experience over the last 6 years has shown that only 6% of our patients have required shunting.

Closure

Beginning distally, the arteriotomy is closed with a continuous 6-0 monofilament (Prolene) suture to below the bifurcation. Another 6-0 monofilament

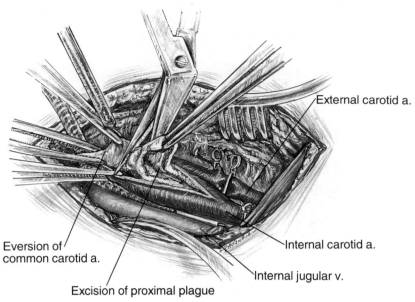

External carotid a.

Eversion of
common carotid a.

Internal carotid a.

Internal jugular v.

Excision of proximal plague

Figure 7. The proximal portion of the plaque is excised using Pott's scissors, allowing the lesion to be grasped and pulled superiorly with a gentle traction so that further dissection in the correct plane is accomplished.

is used starting proximally on the common carotid artery. When the arteriotomy is almost complete and prior to tying the two sutures, backbleeding of the internal and external carotid arteries is accomplished by briefly opening the temporary aneurysm clips. The quality and extent of the backbleeding from the internal carotid artery are important. Poor or no flow often indicates thrombosis at or distal to the operative site. This situation requires immediate reexploration and is usually caused by an unrecognized or insufficiently re-

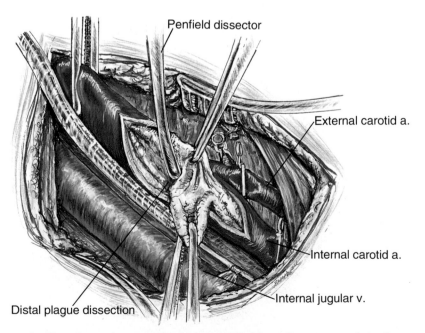

Penfield dissector

External carotid a.

Internal carotid a.

Internal jugular v.

Distal plague dissection

Figure 8. The plaque is everted and transected from its entrance into the superior thyroid and external carotid arteries. The remaining distal portion in the internal carotid artery is dissected free and removed with the intent of creating a smooth or feathering distal transition, avoiding the formation of an intimal flap.

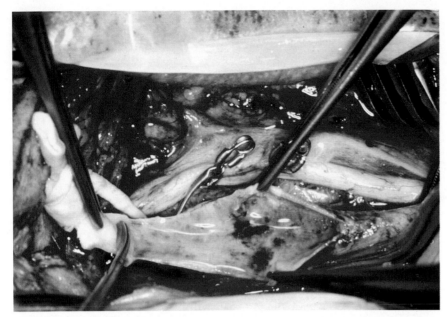

Figure 9. A view through the operating microscope shows the distal plaque in the final stages of removal and the excellent visualization of the luminal surface provided by the superior lighting and magnification of the operating microscope.

paired intimal flap or by a suture grabbing both the anterior and posterior walls of the artery. The superior vision afforded by the operating microscope, however, has made this technical mistake exceedingly rare. In our experience, it occurs significantly less than 1% of the time. Failure to restore acceptable backflow once the sutures are removed implies distal internal carotid artery thrombosis and may necessitate balloon catheter thrombectomy (see Chapter 8).

The common carotid clamp is also opened momentarily to permit any thrombotic or atheromatous material to be expelled through the open lumen. The superior thyroid artery clip is removed permanently. Consequently, the slow, continuous backbleeding pushes trapped air out through the arteriotomy opening or through the small spaces between the sutures. All microsutures must be handled delicately, and crimping must be avoided. Multiple throws are required to hold the knot of this suture. Including only 1 or 2 mm of the cut edge of the artery permits only small bites with each suture to avoid kinking of the vessel (Fig. 10).

After the arteriotomy has been closed, the vessels are deoccluded with a specific rationale in mind (Fig. 11). The external carotid artery is opened first. The common carotid clamp is opened temporarily to permit atheromatous debris, thrombus, or air to wash up the external carotid artery distribution and away from the hemispheric blood supply. Next, the internal carotid artery clip is released momentarily to allow any debris accumulated between the endarterectomy site and the distal internal carotid artery clip to travel by retrograde flow into the external carotid system. The common carotid clamp is permanently removed, finally restoring anterograde flow through the internal carotid artery.

The arteriotomy suture line should be hemostatic except for slight oozing through needle holes or between sutures. Any source of pumping blood or area that does not immediately stop is closed with single, interrupted 6-0 monofilament sutures. Complete hemostasis is attained, and a topical hemostatic agent (Avitene) may be applied to the wound after copious irrigation with a topical antibiotic solution. The blood pressure is brought to or very

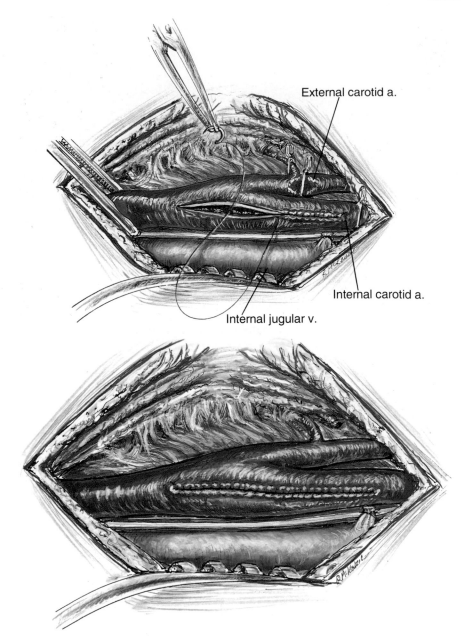

Figure 10. Following completion of the arteriotomy closure, backbleeding and deocclusion is accomplished in the correct manner in an attempt to expel any air or debris either out the lumen or into the external (not internal) carotid artery distribution.

near normal to avoid hypertension-induced intracerebral hemorrhage in a dysautoregulated cerebral hemisphere. The systemic heparinization is not reversed. The wound is closed in two layers with absorbable sutures, and Steristrips are used for the skin.

IMMEDIATE POSTOPERATIVE PERIOD

In the recovery room and during the patient's overnight stay in the intensive care unit, blood pressure must be controlled to avoid hypertension. Hypertension can lead to intracerebral hemorrhage. Conversely, hypoten-

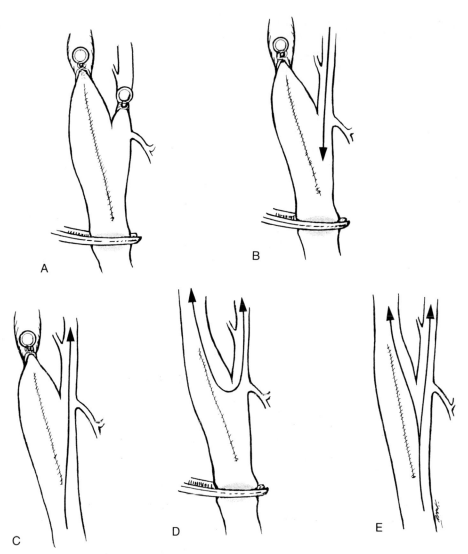

Figure 11. Following arteriotomy completion, deocclusion is best accomplished by the following method. **A:** Careful attention is paid so that the suture line is not handled with forceps and any bipolar coagulation of adventitial bleeding points does not occur near the sutures. In addition, the temporary aneurysm clip on the superior thyroid artery has been previously removed just prior to arteriotomy closure, which causes a constant, low-volume blood backflow through the arteriotomy site. This helps to maintain a full column of fluid and to expel air bubbles. **B:** The external carotid artery is opened to allow any trapped thrombotic or atherosclerotic debris as well as air bubbles caused by retrograde flow to be at least partially removed through the arteriotomy. In addition, this retrograde flow will often reveal any sources of significant leaks in the arteriotomy closure. **C:** With the internal carotid artery still occluded by a temporary aneurysm clip, the vascular clamp on the common carotid artery is opened, allowing a few moments for blood and any proximal debris to flow out through the external carotid system. **D:** With the proximal common carotid artery again temporarily occluded, the clip on the distal internal carotid artery is released, allowing any debris distal to the internal carotid clip to travel back into the external carotid artery by retrograde flow. The maneuver in C is then briefly repeated. **E:** All clips are removed and the common carotid artery is opened, establishing antegrade internal carotid artery flow. Transcranial Doppler monitoring has shown in our experience that embolization into the cerebral circulation is markedly diminished or eliminated by using these maneuvers.

sion can encourage thrombosis at the operative site. Aspirin (650 mg) is administered rectally in the recovery room and then orally each day for an indefinite period. Routine antibiotics are administered for 24 hours.

Invasive cardiac or other monitoring is performed postoperatively as indicated. Many patients who receive intraoperative barbiturates for cerebral protection may experience postoperative respiratory depression, neurologic depression, or both. Usually the latter diminishes rapidly. Even when patients are deeply pharmacologically obtunded, brain stem reflexes are intact, and meaningful movement or a withdrawal pattern to painful stimuli may be seen. Consequently, a basic examination can ordinarily detect focal or localizing findings even at this stage.

In the occasional patient who is initially deeply sedated upon arrival at the recovery room, EEG or transcranial Doppler (TCD) monitoring may be continued until a neurologic examination becomes possible. Of all the methods of postoperative monitoring, TCD gives the earliest warning of impending carotid occlusion, by showing a marked decline in ipsilateral flow velocities (see Chapter 5). Often TCD findings significantly precede other methods of detection, even the clinical neurologic examination, especially in a patient just emerging from a general anesthetic (Fig. 12).

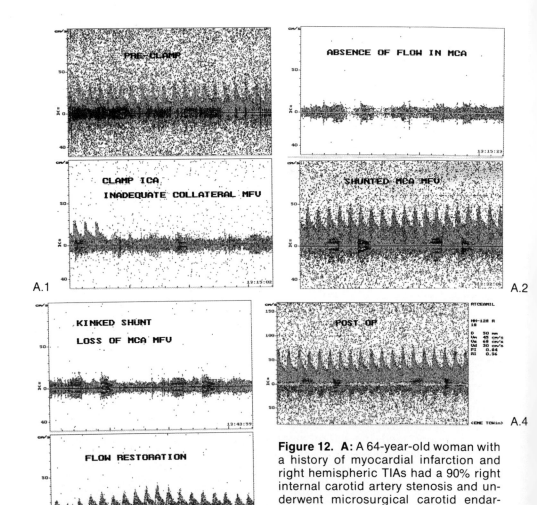

Figure 12. A: A 64-year-old woman with a history of myocardial infarction and right hemispheric TIAs had a 90% right internal carotid artery stenosis and underwent microsurgical carotid endarterectomy. Upon cross-clamping the common carotid artery, an immediate TCD drop occurred from baseline near velocities (right middle cerebral artery preinduction 36 cm/s, postinduction 20 cm/s) to zero measurable flow, indicating grossly inadequate collateral blood supply.

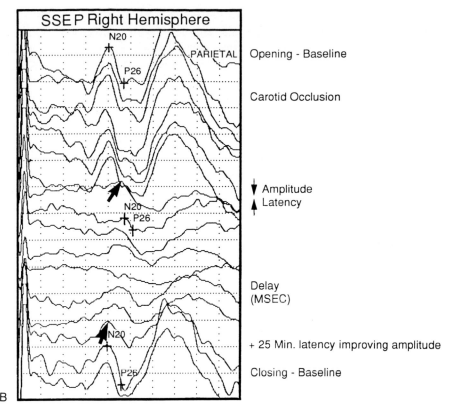

Figure 12. *Continued.* **B:** However, it was not until 5 and 6 minutes later that somatosensory evoked potentials and eight-channel EEG became asymmetric. These early warnings of the TCD allowed preparation for and insertion of an intraluminal shunt. The same technique also readily indicated when external kinking of the shunt occurred, a phenomenon not apparent upon inspection by the surgeon.

Postoperative Care

The postoperative treatment of patients with carotid endarterectomy follows the guidelines for routine postoperative care, but several important aspects are given special consideration. Careful cardiac monitoring and assessment of the patient's cardiac clinical status are stressed in the immediate postoperative period.

We usually maintain the patient in the intensive care unit for at least the first 24 hours after endarterectomy. Invasive monitoring (e.g., arterial blood pressure lines, Swan-Ganz catheters, central venous pressure catheters, saturation monitors) are utilized as indicated (see Chapter 6). Patients who have received significant doses of intraoperative barbiturate (usually more than 1 g of thiopental) are subject to postoperative respiratory depression. This effect usually resolves within several hours. An occasional patient may require intubation and ventilation overnight, and patients are often managed by consulting with specialists in intensive care medicine. Although deep vein thrombosis prophylaxis therapy (subcutaneous heparin) is considered safe for use in the postoperative period, we use it only to treat patients considered to be at high risk.

Patients are mobilized early in the postoperative period and allowed out of bed on the first postoperative day if their general and cardiac condition permits. If patients are otherwise stable, they are transferred from the intensive care unit to a regular care bed on the first postoperative day. Postoperative antiplatelet therapy is continued indefinitely (650 mg aspirin daily), and the patient is allowed a general diet and full ambulatory activity.

During the next 2 days, blood pressure must be monitored closely, particularly as patients become fully ambulatory. Postoperative hypertension, even if mild, should be considered for aggressive treatment. Early postoperative hypertension, especially in patients with preoperative tight carotid stenotic lesions, may predispose patients to postoperative intracerebral hemorrhage. Symptoms such as severe ipsilateral headache, facial pain, or seizures may also herald a cerebral hyperperfusion syndrome and possible intracerebral hemorrhage. During these first postoperative days, the wound is carefully inspected for any evidence of hematoma or infection. If no complicating or extenuating events have occurred, the patient is discharged on the third or fourth postoperative day and followed closely as an outpatient.

CONTROVERSIES IN CAROTID ENDARTERECTOMY

Carotid endarterectomy has been employed widely and has benefited many thousands of patients. It has also been in the center of controversy since its implementation 40 years ago. Recent cooperative studies, particularly the North American Symptomatic Carotid Endarterectomy Trial (NASCET), Veteran Affairs (VA), and European reports, have further defined the role of this procedure and the population it best serves. In particular, symptomatic patients with a high-grade stenosis benefit by a reduction in strokes (28,56,64) (Fig. 13). Nonetheless, surgical complications must be minimized in order for the procedure to improve upon the natural history of the carotid atherosclerotic disease. Patients with cerebral or acute ischemic symptoms originating from the carotid artery are faced with a 7% annual incidence of stroke (48,99,103). The surgical results of the NASCET study included 18 (5.5%) perioperative cerebrovascular events: 12 (3.7%) minor events, 5 (1.5%) major events, and 1 (0.3%) death (64).

Accordingly, many facets of this seemingly straightforward operation have generated debate. These facts can be divided into operative technique variables and differences in perioperative medical and anesthetic management. The following discussion addresses areas of concern, controversy, and vital importance in performing successful carotid endarterectomy.

Carotid Patch Graft

The primary materials that have been used for carotid patch angioplasty are saphenous vein, Dacron, or polytetrafluoroethylene. Autogenous saphenous vein has been the preferred material because of its ease in handling; its relatively antithrombotic properties; and its size, tensile strength, and resistance to infection. Proponents of vein patch carotid angioplasty suggest that this technique enlarges the endarterectomized segment and restores normal contour to the carotid bulb. Immediate postoperative and subsequent flow disturbances are thereby minimized (18,100). It is also thought to prevent intimal hyperplasia (39,97). The saphenous vein interposition graft contains viable endothelium that may reduce thrombogenicity, compared with the otherwise denuded surface present following conventional endarterectomy (94).

Many surgeons have advocated the routine use of saphenous vein patch grafts during carotid endarterectomy to reduce the incidence of postoperative restenosis, which has ranged from 1% to 49% (23,44,89,95). Sundt et al. (89,94) regularly employed saphenous vein interposition graft with excellent success. They believed that the vein angioplasty enlarged the endarterectom-

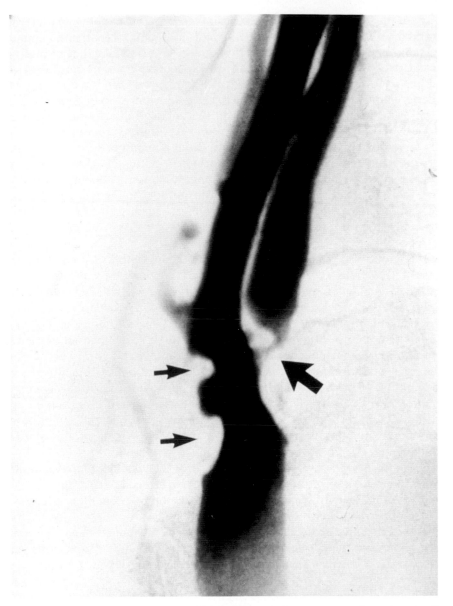

Figure 13. Lateral common carotid angiogram shows a complex ulcer in the distal common carotid and proximal internal carotid origin, resulting in a 95% ulcerative stenosis in a symptomatic patient *(arrows)*.

ized segment and improved the blood flow in this region of the carotid bifurcation. It has been theorized that the saphenous vein interposition graft reorients the configuration of the bifurcation. Consequently, the internal carotid artery becomes the primary extension of the common carotid artery, improving the rheologic characteristics at the operative site (94).

A saphenous vein interposition graft may be most beneficial in the immediate postoperative period, when the potential for thrombosis is highest. Little et al. (53) compared early postoperative intravenous digital subtraction angiograms of 70 cases of conventional carotid endarterectomies with 50 patients who underwent saphenous vein interposition graft endarterectomy. By postoperative angiography, internal carotid artery was consistently larger and the incidence of postoperative thrombosis at the operative site was less in the 50 patients treated with saphenous vein interposition graft endarterectomy. In the conventional endarterectomy group, four patients had internal carotid artery occlusions; two patients had internal, external, and common carotid artery occlusions; and nine patients had various degrees of internal carotid artery stenosis. No patients with saphenous vein interposition graft had postoperative occlusion and only two had stenosis. In the conventional endarterectomy patients with postoperative occlusions who underwent reexplorations, thrombosis was revealed in the angiographically nonvisualized arteries, but no obvious causes were found. Overall, of the six patients in the conventional endarterectomy group, three patients had infarctions that were the main cause of postoperative morbidity. With no occlusions present in the saphenous vein interposition graft endarterectomy patients, the difference was statistically significant and led the authors to recommend the routine use of saphenous vein interposition graft. In this study, the surgical microscope was not used and heparinization was neutralized at the end of the procedure (53).

Other authors have reported similar encouraging benefits from the routine use of a saphenous vein interposition graft, believing that it prevents early thrombosis and late recurrent stenosis (23,44,65,89,94,100). Rosenthal et al. (76), however, retrospectively studied 1,000 consecutive patients who underwent endarterectomy. The patients were divided into four equal groups: 250 patients had a conventional endarterectomy closure, 250 had an expanded polytetrafluoroethylene patch, 250 had a Dacron patch, and 250 had saphenous vein interposition graft. Postoperative patency was documented by B-mode ultrasonography. The difference in the incidence of early or late postoperative stroke and restenosis was not statistically significant among the various methods of arterial closure. The authors recommended saphenous vein interposition graft angioplasty for patients with small arteries and for habitual smokers (76).

By contrast, Hans (39) reported a series of 90 carotid endarterectomies using saphenous vein interposition graft. He performed arteriography at both intermediate (21 months) and late (55 months) follow-up periods. He documented recurrent stenosis in three patients and carotid occlusion in five patients at the intermediate follow-up and recurrent stenosis in an additional three patients at the late follow-up. He thus concluded that saphenous vein interposition graft did not uniformly prevent either early or late postoperative carotid stenosis.

Although studies support both primary suture closure for endarterectomy or saphenous vein interposition graft, the consensus suggests that specific groups of patients may benefit most from saphenous vein interposition graft: patients undergoing reoperation for postoperative recurrent carotid stenosis, patients with unusually small internal carotid arteries (primarily women), patients who have had cervical radiation treatments, patients who are habitual heavy smokers, and patients whose external arterial walls hold sutures poorly. A saphenous vein interposition graft does, however, have disadvantages. It increases operative and carotid cross-clamp time. Postoperatively, the angioplasty segment can balloon, slowing blood flow or causing eddy currents. Such a blood flow pathway can predispose the patient to the formation of mural thrombi and pseudoaneurysms. Vital lower extremity veins, which may later be needed for other arterial reconstruction (e.g., coronary artery bypass) procedures, are often utilized and thus sacrificed. The most dreaded complication of saphenous vein interposition graft angioplasty is rupture of the vein patch, which has been reported in 0.4% to 4.0% of patients. This catastrophic event most often occurs in the first few days after the procedure. Its incidence is increased with hypertension. The associated morbidity and mortality rates, which are high, follow hemorrhagic shock, cerebral ischemia, or airway compression (47,65,74,100).

Our experience suggests that the routine use of saphenous vein interposition graft is unnecessary for microsurgical carotid endarterectomy (86). Although not regularly performed in our patients, postoperative angiography has demonstrated a slight enlargement, not a narrowing, of the endarterectomized segment (Fig. 14). Our low symptomatic early stroke rate of 1% suggests that postoperative patency rates are excellent. It is doubtful that these rates could be improved by saphenous vein interposition graft or synthetic graft angioplasty. We do recommend saphenous vein interposition graft in operations for recurrent carotid stenosis and in extraordinary circumstances such as after cervical radiation for malignancy (Fig. 15).

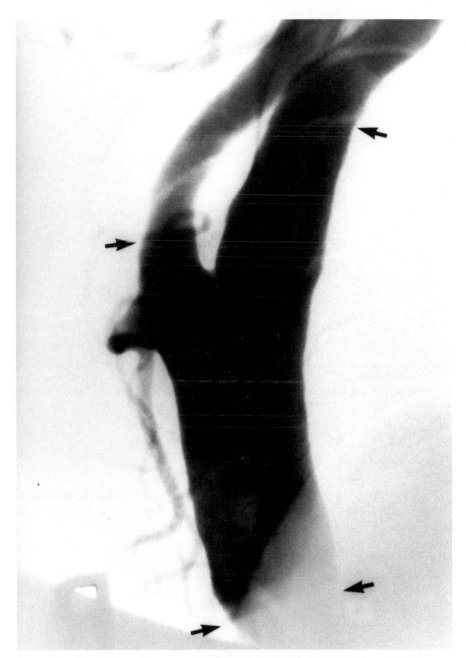

Figure 14. Lateral carotid postoperative angiogram following neurosurgical endarterectomy. By using fine suture and including just the edge of the vessel in the closure, enlargement of the artery is seen postoperatively. The limits of the endarterectomized segment are indicated by the *arrows*. From Spetzler et al., *J Neurosurg* 1986;65:63–73, with permission.

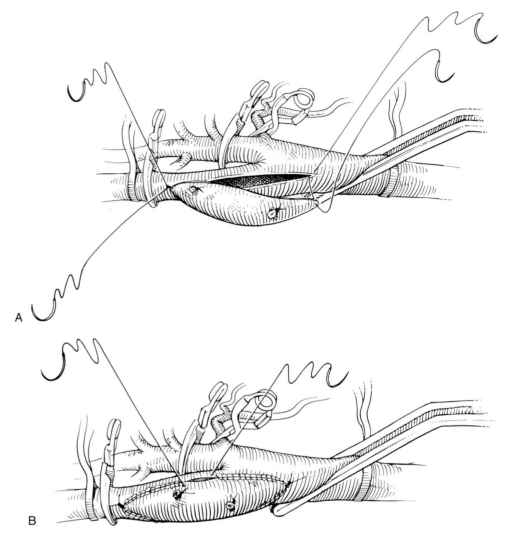

A

B

Figure 15. Although seldom necessary in our series, saphenous vein patch grafts are occasionally necessary, most commonly in redoendarterectomy in our experience. The customary method of inserting a vein patch graft is illustrated here.

Intraoperative Carotid Shunt

The indications for placement of a carotid artery shunt during the period of carotid cross-clamping are also controversial. Many authors believe that the cerebral ischemia induced during the period of carotid cross-clamping is the primary reason for the morbidity associated with the procedure of carotid endarterectomy. Others argue that embolic rather than hemodynamic events cause most cerebral ischemic episodes during carotid endarterectomy. Many surgeons have reported excellent results with the use of intraluminal shunting, believing that the hemodynamic intolerance to carotid cross-clamping is very common (38,72).

During the years that carotid endarterectomy has been performed, surgeons have used various criteria to help determine the need for shunt placement. Sundt et al. (90) measured intraoperative regional cerebral blood flow using extracranial detection of intra-arterially injected xenon 133. Their protocol used shunt insertion for all patients with an occlusion pressure of less than 18 ml/100 g/min. They concluded that with intraoperative carotid occlusion the critical regional cerebral blood flow is approximately 15 ml/100 g/min. Blood flow less than 10 ml/100 g/min during occlusion, which was seen in 8% of their patients, always produced rapid changes in the EEG pattern. Others have used intraoperative measurement of internal carotid artery stump pressures as an indication for shunting; significant ischemia is believed to occur with a mean blood pressure of less than 25 mmHg (45).

Intraoperative temporary carotid shunting is controversial and not without risk. Like many others, we believe that a shunt can produce more problems than benefit (Fig. 16). An intraluminal shunt has several major drawbacks. First, the shunt may allow the embolization of atherosclerotic debris, thrombotic material, or air into the distal cerebral circulation. This phenomenon is often unrecognized by the surgeon until it is detected by changes in the EEG or by a signal change on TCD. At that point, sometimes little can be done to stop further embolization by this route or to reverse the damaging cerebral effects. Second, when inserted into either the common carotid artery or the distal internal carotid artery, the shunt can injure the intimal surface of these vessels. Such an injury can lead to postoperative thrombosis at the operative site. Finally, the presence of a shunt severely limits the surgeon's ability to expose and dissect the atheroma, especially the distal portion. The creation of an intimal flap or the inability to recognize and repair the intima or to remove all of the atherosclerotic debris can contribute to a poor technical outcome. This is true even when the surgical microscope with its improved visualization is utilized. Furthermore, significant periods of ischemia can occur when the shunt is placed and after it is withdrawn, before the arteriotomy closure is completed and carotid cross-clamping is removed. Instances of shunt occlusion and improper placement leading to potential upper extremity ischemia have also occurred (37,101).

Ott et al. (68) conducted a prospective study of 240 patients to determine the effectiveness of carotid endarterectomy performed without shunting. The

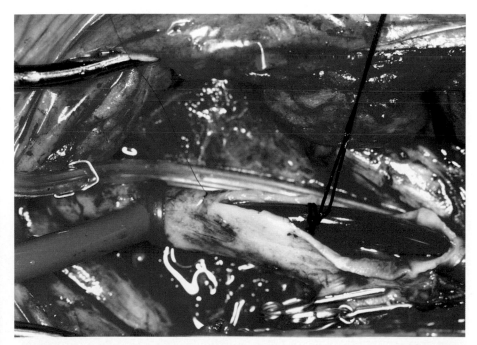

Figure 16. Although seldom utilized during our procedures, carotid artery shunting is vital to successful outcome in cases selected by intraoperative encephalography, TCD, or both. Either external (Javid) or internal (Sundt) shunts are used, the latter pictured here.

incidence of perioperative stroke was 1.3% and the mortality rate was 0.64%, the latter caused by myocardial infarction in two patients. The incidence of permanent neurologic deficit compared favorably with other published series, regardless of whether shunting was used. Furthermore, none of their 102 patients who had either partial or complete occlusion of the contralateral internal carotid artery experienced a postoperative stroke.

Bland et al. (12) reported a series of 280 consecutive carotid endarterectomies performed without using EEG monitoring or an intraluminal shunt. A third of their patients had contralateral stenosis or internal carotid artery occlusion. They believed that adequate cerebral protection was provided by general anesthesia and moderate induced hypertension. Their carotid occlusion time, however, was an average of only 10 minutes. They reported no operative mortality, no strokes in the immediate postoperative period, and only three (1.1%) strokes during the first postoperative month. They concluded that intraluminal shunts and intraoperative monitoring such as EEG and carotid stump pressures are unnecessary, reinforcing the concept that most intraoperative strokes during carotid endarterectomy are embolic in origin.

In 282 consecutive carotid endarterectomies, Ferguson et al. (30) reported that intraoperative stroke occurred in four (1.4%) patients, all of whom were in a small subgroup with a major EEG change and a mean carotid stump pressure of less than 25 mmHg. They concluded that this subgroup of patients is at high risk for hemodynamic stroke and could benefit from shunting.

Halsey (38) reported a multicenter, retrospective study of 1,495 carotid endarterectomy patients in which EEG, regional cerebral blood flow, and TCD were used to determine the ischemic threshold during the period of carotid cross-clamping. The routine use of carotid shunting offered no benefit in neurologic outcome, and he concluded that intraoperative monitoring (TCD less than 40% of baseline flow velocities) could be used to determine the need for selective shunt placement. Sandmann and colleagues (77) conducted a multicenter, randomized, prospective study in 503 patients to assess the need or benefit for routine carotid shunting during endarterectomy. Their overall stroke rate was 4.0%, with the incidence of perioperative stroke not differing significantly between patients who were routinely shunted (4.2%) and those whose endarterectomy was performed without a shunt (3.3%).

Regardless, carotid shunting is an answer to only one problem associated with carotid endarterectomy, that is, cerebral hemodynamic insufficiency. Many other factors, such as technical, embolic, thrombotic, anesthetic, systemic, and experience play a major role besides global cerebral blood flow alone (104).

We believe that in a small subpopulation of carotid endarterectomy patients, temporary carotid artery occlusion will cause hemispheric hypoperfusion that will result in cerebral infarction, and can be corrected by shunt placement. Many patients, however, will respond to moderate induced hypertension, which increases collateral flow. We use a major change in EEG and, more recently, in TCD (mean ipsilateral middle cerebral artery velocity reduced to less than one-third of the preocclusion value) as indications for selective carotid intraluminal shunting, if no response to induced hypertension is seen (38). A recent series by Jansen et al. (46) found that TCD may be more sensitive than EEG in detecting subcortical ischemia and embolic phenomena.

Since instituting this criterion, about 7% of our patients have required intraoperative shunts. None of these patients have experienced a permanent cerebrovascular accident postoperatively. We believe strongly that EEG monitoring, when available, should be used and agree with others that it predicts postoperative deficits accurately (36,93).

OPERATING MICROSCOPE

The operating microscope, which has revolutionized neurologic surgery with its unparalleled visualization and wide range of magnification, is the cornerstone of microsurgical carotid endarterectomy. The size of the operating field can be varied by as much as 12 times that of ordinary operating surgical loupes. The ability to zoom to higher magnification to inspect fine details and to retreat to low degrees of magnification for portions of the procedure such as tying sutures, makes this flexible instrument a mainstay in our surgical protocol. In addition, the operating microscope provides excellent illumination, even in the depths of a wound and in the intraluminal area of the carotid artery.

We use the operating microscope once the gross portion of the atheromatous plaque and intraluminal thrombotic material has been removed. The microscope is then positioned, and the remaining portions of the atheromatous material are removed under high power. The view is unequaled and the luminal surface can be assessed in detail.

Findlay and Lougheed (32) described their technique and results in 60 consecutive patients with symptomatic carotid stenosis who underwent microsurgical carotid endarterectomy. Only one (1.7%) patient suffered a perioperative stroke after common carotid artery occlusion without an obvious cause. Two patients had wound hematomas and three patients had temporary cranial nerve palsies. With an average follow-up of 18 months, no patient experienced a postoperative hemorrhagic or ischemic stroke. One patient died from myocardial infarction 8 months after the endarterectomy. They believed that using the surgical microscope helped to minimize difficulties with the surgical technique (32) (Fig. 17). The benefits of the surgical microscope in the performance of carotid endarterectomy have also been empha-

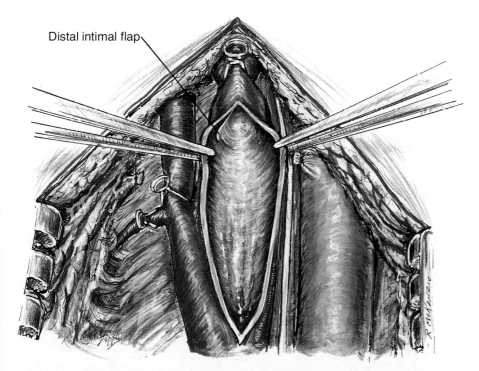

Distal intimal flap

Figure 17. The superior lighting and magnification of the surgical microscope best visualizes the distal transition zone, where an intimal flap usually occurs *(arrows).*

sized by other neurosurgeons (5,34,66,79,86). A previously reported series by the senior author from the Barrow Neurological Institute included 200 consecutive endarterectomies performed in 180 patients using a defined protocol of microsurgical endarterectomy (Fig. 18). Barbiturate protection was used during carotid cross-clamping, the period of potential focal cerebral ischemia. The protocol also included preoperative antiplatelet therapy, barbiturate anesthesia, avoidance of an internal shunt, and strict postoperative control of blood pressure. On the fifth postoperative day, one patient died from a hypertensive cerebral hemorrhage, and two patients suffered postoperative cerebrovascular accidents. The combined permanent morbidity and mortality rate was 1.5% (86). This original series has been expanded, and the results have upheld our opinion that using the operative microscope greatly improves the technical result and ultimate clinical outcome of carotid endarterectomy. The utility of the operating microscope and its ability to improve the manipulation of the diseased artery is highlighted when one realizes that embolic events and technical errors are probably the two leading causes of neurologic morbidity with carotid endarterectomy.

Rosenthal et al. (76) found that two-thirds of the postoperative strokes in their series reflected technical failure: intimal flaps, lateral carotid tears, or carotid clamp injury. The remaining strokes were caused by embolic occlusion of intracranial vessels. Moore et al. (60) described three patients who developed a postoperative neurologic deficit from thromboembolic propagation that originated from an external carotid artery intimal flap. Thrombotic material accumulated in the external carotid artery and passed through the internal carotid artery into the cerebral distribution. This report emphasizes the potential of interaction between the external carotid circulation and the intracranial circulation.

The magnification and illumination of the operating microscope improves the ability to inspect the luminal surface of the external carotid artery. Blaisdell et al. (11) reported that after routine utilization of intraoperative angiography, approximately 25% of the endarterectomized carotid arteries demon-

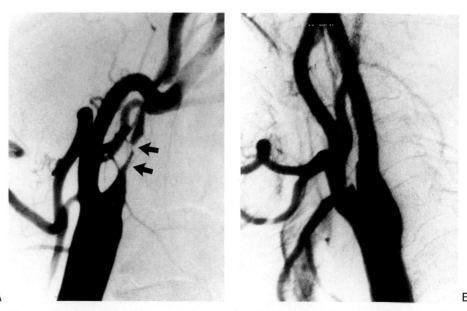

A   B

Figure 18. A: Preoperative angiogram showing a severe long segment stenosis in the proximal internal carotid artery and distal common carotid artery *(arrows)*. **B**: Following microendarterectomy, the postoperative angiogram shows excellent resolution of the severe lesion.

strated a significant technical abnormality that would not have been noted without the operating microscope. They believed that correction of these deficits at the time of the angiography resulted in a 100% late patency rate of their endarterectomy series.

COMPLICATIONS

Postoperative Thrombosis

Thrombosis at the operative site of carotid endarterectomy can occur in the absence of technical errors and can be responsible for serious ischemic complications. The thrombogenic nature of the fresh luminal surface after endarterectomy makes it susceptible to mural thrombosis and/or subsequent embolization. Removal of the atherosclerotic plaque exposes the underlying media and occasionally portions of the adventitial layer. When flow is restored, platelets actively adhere to the underlying collagen (4). Eventually, a pseudoendothelial monolayer of platelets, which is thought to be nonthrombogenic, forms (7,27,70). The adhering platelets release vasoactive substances including adenosine diphosphate and thromboxane A_2, both potent platelet aggregators. Factor XII is activated by the exposed collagen and also initiates the hemostatic cascade that forms a fibrin clot. Platelet factor III, released by the activated platelets, dissipates in the activation of the intrinsic coagulation system (24,50,62). The combination of aggregated platelets, fibrin, and red blood cells constitutes a thrombus at the operative site. This thrombus can fragment with distal embolization. The size of the clot can also continue to increase locally until the vessel is occluded. The clot can also propagate distally. Systemic heparinization prevents the formation of thrombus. Heparin is routinely administered before carotid cross-clamping to prevent intravascular thrombosis and thromboembolism of areas of stasis caused by the carotid occlusion (2,34,36,93). The half-life of heparin is only 90 minutes, and it appears that results are superior if heparinization is not neutralized, because the platelet monolayer can form to protect the exposed elements in the media (24). Some authors have recommended the routine use of postoperative heparin infusion (36). Such a regimen, however, has the potential to cause postoperative hematomas at the operative site and is probably unnecessary.

Platelet inhibitors such as aspirin interfere with normal platelet function by inhibiting the formation of thromboxane A_2 in adenosine diphosphate-induced platelet aggregation (4). Findlay et al. (33) administered a combination of aspirin and dipyridamole or a placebo perioperatively to patients undergoing carotid endarterectomy. Autologous indium III-labeled platelets were injected postoperatively, and platelet collection and deposition were measured at the endarterectomy site. The degree of platelet aggregation and accumulation in the treatment group was significantly reduced compared with the placebo group. Two patients in the control group had postoperative strokes. In one of these patients, a thick, white, mural thrombus, indicative of a platelet clot, was found upon reexploration. None of the patients had a postoperative wound hematoma. They recommended aspirin at a dosage of 300 mg every 8 hours and dipyridamole 75 mg every 8 hours.

Aspirin inhibits the cyclooxygenase system. Dipyridamole interferes with the platelet phosphodiesterase system, elevating the cyclic adenosine monophosphate levels in a synergistic fashion. We have utilized aspirin alone with excellent results. Ercius et al. (27) showed that in canines a single dose of aspirin (10 mg/kg) resulted in the formation of the platelet monolayer, which inhibited thrombus formation at the endarterectomy site. By contrast, doses in the range of 0.5 mg/kg were ineffective.

Antiplatelet treatment may prevent recurrent carotid artery stenosis after an endarterectomy. Degranulated platelets release smooth muscle and fibroblast mitogens with subsequent migration of these elements to the underlying neointima. In many cases, exaggerated or exuberant growth of layers of this neointima may be the origin of recurrent stenosis. This growth is known by terms such as neointimal hyperplasia or fibromuscular hyperplasia (58,96,105). A recent report suggests that aspirin plus dipyridamole was ineffective in reducing the incidence of carotid restenosis when evaluated at 1-year follow-up (41). Hansen et al. (40) likewise noted no difference between treatment with low doses of aspirin (75 mg daily) and a placebo 1 year after carotid endarterectomy. Two months after surgery, 39% of the patients had recurrent carotid artery stenosis of 30% or greater; it also recurred in 42% of patients 6 months after surgery. Greater than 50% stenosis was seen in 9% of patients and 2% had occlusion at the 6-month follow-up.

Bischoff et al. (10) compared antiplatelet therapy with anticoagulation in 328 patients who underwent carotid endarterectomy with a subgroup of patients treated without medication and found no statistically significant difference between the two groups. No difference was seen in their cause of death or in incidence of intracerebral hemorrhage. They concluded that long-term antiaggregant and anticoagulant therapy did not affect the rate of complications or survival after carotid endarterectomy; however, survival was increased in the treated group because the incidence of postoperative myocardial infarction was reduced.

We believe strongly in perioperative antiplatelet therapy. We primarily rely upon aspirin administered about 1 week before surgery and extended indefinitely throughout the postoperative period. As mentioned, aspirin is also administered to the patient rectally in the recovery room immediately after the procedure.

Intracerebral Hemorrhage

Intracerebral hemorrhage is an unusual, although devastating, complication of carotid endarterectomy (8,17,19,93). Postoperative intracerebral hemorrhage, which usually occurs several days after the operation, has been the source of significant morbidity and mortality in series in which operative techniques have otherwise demonstrated great improvements in outcome. The incidence of postoperative intracerebral hemorrhage is thought to be less than 1%. In our series, intracerebral hematoma caused one postoperative morbidity and one death. Bruetman et al. (17) reported that intracerebral hemorrhage complicated 6 of 900 (0.67%) endarterectomies. Spetzler et al. (86) in 1986 reported a 0.5% incidence of postoperative intracerebral hematoma, in one case leading to death. Solomon et al. (84) described 8 patients of 1,930 carotid endarterectomies (0.41%) who sustained a postoperative intracerebral hemorrhage.

Originally, postoperative intracerebral hemorrhage was thought to occur only in patients with preexisting cerebrovascular accidents in which reperfusion of cerebral blood flow to that region could cause hemorrhage into or adjacent to the infarcted zone. In their 1978 review, Caplan et al. (19) described 17 reported cases, all of whom had had preoperative stroke. Two of these patients had severe unilateral carotid stenosis and underwent carotid endarterectomy 4 and 5 weeks after cerebral infarction. Most patients with postoperative intracerebral hemorrhage have a profile of a recent antecedent cerebrovascular accident and preoperative hypertension. Postoperative intracerebral hemorrhage usually occurs in the first few days after surgery and is associated with systemic hypertension. In reported series, these hemorrhages occurred an average of 3 days after surgery and were ipsilateral to the carotid endarterectomy in more than 90% of the cases (16,19,103).

Hypertension often accompanies carotid endarterectomy. Lehv et al. (51) found that mean systolic blood pressure was elevated more than 15 mmHg in 15 of 27 (55%) patients undergoing unilateral carotid endarterectomy. Seven of these patients developed neurologic complications and one died. In one-third of these hypertensive patients, blood pressure was extremely elevated—195 to 250 mmHg systolic and 105 to 130 mmHg diastolic. They believed that postoperative hypertension occurred after the normal carotid sinus reflex was interrupted and therefore was common after bilateral carotid procedures. The absence of other systemic (e.g., retinal, renal, or cardiac) signs of hypertension in some patients suggested that preoperative occult or asymptomatic hypertension did not exist and that a new onset of postoperative hypertension can cause capillary breakdown and hemorrhage (19). Besides recent cerebral infarction and hypertension, transient ischemic attacks and anticoagulation have been regarded as steps contributing to postoperative hemorrhage (13,17,85).

In addition to the risk caused by uncontrolled postoperative hypertension, Sundt (88) documented that postoperative cerebral blood flow increased to the cerebral hemisphere ipsilateral to carotid endarterectomy despite the absence of systemic hypertension. It has been suggested that cerebral hyperperfusion may be symptomatic in certain patients, causing severe headache, facial pain, orbital pain, and paroxysmal lateralizing epileptiform discharges (PLEDs) (25,52,57,58). Brick and colleagues (15) reported a case of a patient who 8 days after endarterectomy developed acute confusion, agitation, and headaches. His work-up disclosed that he had PLEDs and severe angiographic cerebral vasoconstriction. These symptoms subsided in 1 week, did not recur, and were thought to be secondary to impaired cerebral autoregulation. Both focal and generalized seizures have been described in patients with negative computed tomography (CT) scans after carotid endarterectomy (49). Akers et al. (1) found that somnolence, clinical depression, and psychiatric disturbances were present in their postoperative endarterectomy patients. These features were characteristic of patients who had high-grade stenoses corrected and were believed to be secondary to a cerebral hyperperfusion syndrome. These phenomena tended to be self-limited within an 8-week period. Ultrasonography by TCD has been shown to be an effective, accurate, and noninvasive method to document and follow such patients with suspected hyperperfusion until it resolves (7).

Of eight patients with postoperative intracerebral hemorrhage after carotid endarterectomy reported by Solomon and his colleagues (84), six had no evidence of a previous cerebral infarction in the area of the subsequent hemorrhage. Most hemorrhages occurred within the first 5 days of surgery and were not associated with postoperative hypertension. They suggested that a cerebral hyperperfusion syndrome existed in these patients in areas where severe, chronic internal carotid artery stenosis had paralyzed autoregulation of cerebral blood flow. This state is reminiscent of and perhaps has a mechanism similar to that underlying normal perfusion pressure breakthrough after an arteriovenous malformation has been resected (85). In this circumstance, a cerebral blood flow steal causes chronic ischemia in the area surrounding the arteriovenous malformation. The surrounding vessels are in a chronic state of maximal dilatation and have lost the capacity for autoregulation. When the arteriovenous malformation is removed, the surrounding cerebral tissue is unable to react with normal vasoconstriction to a normal perfusion pressure. In certain cases, cerebral hemorrhage or edema can result.

A similar phenomenon has been noted in patients undergoing extracranial-intracranial bypass operations for chronic cerebral ischemia (43). Bernstein et al. (8) reported a 56-year-old normotensive man who underwent carotid endarterectomy to correct a high-grade internal carotid artery stenosis. His immediate postoperative course was normal. The day after surgery, however, he began to experience severe orbital frontal and temporal headaches followed by seizures. These symptoms persisted until the sixth postoperative day, when a massive ipsilateral cerebrovascular accident was heralded by worsening of the headache and orbital pain, vomiting, and hemiplegia. At autopsy, a large hematoma was found in the ipsilateral hemisphere. The small arteries and arterioles throughout that hemisphere showed microscopic pathologic changes consisting of swelling, hyperplasia, hypercellularity and mitosis of endothelial cells, and arterial necrosis with extravasation of erythrocytes and fibrin. All of these changes were consistent with malignant hypertension. Because this patient lacked all other risk factors commonly associated with postoperative hemorrhage, Bernstein et al. (8) suggested that this patient suffered from a chronic diminishment of cerebral perfusion pressure in the circulation of the hemisphere ipsilateral to the severe internal carotid artery stenosis.

Aggressive control of normal or almost normal postoperative blood pressure should be considered if a patient experiences symptoms such as severe orbital or cranial pain, or seizures after an endarterectomy for high-grade carotid stenosis. Although not typically considered a risk factor, antiplatelet therapy may contribute to such events and would probably be best discontinued in this setting. Immediate postoperative hypertension was also common in our patients. We advocate aggressive control of postoperative hypertension and favor a constant infusion of an intravenous antihypertensive agent such as sodium nitroprusside. We have often begun infusion in the operating room in patients who had antecedent hypertension and in those who tended to have hypertension during or at the end of the procedure.

CEREBRAL PROTECTION

The many technical and antecedent facets of carotid endarterectomy are directed at providing a good outcome by protecting cerebral tissue either directly or indirectly. Intraoperatively, the threshold for tolerance of cerebral ischemic is increased by pharmacologic agents; the most common are barbiturates. Barbiturates are used widely in cerebrovascular surgery, during both carotid endarterectomy and periods of temporary cerebral arterial occlusion, particularly in aneurysm surgery.

Barbiturates provide cerebral protection because of a reversible, dose-dependent depression of cerebral blood flow and, ultimately, of the cerebral metabolic rate (78,80,92). Once the EEG reaches an isoelectric state, barbiturates have reduced cerebral blood flow and the cerebral metabolic rate of oxygen by about 50%. This effect is more prominent in the nonischemic portions of the brain (78,79,80,92). The vasoconstriction of the normal portions of the brain is thought to improve cerebral blood flow to the ischemic areas (31). Barbiturates may also decrease the rate of edema formation. By reducing cerebral blood flow and cerebral blood volume, barbiturates also reduce intracranial pressure. Barbiturates may also serve as free radical scavengers and reduce the production of free fatty acids from damaged cells (22,81).

Although the exact mechanism of barbiturate cerebral protection in the setting of arterial occlusion is probably multifactorial and incompletely understood, it is clear that these agents can modify or prevent cerebral damage secondary to focal ischemia (61,80). Laboratory experience with a primate model has demonstrated that prior administration of barbiturates provides dramatic cerebral protection for as long as 6 hours of middle cerebral artery occlusion (63,79,80). This degree of cerebral protection far surpasses that provided by other general anesthetic agents. Barbiturates administered after the onset of cerebral ischemia are not believed to provide protection and may, in fact, be deleterious, especially in the presence of a permanent vascular occlusion (20,78).

The disadvantages of barbiturate use are intraoperative hypotension, myocardial depression, and a prolonged wakeup period postoperatively in selected patients. With the use of vasopressor agents and intravenous volume expansion, intraoperative hypotension has not been a problem. In patients with severe myocardial dysfunction, the anesthesiologist may be concerned that the cardiovascular effects of barbiturates could be overwhelming or detrimental. In such cases, we have used etomidate with excellent results. Etomidate is a short-acting intravenous anesthetic agent that induces a reversible, dose-dependent reduction in the cerebral metabolic rate. The EEG effects of etomidate are similar to the characteristics of barbiturates: isoelectric EEG pattern is associated with about a 50% decrease in the cerebral metabolic rate of oxygen. The cardiovascular depressive affects of etomidate are likely insignificant (59). We have used this drug safely and efficaciously during carotid endarterectomy, as others have for temporary cerebral arterial occlusion (6).

We find that the addition of barbiturate therapy for cerebral protection provides an opportunity for the surgeon to perform a precise and relaxed endarterectomy, including the time needed for complicated arterial reconstruction. In our series, the administration of barbiturates was both feasible and safe.

RESULTS IN OUR SERIES

To be successful and efficacious, the results of carotid endarterectomy must exceed the natural history of symptomatic carotid atherosclerotic disease. We believe that our endarterectomy protocol, employed prospectively, has demonstrated this with favorable results including a minimum of neurologic sequelae.

The initial results of the senior author (R.F.S.) were reported in 1986 and included 200 consecutive endarterectomies performed under the protocol emphasizing for the first time the following facets: (a) utilization of the operating microscope to complete the removal of the atherosclerotic plaque and fine suture material to close the arteriotomy without attendant stenosis; (b) nonutilization of an intraluminal carotid shunt except when indicated by a major EEG change; (c) cerebral protection by barbiturate administration during the period of carotid cross-clamping; (d) perioperative aspirin therapy and full systemic heparinization without reversal; and (e) strict control of blood pressure postoperatively to prevent hypertension with its associated risk of intracerebral hemorrhage. The mean age of the patients was 64 years. They had a history of heart disease (64%), hypertension (58%), tobacco use (56%), or diabetes mellitus (12%). Most patients (93%) were symptomatic and presented with either TIAs (81%) or amaurosis fugax (12%). The incidence of transient nonischemic complications was 8% and included recurrent laryngeal nerve palsy (3.5%), 12th nerve paresis (1.5%), wound hematoma (1.5%), parotid fistula (1%), and wound infection (0.5%).

Ischemic complications included two new postoperative strokes (1.0%). In one patient, a Sundt grade 4, the presentation was that of stroke-in-evolution, and an acute complete internal carotid artery occlusion was found at the time of endarterectomy. The internal carotid was patent at the conclusion of surgery; however, poor backflow was seen. Postoperatively, the patient had a completed stroke, and digital subtraction angiography showed a complete occlusion. It was felt that the poor backflow and occlusion was secondary to carotid siphon disease and he was not returned to surgery. The other perioperative stroke in this series was in a Sundt grade 3 patient who had a normal carotid and cerebral angiogram and cerebral CT scan postoperatively (Fig. 19).

Only one death occurred in this initial series, in an elderly, hypertensive patient with a preocclusive carotid lesion and a contralateral complete internal carotid occlusion. Her initial uneventful postoperative course was complicated by a massive ipsilateral hypertensive intracerebral hemorrhage on the fourth day following surgery.

From 1987 to 1993, an additional 327 carotid endarterectomies have been performed at the Barrow Neurological Institute and Allegheny General Hospital using the identical prospective protocol of the microsurgical technique and associated features for brain protection as described above. Most of the patients [275 (84.1%)] were symptomatic for hemispheric, retinal, or both types of ischemia, whereas 52 endarterectomies (15.9%) were performed in asymptomatic patients. Hemispheric dysfunction was seen approximately five times as frequently as retinal ischemic symptoms. Associated medical illnesses included coexistent coronary artery disease in 53%, hypertension in 48%, tobacco use in 45%, and diabetes mellitus in 10% of patients.

Emergency endarterectomies were performed in 42 (12.8%) patients for either progressive neurologic deterioration or a fluctuating neurologic examination. Transient nonischemic complications consisted of recurrent laryngeal palsy in 9 (2.8%) patients, wound hematomas in 6 (1.8%) patients, wound superficial infection in 5 (1.5%) patients, 12th nerve paresis in 4 (1.2%) patients, and parotid fistula in 1 (0.3%) patient.

Transient postoperative neurologic deficit was observed in four (1.2%) patients, consisting of hemispheric dysfunction in two and partial facial weakness in two patients, all of which resolved in the initial postoperative follow-up period. Strokes occurred in four (1.2%) patients in this series of 327 endarterectomies and were detected immediately following surgery in three patients. The fourth patient was a 67-year-old hypertensive woman who had an uneventful operation but who sustained a 2-cm nondominant parietal hemorrhage on the fourth postoperative day. This caused no motor or sensory deficit but seizures were present, requiring long-term anticonvulsant therapy. Intraluminal shunting, recently performed with slightly greater frequency using the sensitive indicator TCD, was used in 23 (7.0%) of patients in this second series. Three postoperative myocardial infarctions occurred, and one of these patients required insertion of an intra-aortic balloon afterload reduction pump device. Four patients in this series died, not of neurologic causes but of underlying cardiopulmonary disease.

Table 1. *Transient nonischemic postoperative complications in Barrow Neurological Institute/Allegheny General Hospital series of 527 carotid endarterectomies*

Complication	Cases	
	No.	%
Recurrent laryngeal palsy	16	3.0
Wound hematoma	9	1.7
Wound infection	6	1.1
12th nerve paresis	7	1.3
Parotid fistula	3	0.6
Total	41	7.8

Table 2. *Ischemic postoperative complications in Barrow Neurological Institute/Allegheny General Hospital series of 527 carotid endarterectomies*

	Cases	
Complication	No.	%
Transient ischemic attack	8	1.5
Cerebrovascular accident	6	1.1
Death, hypertensive bleed 4 days postoperatively	1	0.2
Cardiorespiratory[a]	4	0.8

[a] Nonneurological death.

Combining the recent and earlier series for the authors yields a total of 527 patients done prospectively with this protocol. Ischemic symptoms were seen in 461 (87%) patients, whereas 66 (13%) procedures were done prophylactically. Intraluminal shunting, based primarily on EEG (TCD also in recent cases) indications, was performed in 27 (5.1%) of cases. Forty-one (7.8%) transient, nonischemic complications were seen (Table 1).

Neurologic complications included transient ischemic symptoms in eight (1.5%) patients, all of which resolved without sequelae. Permanent cerebrovascular accident was seen in 6 patients, 1.1% of the total series of 527 patients. Death of neurologic origin occurred in one of the five (0.9%) patients, who died (Table 2).

CONCLUSIONS

Since its inception, carotid endarterectomy has been both popular and controversial. Its efficacy and benefit, however, have been demonstrated by the recently published cooperative studies. The relative risks of the proce-

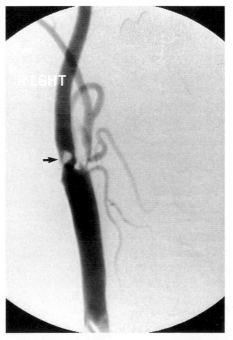

Figure 19. Lateral carotid angiogram in a patient with a minor stroke syndrome shows the appearance of minimal stenosis but a typical angiographic appearance of a thrombus. Despite his stroke several days prior, he underwent successful microsurgical endarterectomy. At the time of surgery, a large thrombus and atherosclerotic plaque were found at the internal carotid artery origin.

Table 3. *Mayo Clinic classification of preoperative risk*

Grade	Features
I	Neurologically stable (no neurologic risk factors)
	No major medical risks
	No angiographically determined risks
	Unilateral or bilateral ulcerative-stenotic disease
II	Significant angiographically determined risks
	Neurologically stable
	No major medical risks
III	Major medical risks
	Neurologically stable
	With/without significant angiographically determined risks
IV	Major neurologic risks
	With/without major medical risks
	With/without angiographically determined risks

Data from Sundt et al., *Adv Neurol* 1977; 16:97–119 and *Mayo Clin Proc* 1975; 50:301–306.

Table 4. *Preoperative risk factors for carotid endarterectomy*

Neurologic	Medical	Angiographic
	Age >70 years	Extensive internal carotid artery involvement
Progressive deficit	Severe hypertension	Opposite internal carotid artery occlusion
Deficit <24 hours	Chronic obstructive pulmonary disease	Internal carotid artery siphon stenosis
	Myocardial infarction within 6 mo	Soft thrombus in ulceration
Multi-infarct deficit Frequent TIAs	Angina pectoris	High bifurcation, thick neck

dure vary, depending on many factors, including the patient's medical and neurologic condition, the status of the carotid, and the direct and collateral cerebral circulation. This latter information is readily determined from preoperative angiography. All these factors are considered within the classification scheme of risk proposed by Sundt (Table 3). Many technical factors such as the patient's size, the level of the carotid bifurcation, and the extent of the atherosclerotic lesion, together with the neurologic, medical and angiographic assessments, help to determine the likelihood of success or failure (Table 4). Besides the many patient factors that influence the risk of carotid endarterectomy and frequency of complicating cerebrovascular accidents, the experience of the operating surgeon, participating nursing personnel, intensive care unit, and supporting staff likewise contribute to the ability to achieve lower morbidity and mortality rates.

We believe that our protocol, as described here (including extensive preoperative medical and cardiac evaluation, the intraoperative use of systemic heparinization without reversal, microsurgical endarterectomy, EEG monitoring with selective shunting for major EEG change, barbiturate cerebral protection, and perioperative antiplatelet therapy), can result in favorable surgical outcomes.

ACKNOWLEDGMENTS

We would like to thank Karl A. Greene, MD, PhD, for his help in putting together the data for this chapter.

REFERENCES

1. Akers DL, Brinker MR, Engelhardt TC, et al. Postoperative somnolence in patients after carotid endarterectomy. *Surgery* 1990;107:684–687.
2. Allen GS, Preziosi TJ. Carotid endarterectomy: a prospective study of its efficacy and safety. *Medicine* 1981;60:298–309.
3. Archie JP, Green JJ. Saphenous vein rupture pressure, rupture stress, and carotid endarterectomy vein patch reconstruction. *Surgery* 1990;107:389–396.
4. Bailes JE, Quigley MR, Kwaan HC, et al. The effects of intravenous prostacyclin in a model of microsurgical thrombosis. *Microsurgery* 1988;9:2–9.
5. Barrow DL, Mizuno J. Carotid endarterectomy: technical aspects and perioperative management. In: Awad IA, ed. *Cerebrovascular occlusive disease and brain ischemia.* Chicago: American Association of Neurological Surgeons; 1992:162–185.
6. Batjer HH, Frankfurt AI, Purdy PD, et al. Use of etomidate, temporary arterial occlusion, and intraoperative angiography in surgical treatment of large and giant cerebral aneurysms. *J Neurosurg* 1988;68:234–240.
7. Baumgartner HR, Haudenschild C. Adhesion of platelets to subendothelium. *Ann NY Acad Sci* 1972;201:22–36.
8. Bernstein M, Fleming JFR, Deck JHN. Cerebral hyperperfusion after carotid endarterectomy: a cause of cerebral hemorrhage. *Neurosurgery* 1984;15:50–56.
9. Bhatti SU, Selman WR, Lust WD, et al. Techniques of cerebral protection. *Neurosurgery* 1992;1:197–213.
10. Bischoff G, Pratschner T, Kail M, et al. Anticoagulants, antiaggregants or nothing following carotid endarterectomy? *Eur J Vasc Surg* 1993;7:364–369.
11. Blaisdell FW, Lim R, Hall AD. Technical result of carotid endarterectomy: arteriographic assessment. *Am J Surg* 1962;114:239–246.
12. Bland JE, Lazar ML. Carotid endarterectomy without shunt. *Neurosurgery* 1981;8:153–157.
13. Bland JE, Chapman RD, Wylie EJ. Neurological complications of carotid artery surgery. *Ann Surg* 1970;171:459–464.
14. Boysen G. Cerebral hemodynamics in carotid surgery. *Acta Neurol Scand* 1973;49[Suppl 52]:59–60.
15. Brick JF, Dunker RO, Gutierreg AR. Cerebral vasoconstriction as a complication of carotid endarterectomy. *J Neurosurg* 1990;73:151–153.
16. Browne TR, Poskanzer DC. Treatment of strokes (first of two parts). *N Engl J Med* 1969;281:594–602.
17. Bruetman ME, Fields WS, Crawford ES, et al. Cerebral hemorrhage in carotid artery surgery. *Arch Neurol* 1963;9:458–467.
18. Callow AD. Discussion of Rosenthal D, Stanton PE, Lamis PA. Carotid endarterectomy: the unreliability of intraoperative monitoring in patients having stroke or reversible ischemic neurologic defects. *Arch Surg* 1981;116:1569–1573.
19. Caplan LR, Skillman J, Ojemann R, et al. Intracerebral hemorrhage following carotid endarterectomy: a hypertensive complication? *Stroke* 1978;9:457–460.
20. Corkill G, Chikovani OK, McLeish I, et al. Timing of pentobarbital administration for brain protection in experimental stroke. *Surg Neurol* 1976;5:147–149.
21. Crowell RM, Ojemann RG. Results and complications of carotid endarterectomy. In Smith RR, ed. *Stroke and the extracranial vessels.* New York: Raven Press; 1984:203–212.
22. Demopoulos HB, Flamm ES, Seligman ML, et al. Antioxidant effects of barbiturates in model membranes undergoing free radical damage. *Acta Neurol Scand Suppl* 1977;64:152–153.
23. Deriu GP, Ballotta E, Bonavina L, et al. The rationale for patch-graft angioplasty after carotid endarterectomy: early and long-term follow-up. *Stroke* 1984;15:972–979.
24. Dirrenberger RA, Sundt TM Jr. Carotid endarterectomy: temporal profile of the healing process and effects of anticoagulation therapy. *J Neurosurg* 1978;48:201–219.
25. Dolan JG, Mushlin AI. Hypertension, vascular headaches, and seizures after carotid endarterectomy. Case report and therapeutic considerations. *Arch Intern Med* 1984;144:1489–1491.
26. Dunsker SB. Complications of carotid endarterectomy. *Clin Neurosurg* 1976;23:336–341.
27. Ercius MS, Chandler WF, Ford JW, et al. Early versus delayed heparin reversal after carotid endarterectomy in the dog. A scanning electron microscopy study. *J Neurosurg* 1983;58:708–713.
28. European Carotid Surgery Trialists Collaborative Group. MRC European Carotid Surgery Trial: interim results for symptomatic patients with severe (70–99%) or with mild (0–29%) carotid stenosis. *Lancet* 1991;337:1235–1243.
29. Ferguson GG. Extracranial carotid artery surgery. *Clin Neurosurg* 1982;29:543–574.
30. Ferguson GG, Blume WT, Farras JK. Carotid endarterectomy: an evaluation of results in 282 consecutive cases in relationship to intraoperative monitoring. Abstract 54, Program of Annual Meeting of the American Association of Neurologic Surgeons, Atlanta, April 23, 1985.
31. Feustel PJ, Ingvar MC, Severinghaus JW. Cerebral oxygen availability and blood flow during middle cerebral artery occlusion: effects of pentobarbital. *Stroke* 1981;12:858–863.
32. Findlay JM, Lougheed WM. Carotid microendarterectomy. *Neurosurgery* 1993;32:792–798.

33. Findlay JM, Lougheed WM, Gentill F, et al. Effect of perioperative platelet inhibition on postcarotid endarterectomy mural thrombus formation. *J Neurosurg* 1985;63:693–698.

34. Giannotta L, Dicks RE, Kindt GW. Carotid endarterectomy: technical improvements. *Neurosurgery* 1980;7:309–312.

35. Green RM, Messick WJ, Ricotta JJ, et al. Benefits, shortcomings, and costs of EEG monitoring. *Ann Surg* 1985;201:785–791.

36. Gross CE, Adams HP Jr, Sokoll MD, et al. Use of anticoagulants, electroencephalographic monitoring, and barbiturate cerebral protection in carotid endarterectomy. *Neurosurgery* 1981;9:1–5.

37. Gumerlock MK, Neuwelt EA. Carotid endarterectomy: to shunt or not to shunt. *Stroke* 1988;19:1485–1490.

38. Halsey JH. Risks and benefits of shunting in carotid endarterectomy. *Stroke* 1992;23: 1583–1587.

39. Hans SS. Late follow-up of carotid endarterectomy with venous patch angioplasty. *Am J Surg* 1991;162:50–54.

40. Hansen F, Lindblad B, Persson NH, et al. Can recurrent stenosis after carotid endarterectomy be prevented by low-dose acetylsalicylic acid? A double-blind, randomized and placebo-controlled study. *Eur J Vasc Surg* 1993;7:380–385.

41. Harker LA, Bernstein EF, Dilley RB, et al. Failure of aspirin plus dipyridamole to prevent restenosis after carotid endarterectomy. *Ann Intern Med* 1992;116:731–736.

42. Hays RJ, Levinson SA, Wylie EJ. Intraoperative measurement of carotid back pressure as a guide to operative management for carotid endarterectomy. *Surgery* 1972;72: 953–960.

43. Heros RC, Scott RM, Kistler JP, et al. Temporary neurological deterioration after extracranial-intracranial bypass. *Neurosurgery* 1984;15:178–185.

44. Hertzer NR, Beven EG, O'Hara PJ, et al. A prospective study of vein patch angioplasty during carotid endarterectomy. Three-year results for 801 patients and 917 operations. *Ann Surg* 1987;206:628–635.

45. Hunter GC, Sieffert G, Malone JM, et al. The accuracy of carotid back pressure as an index for shunt requirements: a reappraisal. *Stroke* 1981;13:319–326.

46. Jansen C, Vriens EM, Eikelboom BC, et al. Carotid endarterectomy with transcranial Doppler and electroencephalographic monitoring. A prospective study in 130 operations. *Stroke* 1993;24:665–669.

47. John TG, Bradbury AW, Ruckley CV. Vein-patch rupture after carotid endarterectomy: an avoidable catastrophe. *Br J Surg* 1993;80:852–853.

48. Kannel WB, Wolf PA, Verter J. Risk factors for stroke. In Smith RR, ed. *Stroke and the extracranial vessels.* New York: Raven Press; 1984:47–58.

49. Kieburtz K, Ricotta JJ, Moxley RT. Seizures following carotid endarterectomy. *Arch Neurol* 1990;568–570.

50. Kinlough-Rathbone RL, Packham MA, Reimers HJ, et al. Mechanism of platelet shape change, aggregation and release induced by collagen, thrombin, or A23, 187. *J Lab Clin Med* 1977;90:707–719.

51. Lehv MS, Salzman EW, Silen W. Hypertension complicating carotid endarterectomy. *Stroke* 1970;1:307–313.

52. Leviton A, Caplan L, Salzman E. Severe headache after carotid endarterectomy. *Headache* 1975;15:207–210.

53. Little JR, Bryerton BS, Furlan AJ. Saphenous vein patch grafts in carotid endarterectomy. *J Neurosurg* 1984;61:743–747.

54. Lord SA, Raj TB, Graham AR. Carotid endarterectomy, siphon stenosis, collateral hemispheric pressure, and perioperative cerebral infarction. *J Vasc Surg* 1987;6:391–397.

55. Lusby RJ, Wylie EJ. Complications of carotid endarterectomy. *Surg Clin North Am* 1983; 63:1293–1302.

56. Mayberg MR, Wilson SE, Yatsu F, et al. for the Veteran Affairs Cooperative Studies Program 309 Trialists Group. Carotid endarterectomy and prevention of cerebral ischemia in symptomatic carotid stenosis. *JAMA* 1991;266:3289–3294.

57. Messert B, Black JA. Cluster headache, hemicrania, and other head pains: morbidity of carotid endarterectomy. *Stroke* 1978;9:559–562.

58. Metke MP, Lie JT, Fuster V. Reduction of intimal thickening in canine coronary bypass vein grafts with dipyridamole and aspirin. *Am J Cardiol* 1979;43:1144–1148.

59. Milde LN, Milde JH, Michenfelder JD. Cerebral functional, metabolic, and hemodynamic effects of etomidate in dogs. *Anesthesiology* 1985;63:371–377.

60. Moore WS, Martello JY, Quinones-Baldrich WJ, et al. Etiologic importance of the intimal flap of the external carotid artery in the development of postcarotid endarterectomy stroke. *Stroke* 1990;21:1497–1502.

61. Moseley JI, Laurent JP, Molinari GF. Barbiturate attenuation of the clinical course and pathological lesions in a primate stroke model. *Neurology* 1975;25:870–874.

62. Mustard JF, Jorgenson L, Hovig T, et al. Role of platelets in thrombosis. *Thromb Diath Haemorrh* 1966;21[Suppl]:131–158.

63. Nehls D, Todd M, Spetzler RF, et al. A comparison of the cerebral protective effects of isoflurane and barbiturates during temporary focal ischemia in primates. *Anesthesiology* 1987;66:453–464.

64. North American Symptomatic Carotid Endarterectomy Trial Collaborations. Beneficial effect of carotid endarterectomy in symptomatic patients with high-grade carotid stenosis. *N Engl J Med* 1991;325:445–453.

65. O'Hara PJ, Hertzer NR, Krajewski LP, et al. Saphenous vein patch rupture after carotid endarterectomy. *J Vasc Surg* 1992;15:504–509.
66. Ojemann RG. Comment on Bland JE, Logan ML. Carotid endarterectomy without shunt. *Neurosurgery* 1981;8:156–157.
67. Ojemann RG, Crowell RM, Roberson GH, et al. Surgical treatment of extracranial carotid occlusive disease. *Clin Neurosurg* 1975;22:214–263.
68. Ott DA, Cooley DA, Chapa L, et al. Carotid endarterectomy without temporary intraluminal shunt. *Ann Surg* 1980;191:708–714.
69. Perdue GD. Management of postendarterectomy neurologic deficits. *Arch Surg* 1982;117: 1079–1081.
70. Plecha FR, Pories WJ. Intraoperative angiography in the immediate assessment of arterial reconstruction. *Arch Surg* 1972;105:902–907.
71. Powers AD, Smith RR. Hyperperfusion syndrome after carotid endarterectomy: a transcranial Doppler evaluation. *Neurosurgery* 1990;26:56–60.
72. Quinones-Baldrich WJ, Moore WS. Intraoperative monitoring and use of the internal shunt during carotid endarterectomy. *Int Surg* 1984;69:207–213.
73. Reith HB, Edelmann M, Reith C. Spontaneous intracerebral hemorrhage following carotid endarterectomy. Experience of 328 operations from 1983–1988. *Int Surg* 1992;77:224–225.
74. Riles TS, Imparato AM, Mintzer R, et al. Comparison of results of bilateral and unilateral carotid endarterectomy five years after surgery. *Surgery* 1982;91:258–262.
75. Riles TS, Lamparello PJ, Giangola G, et al. Rupture of the vein patch: a rate complication of carotid endarterectomy. *Surgery* 1990;107:10–12.
76. Rosenthal D, Archie JJP, Garcia-Rinaldi R, et al. Carotid patch angioplasty: immediate and long-term results. *J Vasc Surg* 1990;12:326–333.
77. Sandmann W, Kolvenback R, Willeke F. Risks and benefits of shunting in carotid endarterectomy [Letter]. *Stroke* 1993;24:1098.
78. Selman WR, Spetzler RF, Jackson D, et al. Regional cerebral blood flow following middle cerebral artery occlusion and barbiturate therapy in baboons. *J Cereb Blood Flow Metab* 1981;1[Suppl 1]:214–215.
79. Selman WR, Spetzler RF, Roessman UR, et al. Barbiturate-induced coma therapy for focal cerebral ischemia. Effects after temporary and permanent MCA occlusion. *J Neurosurg* 1981;55:220–226.
80. Selman WR, Spetzler RF, Roski RA, et al. Barbiturate coma in focal cerebral ischemia. relationship of protection to timing of therapy. *J Neurosurg* 1982;56:685–690.
81. Shiu GK, Nemoto FM. Barbiturate attenuation of brain free fatty acid liberation during global ischemia. *J Neurochem* 1981;37:1448–1456.
82. Sieber FE, Toung TJ, Diringer MN, et al. Preoperative risks predict neurological outcome of carotid endarterectomy related stroke. *Neurosurgery* 1992;30:847–854.
83. Simeone FA, Frazer G, Lawner P. Ischemic brain edema: comparative effects of barbiturates and hypothermia. *Stroke* 1979;10:8–12.
84. Solomon RA, Loftus CM, Quest DO, et al. Incidence and etiology of intracerebral hemorrhage following carotid endarterectomy. *J Neurosurg* 1986;64:29–34.
85. Spetzler RF, Wilson CB, Weinstein P, et al. Normal perfusion pressure breakthrough theory. *Clin Neurosurg* 1978;25:651–672.
86. Spetzler RF, Martin N, Hadley MN, et al. Microsurgical endarterectomy under barbiturate protection: a prospective study. *J Neurosurg* 1986;65:63–73.
87. Strawn DJ, Hunter GC, Guernsey JM, et al. The relationship of intraluminal shunting to technical results after carotid endarterectomy. *J Cardiovasc Surg* 1990;31:424–429.
88. Sundt TM Jr. The ischemic tolerance of neural tissue and the need for monitoring and selective shunting during carotid endarterectomy. *Stroke* 1983;14:93–98.
89. Sundt TM Jr. *Occlusive cerebrovascular disease: diagnosis and surgical management.* Philadelphia: WB Saunders; 1987.
90. Sundt TM Jr, Sandok BA, Whisnant JP. Carotid endarterectomy: complications and preoperative assessment of risk. *Mayo Clin Proc* 1975;50:301–306.
91. Sundt TM Jr, Houser OW, Sharbrough FW, et al. Carotid endarterectomy: results, complications, and monitoring techniques. *Adv Neurol* 1977;16:97–119.
92. Sundt TM Jr, Anderson RE, Michenfelder JD. Intracellular redox states under halothane and barbiturate anesthesia in normal, ischemic, and anoxic monkey brain. *Ann Neurol* 1979;5:575–579.
93. Sundt TM, Sharbrough FW, Piepgras DG, et al. Correlation of cerebral blood flow and electroencephalographic changes during carotid endarterectomy. *Mayo Clin Proc* 1981; 56:533–543.
94. Sundt TM, Whisnant JP, Houser OW, et al. Prospective study of the effectiveness and durability of carotid endarterectomy. *Mayo Clin Proc* 1990;65:625–635.
95. Tempelhoff R, Modica PA, Grubb RL, et al. Selective shunting during carotid endarterectomy based on two-channel computerized electroencephalographic/compressed spectral array analysis. *Neurosurgery* 1989;24:339–344.
96. Thomas M, Otis SM, Rush M, et al. Recurrent carotid artery stenosis following endarterectomy. *Ann Surg* 1984;200:74–79.
97. Thompson JE. Carotid endarterectomy. In Najarian JS, Delaney JP, eds. *Vascular surgery.* New York: Stratton; 1988:333–341.
98. Thompson JE, Austin DJ, Patman RD. Carotid endarterectomy for cerebrovascular insufficiency: long-term results in 592 patients followed up to thirteen years. *Ann Surg* 1970; 172:663–679.

99. Toole JF, Janeway R, Choik, et al. Transient ischemic attacks due to atherosclerosis. A prospective study of 160 patients. *Arch Neurol* 1975;32:5–12.
100. Van Dammer H, Grenade T, Creemers E, et al. Blowout of carotid venous patch angioplasty. *Ann Vasc Surg* 1991;5:542–544.
101. Waring PH, Kraftson DA. Another complication of carotid artery shunting during endarterectomy [Letter]. *Anesthesiology* 1990;72:1099.
102. Whisnant JP, Matsumoto N, Elveback LR. Transient cerebral ischemic attacks in a community. Rochester, Minnesota, 1955 through 1969. *Mayo Clin Proc* 1973;48:194–198.
103. Wylie EJ, Hein MF, Adams JE. Intracranial hemorrhage following surgical revascularization for treatment of acute strokes. *J Neurosurg* 1964;21:212–215.
104. Zampella E, Morawetz RB, McDowell HA, et al. The importance of cerebral ischemia during carotid endarterectomy. *Neurosurgery* 1991;29:727–731.
105. Zierler R, Bandyk DF, Thiele BL, et al. Carotid artery stenosis following endarterectomy. *Arch Surg* 1982;117:1408–1412.

8

Management of Total Carotid Occlusion

Robert F. Spetzler, Julian E. Bailes, and
Patrick W. McCormick

Although most occlusions of the internal carotid artery (ICA) are discovered incidentally and are apparently asymptomatic, those patients with associated signs and symptoms of stroke or transient ischemic attacks (TIAs) may benefit from aggressive medical and surgical management. Operative treatment is recommended for patients with acute blockages but no major neurologic deficits. In such patients, ICA occlusions can be opened successfully with minimal morbidity and mortality. Patients with a chronic occlusion may have symptoms resulting from embolization from the proximal segment (stump) of the internal carotid artery. We present our experience with patients who have symptomatic ICA occlusion as well as that reported in the literature. A treatment algorithm for management of these patients is presented.

NATURAL HISTORY

The natural history of ICA occlusion has been analyzed in various retrospective and prospective clinical series. Early studies failed to provide specific data on the vascular territory responsible for infarction and included patients with substantial neurologic deficits. These patients thus had a limited

R. F. Spetzler: Division of Neurological Surgery, Barrow Neurological Institute, Phoenix, Arizona 85013.

J. E. Bailes: Department of Neurological Surgery, Allegheny General Hospital, Pittsburgh, Pennsylvania 15212.

P. W. McCormick: The Toledo Hospital, Toledo, Ohio 43608.

ability to withstand a stroke or have a subsequent stroke detected. Different forms of therapy were also applied without analyzing the specific complications and outcome associated with the treatments (Tables 1 and 2).

Hardy et al. (16) presented 153 patients with complete common carotid artery or ICA occlusion. Eighty patients presented with the sudden onset of symptoms, and 52 patients presented with episodic symptoms that persisted for 5 days to 7 years, with an average of 11 months between the onset of the TIAs and a final stroke. In 15 patients, the onset of neurologic symptoms was progressive and evolving; overall, this group had the poorest outcome. Six patients presented with minor symptoms such as tinnitus, headaches, subjective bruit, blurry vision, or seizures. Overall, 62% of the patients died within 1 year, with an average of 4.5 months between symptom onset and a completed stroke. Cerebrovascular accident was the cause of death in 77% of the patients who died.

Dyken et al. (7) reported 43 patients who presented with total ICA occlusion. Thirty (70%) patients presented with moderate-to-severe neurologic deficits and had cerebrovascular accidents. Six (14%) patients experienced TIAs and two patients each presented with an organic brain syndrome and vascular headaches. Twelve (28%) patients had more than 70% stenosis of either the contralateral carotid artery or one vertebral artery. Complete occlusion of one ICA or even varying combinations of occlusion of the carotid and vertebral arteries was not necessarily associated with a cerebral infarction. However, the more severe the atherosclerosis and widespread the occlusive disease, the initial insult appeared to be worse and recovery less likely.

McDowell et al. (25) studied 57 patients with total ICA occlusion; about 40% had TIAs and 50% had a neurologic deficit. The in-hospital mortality was 35%, and 30% of patients had subsequent neurologic symptoms—either cerebrovascular accidents or TIAs. After surviving the acute period of hospitalization, 7% of the patients had later strokes and 5% had died at the 2-year follow-up, similar to the results of Dyken et al. (7).

More recent studies have shed light on the outcome of patients with symptomatic, atherosclerotic ICA occlusion. Grillo and Patterson (13) reported 44 patients with symptomatic atherosclerotic ICA occlusion, 2 of whom had bilateral ICA occlusion. Of the 44 patients, 8 died after an ipsilateral infarction, 7 of which caused the initial presenting symptoms. During the study's follow-up, one patient sustained a fatal stroke, and four had nonfatal strokes, all located in the contralateral hemisphere. The authors concluded that pa-

Table 1. *Prognosis of carotid artery occlusion—I[a]*

Reference	No. of patients	Type of study	Patient population	Mean period of follow-up (months)	Strokes during follow-up [no. (%)]	Deaths during follow-up [no. (%)]
McDowell et al. (25) (1961)	38	Retrospective	Major completed strokes included	24	3 (8)	5 (13)
Hardy et al. (16) (1962)	133	Retrospective	Major completed strokes included	48	30 (23)	51 (39)
Dyken et al. (7) (1974)	43	Prospective	Half of patients with moderate-to-severe deficit	16.5	3 (7)	6 (14)
Fields et al. (8) (1976)	359	Prospective	Significant number of patients with initial severe deficit	44	89 (25)	155 (43)

[a] The above studies give an overall stroke rate with no or incomplete reference to vascular territory involved.

Table 2. *Prognosis of carotid artery occlusion—II[a]*

Reference	No. of patients	Type of study	Patient population	Mean period of follow-up (months)	Strokes during follow-up [no. (%)]	Deaths during follow-up [no. (%)]
Grillo and Patterson (13) (1975)	37	Retrospective	Majority having TIA or stroke	36	6 (16)[b]	10 (27)
Samson et al. (31) (1977)	7	Prospective	TIA or minor stroke	17	2 (28)[c]	0
Barnett (1) (1978)	25	Prospective	TIA or minor stroke	24	7 (28)[c]	—
Furlan et al. (11) (1980)	138	Retrospective	TIA or minor stroke	60	11 (8) 6 (4)[b]	30 (21)
Heyman (1982)	13	Prospective	TIA	24	7 (54)[c]	2 (15)
Bogousslavsky et al. (2) (1981)	23	Retrospective	Majority having TIA or minor stroke	27	0	0
Cote et al. (3) (1983)	47	Prospective	TIA or minor stroke	34	7 (15)[c] 4 (8.5)[b]	4 (8.5)

[a] These studies give stroke rate ipsilateral to occluded artery.
[b] Stroke in other vascular distribution.
[c] Ipsilateral stroke.

tients with ICA occlusion either did well or became imminently symptomatic, suffering stroke and death. Patients who tolerated their initial presentation with ICA occlusions were more apt to die later of myocardial infarction rather than neurologic events. This study supports the contention that acute symptomatic ICA occlusion—in the absence of a major, completed stroke—should be approached with the intent of emergent deocclusion and restoration of flow to that hemisphere (13).

In several retrospective series, the incidence of subsequent stroke or TIAs after complete ICA occlusion varied between 0% and 23% (7,11,14). Prospective series, which may be a more sensitive indicator when minor syndromes are considered, have found between 7% and 54% incidence of subsequent stroke, with a mean of 23.6% (3,8,36). In about two-thirds of the patients, the strokes occurred ipsilateral to the carotid occlusion and in one-third strokes were located in a contralateral distribution. Fields and Lemak (8) followed 359 patients for a mean period of 44 months. New strokes occurred in 25% of the patients, and 64% of the strokes were ipsilateral to the occluded ICA. Furlan et al. (11) reported a 3% annual stroke rate following angiographically proven ICA occlusion; one-third occurred on the contralateral side.

Cote et al. (3) reported a series of 47 patients with ICA occlusion associated with TIAs or minor strokes. In a mean follow-up period of 34 months, 7 (15%) patients had an ipsilateral stroke. Four (8.5%) patients had a stroke in other vascular distributions, three of which were in the contralateral hemisphere and one of which was in the vertebrobasilar distribution. Of the 47 patients, 24 (51%) continued to have TIAs in the vascular distribution distal to an ICA occlusion. Their observed annual stroke rate distal to the ICA occlusion was 5%.

Hennerici et al. (17) prospectively followed 49 patients with an asymptomatic ICA occlusion for a mean of 31.2 months to determine the natural history in patients without initial neurologic involvement. Eight (16%) patients sustained a stroke, five of which were ipsilateral to the occluded carotid artery. Four (8%) patients experienced TIAs ipsilateral to the occlusion. They concluded that asymptomatic ICA occlusion is not a stable situation and is associated with a significant incidence of subsequent transient or permanent ischemia (15). Nearly one-half of their patients died during the period of followup, with most succumbing to coexisting cardiac disease. Wade et al. (36) studied 34 patients with bilateral ICA symptomatic occlusion prospectively for a mean of 42 months. Isolated TIAs occurred in 7 (20.6%) patients and stroke occurred in 11 (32.4%) patients. Deaths occurred at a rate of 3 (8%) a year.

SURGICAL TREATMENT

The morbidity and mortality rates associated with the operative treatment of complete ICA occlusion have declined since the earliest reports. In 1965, Murphey and Maccubbin (27) described the results of operative treatment of 165 patients for 194 diseased ICAs, 80 of which were totally occluded. The overall morbidity associated with angiography and surgery was 16.4% (27 patients), and 15.7% (26 patients) patients died. Of 80 patients with complete ICA occlusion, 35 (43.7%) had successful deocclusion of the vessel; however, almost half later rethrombosed. The authors stressed, as had DeBakey et al. (5) had earlier, that vessel patency can often be restored if an operation is performed within 48 hours of occlusion. Surgical intervention carried significant risk, however, if signs of completed stroke (e.g., hemiplegia, dysphasia) were present preoperatively.

Thompson et al. (35) described 118 operations with a 6.2% operative mortality rate, and Hunter et al. (19) reported a surgical morbidity and mortality rate of about 15% in 21 patients. These reports demonstrate that the surgical morbidity and mortality rate is high if all patients with ICA occlusion undergo surgery. A subgroup, however, fared better than the group as a whole. This subgroup included patients who presented early without ''profound'' neurologic deficits.

Hunter et al. (19) reported their experience with 21 patients who had acute neurologic deficits caused by severely stenotic or occlusive ICA lesions. They believed that deocclusion should not be attempted in patients with a severe neurologic deficit and complete occlusion. This theory is widely accepted. Although the period considered crucial for significant ischemia has varied between 2 and 48 hours, few surgeons would argue that thromboendarterectomy should be undertaken in the presence of an acute severe neurologic deficit.

In 1971, Najafi et al. (28) studied 32 patients who had emergency procedures for ICA occlusion. Fifteen patients had postangiographic ICA occlusion, ten had spontaneous carotid thrombosis, and seven had developed a postoperative occlusion after carotid endarterectomy. The ICAs were reopened successfully in more than half of the patients with acute occlusions. Consequently Najafi et al. (28) concluded that blood flow must be restored within 1 hour to achieve an optimal result.

Kwann et al. (22) compared immediate surgery for three patients who experienced acute postoperative occlusion after carotid endarterectomy with six other patients in whom deocclusion was delayed for more than 3 hours because angiography was performed. Of the patients who underwent immediate reexploration and restoration of blood flow, two recovered completely and the third patient's neurologic deficits partially resolved. They concluded that surgery must be performed within 1 hour. Consequently they advocated that no angiogram should be performed for documentation to avoid losing valuable time (12).

Thompson et al. (35) reported the outcome of 118 operations for complete

ICA occlusion in 112 patients. Blood flow was reestablished in 48 instances (40.7%), and 7 (6.2%) operative mortalities occurred. They recommended emergency thromboendarterectomy if patients presented within 6 to 12 hours of the onset of ICA occlusion. They believed the operation was too risky for patients who presented any later. When patients with neurologic deficits were excluded, the operative mortality rate associated with carotid endarterectomy decreased from 6.2% to 1.1%. On the subject of ICA reopening, they felt that clinical consideration of stroke *per se* was the most important issue determining operability. If patients had acute, dense neurologic deficits of 12 hours' duration or more, operation was not recommended because of the prohibitive mortality. They questioned whether one should operate on such a patient if the patient was seen within 6 hours of onset of symptoms. If the neurologic deficit was mild and improving rapidly, or if a previously audible carotid bruit suddenly disappeared, they recommended that the operation ''be done immediately to effect restoration of internal carotid blood flow'' (35).

In 1986, Meyer et al. (26) described their experience with 34 patients treated by carotid thromboendarterectomy for acute ICA occlusion. All of these patients except one experienced changes in their level of consciousness and major neurologic deficits that began while they were hospitalized. Nine (26.5%) patients returned to normal, four patients (11.8%) were left hemiplegic, and seven (20.6%) died. Walters et al. (37) performed emergency carotid endarterectomies in 64 patients, 16 of whom had presumed acute, complete occlusion (some of whom were later proved to have pseudo-occlusions). Blood flow through the ICA was reestablished in all cases. Postoperatively, 14 patients were unchanged or improved, one patient's neurologic status deteriorated, and one patient died from cardiopulmonary arrest on the 24th postoperative day.

Two groups of investigators have reported their results with surgical thromboendarterectomy for ICA occlusion in patients who presented early, without profound deficits. This category of patients was the one most likely to benefit from surgery. Hugenholtz and Elgie (18) excluded patients with drowsiness, major neurologic deficits, and tandem lesions distal to the internal carotid artery occlusion. With these criteria, they reduced the surgical morbidity rate to 10% and the surgical mortality rate to 0% in a group of 35 patients. Using similar selection criteria in 47 patients, Hafner and Tew (15) achieved surgical mortality and neurologic morbidity rates of 0%. Kusunoki et al. (21) studied two groups of patients: those with neurologic, medical, and angiographic risk factors and those without. The latter group of 14 patients had no operative mortality. Clearly, case series that excluded patients with severe neurologic deficits demonstrate that restoring blood flow in the ICA is beneficial.

Despite the identification of a subgroup of patients expected to benefit from restoring blood flow through the ICA, as well as the publication of two clinical series showing favorable surgical morbidity and mortality rates in this group, a recent poll indicated that, according to expert opinion, ICA occlusion was a contraindication to ICA surgery (39). In fact, after reviewing 1,000 carotid endarterectomies, the responders categorized the 60 endarterectomies (6%) performed for complete ICA occlusion as inappropriate.

As this review indicates, the optimal treatment of carotid occlusion, especially surgical intervention, is controversial. The controversy partially reflects the difficulties in defining the population best suited for surgical intervention and in performing prospective studies to determine the outcome of different treatment groups. There does appear to be a subgroup of patients who fare well if they can be diagnosed and treated expeditiously before significant cerebral infarction occurs.

OUR CLINICAL EXPERIENCE

At the Barrow Neurological Institute, 42 patients with angiographically documented internal carotid artery occlusion were evaluated over a 6-year period. All patients were diagnosed by the same protocol including computerized tomography (CT) of the brain at the time of presentation to exclude the presence of a major infarction, hemorrhage, or other lesions. Four-vessel cerebral angiography was performed immediately in all patients using selective catheterization, image subtraction, and image magnification techniques. In all patients, a complete occlusion of the ICA was documented (Fig. 1). No patients with evidence of a ''string sign'' or delayed anterograde filling through an apparently occluded vessel segment, indicative of near-total or pseudo-occlusion were included (Fig. 2). The site of atherosclerotic occlusion was the origin of the ICA and carotid bifurcation in all cases. All patients exhibited complete occlusion of the ICA ipsilateral to the symptomatic hemisphere. Heparin was administered intravenously in 21 patients while they were prepared for surgery. Surgery was performed emergently on every patient with appropriate symptoms. Patients with profound neurologic deficits or intracerebral hemorrhage visualized on CT or patients with docu-

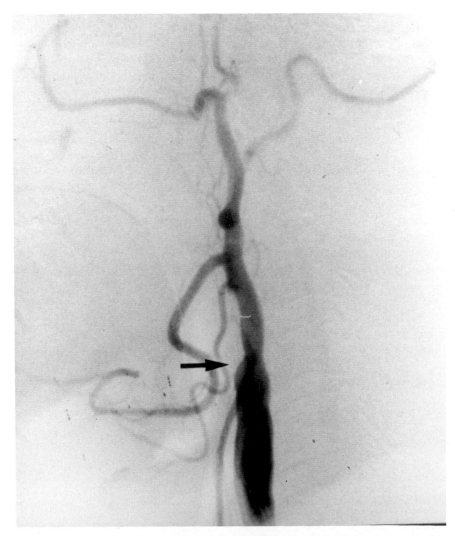

Figure 1. Lateral carotid angiogram demonstrating complete occlusion of the ICA at its origin with filling of the external carotid artery branches.

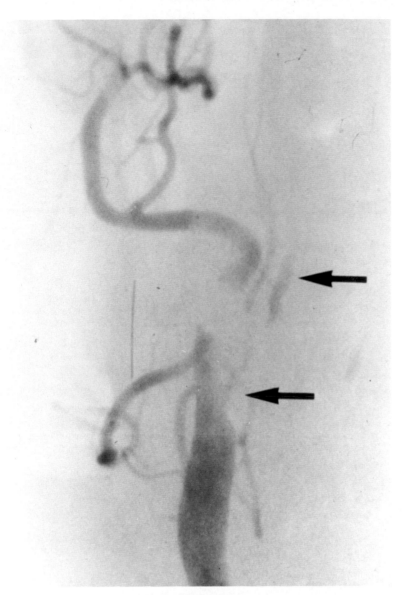

Figure 2. Lateral common carotid injection with delayed films shows what initially appeared to be an ICA occlusion but actually was a pseudo-occlusion with a small amount of contrast dye flowing past the bifurcation and proximal internal carotid regions *(arrows)*. This patient presented with symptoms of stroke-in-evolution. The angiogram suggested that he was a good candidate for endarterectomy, which was successfully performed because complete thrombosis with organized clot had not occurred.

mented chronic ICA occlusion without reflux of the petrous ICA were excluded. Only patients with symptomatic ICA occlusion were included in this study, since most such lesions are incidentally discovered (Fig. 3).

Surgical Technique

A standard carotid endarterectomy longitudinal incision was made along the medial border of the sternocleidomastoid muscle, through the platysma muscle and cervical fascia, to expose the carotid sheath. After the carotid artery was isolated above and below the level of the bifurcation, the vessel

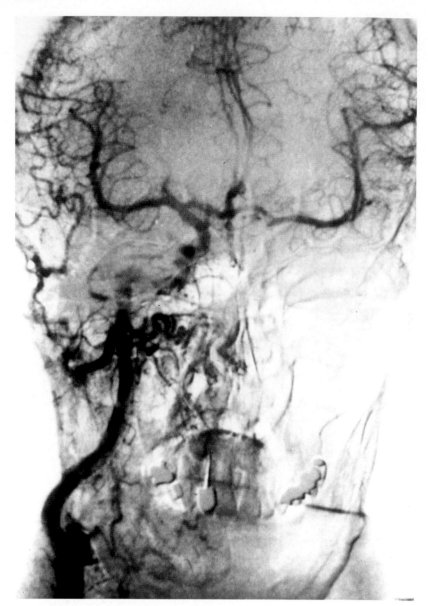

Figure 3. Right anteroposterior angiogram in a patient with complete left ICA occlusion shows excellent filling of the left hemisphere via a patent anterior communicating artery. Internal carotid artery occlusion is usually chronic, tolerated in approximately 95% of patients, and often found incidentally.

was inspected to determine its size and external appearance. If the ICA was small, thin, and fibrotic, no attempt was made to reopen it, and surgery was directed toward performing a stumpectomy if otherwise indicated. Before cross-clamping the common carotid artery, thiopental sodium (125 to 250 mg) was administered intravenously to achieve 15- to 30-s burst suppression on the electroencephalogram (EEG) (34). Dissection was completed to expose the common, internal, and external carotid arteries, and care was exercised to avoid manipulating the occluded ICA.

A small arteriotomy was made on the lateral ICA distal to the obvious atheromatous disease. At this point, one of three phenomena occurred: (a) the clot spontaneously expressed itself with good backflow, (b) the clot did not spontaneously exit and backflow was not observed, or (c) a small amount of clot exited and was followed by poor backflow. In the first instance, standard cross-clamping of the vessels was performed followed by an endarterectomy. In the case of the latter two events, a 2-F Fogarty catheter with a 0.2-ml balloon was passed up the ICA with very gentle pressure to near (10 to 12 cm) the carotid siphon. The balloon was inflated with saline and gently withdrawn. In cases of acute or subacute thrombosis, especially where collateral flow had kept the distal ICA patent, it was possible to remove the clot (Fig. 4). Brisk bleeding from the distal ICA was then immediately encountered. After good retrograde flow was established, the distal ICA was rapidly occluded, in addition to the external and common carotid arteries. The endarterectomy was then completed in the standard fashion by extension of the arteriotomy into the common carotid artery. Shunting was not performed unless indicated by major EEG changes as described in our standard endarterectomy protocol (see Chapter 7). If the ICA could not be reopened by passing the catheter three times, the attempt to reopen was aborted (Fig. 5).

If the ICA could not be reopened or was atretic upon inspection, as described earlier, a proximal remnant angioplasty (stumpectomy) and an external carotid endarterectomy were performed if indicated. Proximal remnant angioplasty was performed by closing the ICA flush at its origin with a large vascular clip, dissecting along the posterior wall of the internal carotid artery, and transecting it from the distal portion (Fig. 6). These maneuvers avoided angulation as flowing blood passed into the external carotid artery. This maneuver may reduce the propensity for stagnated blood, eddy currents, and embolic material to form in the area of the ICA origin.

In our series, patients were maintained throughout the surgical procedure with EEG burst-suppression by means of titrated doses of barbiturate. Blood pressure was maintained in a normotensive or slightly hypertensive range

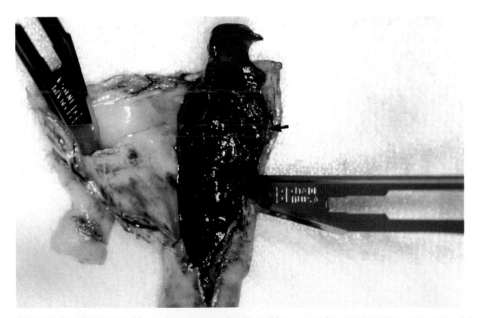

Figure 4. This specimen was taken from a 74-year-old woman who presented with stroke-in-evolution and was found to have an acute ICA occlusion on angiogram. Retrograde flow through orbital and cavernous collaterals maintained good retrograde flow through the distal internal carotid artery into the petrous segment, allowing successful thromboendarterectomy. This specimen demonstrates an acute organized thrombus *(arrow)* at the region of the cervical carotid bifurcation; however, the portion of the thrombus distal to the bifurcation was soft, nonorganized, and extractable, as can be appreciated here.

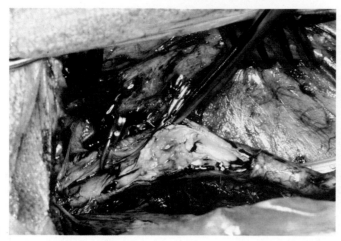
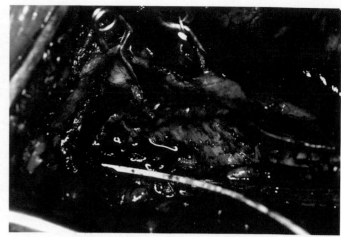

A   B

Figure 5. A: Intraoperative appearance of the atherosclerotic lesion and proximal ICA thrombus *(arrow)* in a patient presenting with acute carotid occlusion. **B:** Balloon catheter extraction of the initial portion of the thrombus *(arrow)* in a patient with acute, complete ICA occlusion.

during carotid cross-clamping. In patients who received heparin preoperatively, its administration was continued throughout the operative procedure until the arteriotomy closure was completed. All patients received perioperative aspirin. Vessel shunting was employed on one occasion when an asymmetric EEG burst-suppression pattern developed during the endarterectomy.

Patient Population

Of the 42 patients in our series, 29 (70%) were men. The average age was 61.4 years. Associated medical conditions included smoking in 67%; essential hypertension in 72%; and previous myocardial infarction, stable angina, or both in 26%. Clinical presentations included focal cortical TIAs in 68%, amaurosis fugax in 28%, new fixed neurologic deficits in 28%, and stroke-in-evolution in 9%. For patients who presented initially to our institution for treatment, the mean time from the neurologic event to the first surgical procedure was 42 hours.

Computed tomography scans of the brain obtained within 4 hours of presentation demonstrated remote cerebral infarctions in 19%, lacunar infarctions in 17%, and new ischemic changes in 15%. In the last group, four patients had watershed distribution infarcts. More than half (56%) of the CT scans were normal.

Results

Forty-six operations were performed on the 42 patients, including 24 (52%) successful vessel reopenings, 9 (20%) stumpectomies with associated external carotid endarterectomies, and 4 (9%) stumpectomies with external carotid endarterectomies that eventually required extracranial-intracranial (EC-IC) bypass. Three (7%) patients experienced transient surgical morbidity: a postoperative seizure in one, vocal cord paralysis in one, and a mild contralateral hemiparesis in one. One (2%) patient's hemiparesis worsened after restoration of blood flow in the ICA. Postoperative TIAs occurred in four patients who initially underwent stumpectomy and external carotid endarterectomy. In compliance with our treatment algorithm, these patients

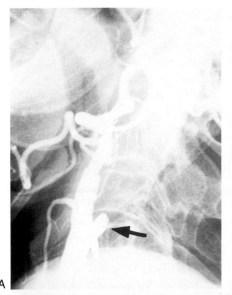

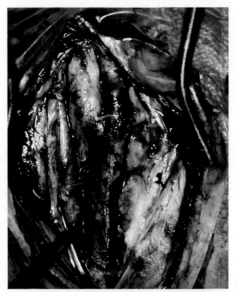

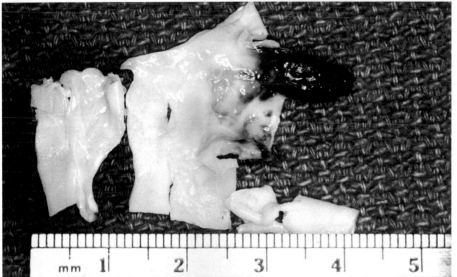

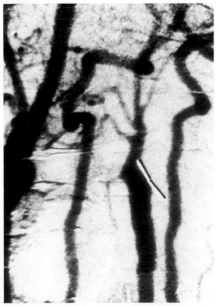

Figure 6. A: Lateral carotid angiogram showing complete ICA occlusion distal to the cervical bifurcation. A symptomatic remnant (stump) is visualized *(arrow).* **B:** Intraoperative view of a patient with chronic ICA occlusion and symptomatic proximal remnant. Two large vascular clips have been placed flush with the carotid bifurcation to obliterate the stump, and an external carotid endarterectomy has been performed to optimize blood flow through the external carotid system. **C:** Specimen removed from this procedure shows the atherosclerotic plaque from the external carotid and common carotid arteries and the organized thrombus with associated platelet matter that extended into the ICA remnant and was responsible for the embolic events. **D:** Postoperative angiogram shows obliteration of the proximal remnant using vascular clips with a smooth transition and straightening of the bifurcation region to allow improved blood flow through the external carotid artery system.

subsequently underwent an EC-IC bypass procedure. No operative deaths occurred in the series.

Long-term arterial patency was assessed in 17 (73%) of the 24 patients. Carotid Doppler ultrasound studies were performed a mean of 28 months after surgery. In 15 (88%) of these patients, the ICAs were widely patent. Of the other two, one had more than 70% stenosis and one had reocclusion. The restenosed vessel was operated on again, and a vein patch was placed.

Three patients were lost to follow-up, which for the remaining 39 patients was an average of 40 months after their last operation. Five (13%) patients died, two of cancer and three of myocardial infarction. Four (10%) patients experienced neurologic events: TIAs in two and vertebrobasilar insufficiency in two. Six (15%) patients had new myocardial infarctions or new-onset angina. The outcome for patients with successful restoration of ICA flow was not significantly different from that of patients who were treated until asymptomatic with the alternative surgical strategies described. No patient had a subsequent stroke during the follow-up period, and the rates for neurologic transient events (TIAs and vertebrobasilar insufficiency) for both groups were comparable with the expected natural history for completed stroke in nonsurgically treated patients.

These data further strengthen the conclusion that a subgroup of patients, chosen primarily from their presenting neurologic examination, will have low surgical morbidity and mortality rates from restoration of ICA flow (23). The issue of timing of surgery remains unclear. The precise timing between ICA occlusion and attempted restoration of flow is known in few series. These include postangiographic or postsurgical occlusions that represent a pathophysiology other than spontaneous occlusion associated with atherosclerotic disease. The impression of those reporting such series is that the earlier surgery is performed, the better patients fare.

OPERATIVE STRATEGY

Certain methodologic considerations concerning restoration of blood flow in the ICA deserve emphasis. Preoperatively, patients should be started on aspirin therapy, which can be given by suppository if necessary. Heparinization seems to be a logical medical treatment for symptomatic ICA occlusion before surgery, but no strong efficacy data are available. Distal embolization can occur and is associated with a poor outcome. In patients receiving heparin (partial thromboplastin time 1.5 × control), we continue heparin administration throughout the operation until the arteriotomy closure is completed.

During induction of anesthesia, great care must be taken to keep the patient's blood pressure normotensive. Reduction in blood pressure can decrease collateral flow to compromised vascular territories. Intravenous thiopental titrated to maintain the patient in EEG burst-suppression reduces the metabolic requirements of ischemic neurons. Careful use of this technique will protect the brain from fluctuations in collateral blood flow during surgical manipulation.

It is important to monitor a parameter sensitive to cerebral oxygen delivery during the operation to assess the adequacy of collateral flow. Under barbiturate cerebral protection, this can be accomplished by observing the symmetry of the burst-suppression pattern between hemispheres or by direct assessment of cerebral oxygen saturation (24,34). In our experience with ICA occlusion, cross-clamping the external carotid artery may sometimes cause EEG asymmetries.

When the arteriotomy is made, the clot should be given time to decompress spontaneously (Fig. 7). Only if it fails to do so should an attempt be made

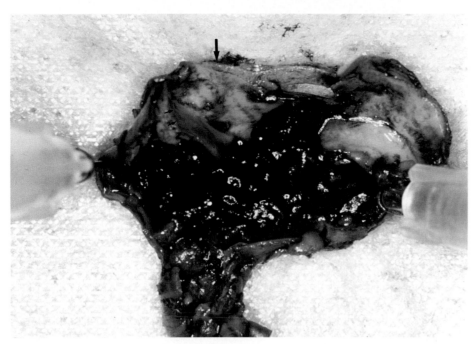

Figure 7. A magnified view as taken through the operating microscope showing the complexity of a carotid atherosclerotic lesion. The cholesterol, lipid, and calcium-containing atherosclerotic plaque *(arrow)* has a superimposed intramural hemorrhage with a raised intimal flap *(small arrows)* along with an acute thrombosis. This thrombus is composed of soft platelet components *(open arrow)* and the darker thrombus, consisting of fibrin and erythrocytes.

to pass a Fogarty catheter, a maneuver that requires experience and judgment. Low neurologic morbidity and mortality rates are associated with a 50% to 60% successful restoration of flow. Attempts to reopen a vessel may result in a poor surgical outcome due to intimal injury, dissection, distal embolization, or hemorrhage. Vessels that are small and atretic should not be subjected to attempts to restore flow with a catheter technique.

As early as 1930, techniques to reopen an occluded ICA included the procedure of retrograde flushing, which was modified to the technique of retrograde "milking (Table 3)." Several methods were subsequently implemented in attempts to reopen totally occluded carotid arteries. Originally, catheter suction and irrigation were used to remove thrombotic material. In peripheral arteries such as the popliteal and brachial, distal arteriotomy with retrograde flushing was often successful. As a thrombus begins to organize in the first several days after its formation, it becomes increasingly difficult to extract because it adheres to the arterial wall. In 1960, Shaw (32) developed an instrument consisting of a wire with a helical portion on one end that could successfully extract the distal portion of a clot without distal arteriotomy. This instrument became known as the corkscrew device (28) (Table 3).

In 1963, Fogarty et al. (10) developed a new catheter with an inflatable

Table 3. *Techniques for thrombus extraction*

Retrograde flushing (Lerman et al., 1930)
Retrograde "milking technique" (Keley and Rooney, 1951)
Corkscrew device [Shaw, 1960 (32)]
Balloon catheter [Fogarty et al., 1963 (10)]

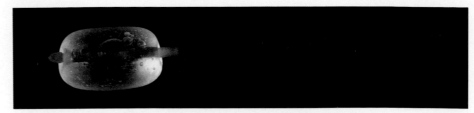

Figure 8. Magnified view of a #2 Fogarty catheter with balloon inflated.

distal balloon that provided a simple but superior technique in distal clot extractions because it was generally safe, effective, and obviated distal arteriotomy (Fig. 8). In 1967, Davie and Richardson (4) reported the first case of carotid-cavernous fistula occurring as a complication of Fogarty catheter use. Subsequently, several authors described similar phenomena associated with extraction of thrombus using Fogarty catheters (A. Heyman, personal communication). Other iatrogenic complications associated with the use of such catheters include intimal and medial tears with immediate or delayed dissection or pseudoaneurysm formation, complete transmural arterial tears, intracranial hemorrhage, and embolization (12,18,19,22,38,39). Animal studies have shown on the microscopic level that from the use of these catheters, a transmural injury is associated with internal elastic lamina disruption and endothelial proliferation (12). We have found the use of balloon thrombectomy catheters to be safe and have had no known complications associated with their use; we limit the number of passes to three (Table 4).

Proper technique when using Fogarty catheters cannot be overemphasized, particularly gentle insertion and withdrawal (Fig. 9). Overinflation of the balloon must also be avoided. In addition, the optimal size of balloon must be chosen. Another key factor in the safe and effective use of these catheters is limiting how far they are advanced distally into the ICA. To avoid creating a carotid-cavernous fistula, the surgeon should not pass the catheter tip beyond the junction of the petrous and cavernous portions of the ICA. In adults, the distance from the carotid bifurcation varies between 14 and 8 cm, averaging 10.6 cm.

If the ICA cannot be reopened and extracranial surgical procedures do not prevent subsequent neurologic symptoms, surgical augmentation of cerebral collateral blood flow has been successful. Four patients in our series had anterior circulation TIAs following stumpectomy and external carotid endarterectomy; therefore a superficial temporal-to-middle cerebral artery bypass was performed. One patient died 2 years later of a myocardial infarction and three remained asymptomatic at an average of 37 months after surgery. This select group of patients is believed to have hemodynamic ischemic symp-

Table 4. *Potential complications of Fogarty catheter use in internal carotid thromboendarterectomy*

Arteriovenous fistula
Intimal/medial tear
   Immediate dissection
   Delayed dissection
   Pseudoaneurysm
   Thrombosis
Complete transmural tear—hemorrhage
Intracranial embolization
Intracranial hemorrhage

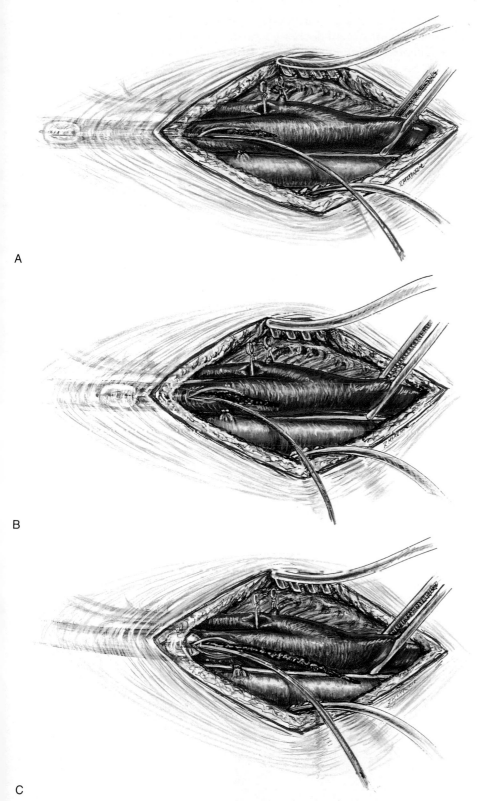

A

B

C

Figure 9. The soft tip of the Fogarty catheter may be advanced through a thrombus with the balloon deflated, followed by inflation of the balloon and withdrawal of the catheter and thrombus in a retrograde fashion. This maneuver, however, is extremely dangerous and should only be undertaken as a last resort when other conventional measures such as microdissection and suction do not deocclude the artery. Despite its relatively soft tip, during advancement through the wall vessel perforation may still occur and this possibility must be constantly guarded against. We utilize a maximum of three passes of the catheter before aborting the procedure of thrombectomy.

toms; their xenon CT cerebral blood flow studies or positron emission tomography scan demonstrated decreased perfusion worsened by the administration of Diamox, which explains their response to bypass surgery.

Angiographic Assessment

Branches of the internal maxillary artery anastomose with the first intracranial carotid branches, which are the caroticotympanic artery and the pterygoid artery. The meningohypophyseal artery arises from the cavernous portion of the ICA as do the inferior cavernous sinus artery and a variable number of capsular arteries. The vertebral, external carotid, and ophthalmic arteries all give rise to meningeal branches that anastomose with cavernous carotid artery branches. In cases of atherosclerotic ICA occlusion, antero-

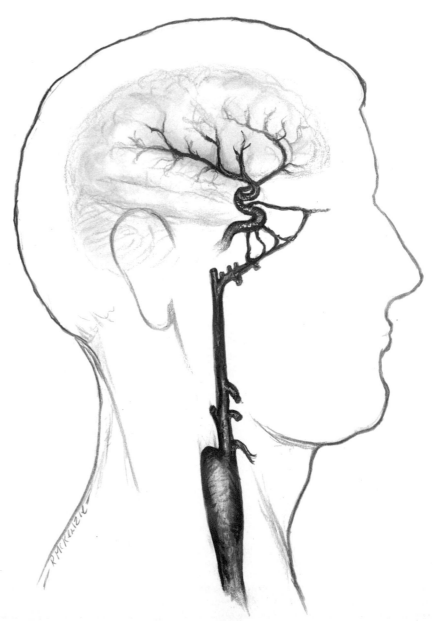

Figure 10. Artist's drawing demonstrating the common extracranial-intracranial communications that may become viable in instances of ICA occlusion: superior ethmoidal, ophthalmic, and cavernous arterial branches.

grade flow within the ICA is most commonly supplied by collaterals filling via the ophthalmic artery in a retrograde fashion. It is believed that the artery of the inferior cavernous sinus largely contributes to the opacification of the cavernous and precavernous segments of the ICA seen in these situations (Fig. 10). The extensive arterial anastomoses existing between the cavernous portion of the ICA and the external carotid artery are not usually seen in the normal situation. They may enlarge to have a functional role and be radiographically visible when they act to fill the ICA in a retrograde fashion (Fig. 11). With the use of detailed arteriographic technique, it is often possible to detect slight antegrade blood flow in a severely stenotic but not completely occluded ICA. In this situation the artery is still open and a slight luminal channel persists. Usually the artery is readily treatable by standard thromboendarterectomy. This sort of pseudo-occlusion pattern was excluded from our series. An important observation in our series was the correlation between the extent of reflux visualization of the occluded ICA by angiography and the ability to reopen the ICA. Although other authors have mentioned this relationship, labeled "collateral filling," it probably does not represent true collateral filling for two reasons (5,7,33). Minimal collateral supply exists to the petrous carotid artery and no such supply to the cervical carotid artery. The vessel fills retrogradely on delayed-sequence films, and the vessel has no pressure differential across it, especially in the retrograde direction. In our opinion, the vessel fills with contrast medium in a delayed fashion as a result of reflux of contrast medium into the distal portion, possibly aided by turbulent flow patterns in this region.

The amount of angiographic reflux in the ICA on preoperative angiograms was found to correlate with the ability to reopen an occluded ICA successfully (Fig. 12). We evaluated the angiographic data in 26 patients with delayed selective digital subtraction studies to access the retrograde reflux visualization of the occluded ICA. Based on the Hugenholtz and Elgie grading system (18), reflux to the supraclinoid segment only (grade 2) occurred in four

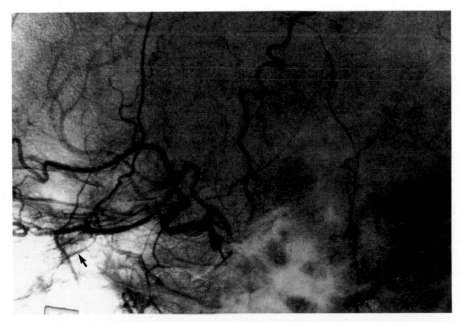

Figure 11. Lateral carotid angiogram, late cerebral phase, indicating a total occlusion of the ICA with terminal branches of the external carotid artery filling. The distal ICA is being reconstituted by retrograde flow via the superior ethmoidal artery *(arrow)*, ophthalmic artery, and cavernous carotid branches. The ICA is filled by retrograde flow back to the petrous carotid artery.

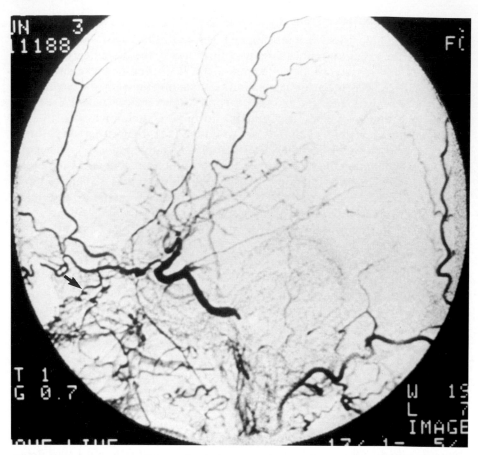

Figure 12. Lateral carotid cerebral phase angiogram in a patient with a complete ICA occlusion. Reconstitution of the distal ICA and cavernous carotid region is done from retrograde ophthalmic artery and cavernous arterial branches resulting in retrograde filling through the proximal carotid siphon area. This patient would have a 50% or greater chance for restoration of flow, due to the retained patency proximal to the cavernous carotid region.

patients, with successful reopening in one patient, for a success rate of 25%. Reflux to the cavernous portion of the ICA (grades 3 and 4) occurred in eight patients with successful reopening in four, for a success rate of 50%. Reflux to the petrous ICA occurred in 14 patients, with successful reopening in 10, for a success rate of 71%.

Hugenholtz and Elgie (18) described a five-tier classification system for grading this reflux pattern but were unable to conclude if such a detailed classification was necessary. We have reduced the classification system to three tiers and have shown in our series that the further the refluxing of contrast medium into the vessel, the greater the likelihood of restoration of flow. Filling of the petrous vessel was associated with a 71% success rate for restoration of flow. This finding is important because it facilitates preoperative surgical planning and patient counseling. Patients with symptomatic chronic ICA occlusion and petrous vessel reflux are candidates for thromboendarterectomy. Furthermore, if a reflux pattern is not encouraging, an intraoperative decision to abort attempts at restoration of flow with a Fogarty catheter can be reached earlier.

Outcome of Surgical Treatment

The permanent surgical morbidity rate for attempted ICA reopening in the 42 operations in our series was 2%, and the 30-day surgical mortality rate

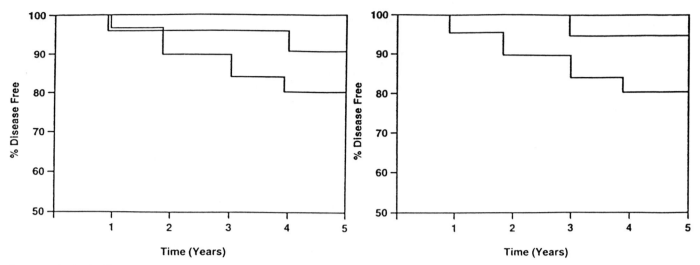

Figure 13. **Left:** Graph showing the long-term outcome for patients with successful restoration of flow in the internal carotid artery for the end points of stroke, transient ischemic attacks, and stroke death *(upper line)* and the expected stroke event in patients left untreated *(lower line)*. **Right:** Same analysis for patients who did not have successful reopening but who were surgically treated with stumpectomy, external carotid endarterectomy, or extracranial-intracranial bypass until their symptoms resolved *(upper line)* and for patients left untreated *(lower line)*. Reprinted with permission from *Journal of Neurosurgery*.

was 0% (Fig. 13). These outcomes compare well with the anticipated morbidity and mortality rates of ICA occlusion even in this select group (those with profound deficits were excluded by our protocol) of patients. In an average follow-up period of 40 months, no patient with successful restoration of flow in our series had a stroke. In addition, no patients treated with alternative surgical approaches until their symptoms resolved had subsequent strokes.

The literature concerning thromboendarterectomy of spontaneously occluded symptomatic ICAs consistently demonstrates a subgroup of patients who have successful restoration of flow with little morbidity and mortality (Fig. 14). This subgroup is best defined as those without severe neurologic deficits, a decreased level of consciousness, or intracerebral hemorrhage. Clinical experience with such patients at our institution and others shows a low surgical morbidity and mortality rate associated with carefully performed

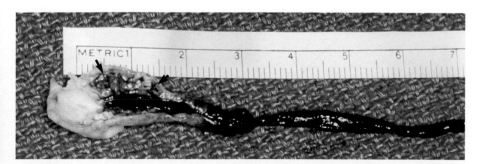

Figure 14. This atherosclerotic lesion was removed following a thromboendarterectomy in a 65-year-old man who presented with a fluctuating hemispheric deficit. Angiography disclosed an acute ICA occlusion, which, combined with his symptoms, suggested an impending cerebrovascular accident. At operation, the large atherosclerotic lesion had the typical, acute thrombus with a white head, composed primarily of platelets *(arrows)* and a red tail, composed of erythrocytes and fibrin extending 6 cm distally into the ICA. This thrombus was successfully extracted using a Fogarty balloon catheter.

Table 5. *Outcome of patients selected for surgical restoration of ICA flow in four series[a]*

Authors and year	No. of cases	Exclusion criteria	Morbidity	Mortality	Successful reopening
Kusunoki et al. (21) (1978)	14	Profound deficit, major medical problem, severe angiographic disease	1 (7)	0	NA
Hugenholtz and Elgie (18) (1980)	35	ICH, drowsy, major deficit	4 (11)	0	19 (54)
Hafner and Tew (15) (1981)	47	Profound deficit, ICH, symptoms >45 days	0	0	32 (68)
McCormick et al. (23) (1992)	43	Profound deficit, ICH, chronic disease with poor reflux	1 (2)	0	24 (56)
Total	139		6 (4.3)	0	75 (59)

[a] All four series used similar exclusion criteria. Numbers in parentheses are percentages of the total in each study.
ICA, internal carotid artery; ICH, intracerebral hemorrhage; NA, not available. Reprinted with permission from Journal of Neurosurgery.

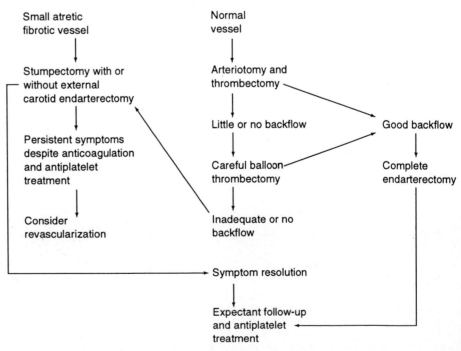

Figure 15. Flowchart for treatment of carotid occlusion.

thromboendarterectomy of the ICA. During long-term follow-up review, the vessels remained patent and the patients had fewer strokes than would be anticipated from natural history data (Table 5). Our patients followed a prospectively designed diagnostic, anesthetic, and surgical protocol. Their evaluation and treatment were interdisciplinary. The data, however, were collected retrospectively and no simultaneous control group was available for comparison. This experience cannot definitively establish the efficacy of surgical management for ICA occlusion. However, based on the available data, we currently recommend surgery for patients with acute symptomatic ICA occlusion who do not have a major neurologic deficit or hemorrhage on CT scan (Fig. 15).

CONCLUSIONS

The natural history of carotid occlusion has been ill defined, and its treatment is controversial. Even when presenting initially in an asymptomatic fashion, probably as many as one-fifth of patients may suffer a cerebral infarction ipsilateral to the occluded carotid artery within 3 years (17). This likelihood suggests that initially asymptomatic ICA occlusion may not be as benign or stable as originally believed. The determination that an occlusion of the ICA is of recent onset is not always made with certainty. Patients with a documented ICA occlusion that is symptomatic are not uncommon and often pose difficulty with recommending optimal treatment. Internal carotid artery occlusion may present with either acute, transient, or evolving cerebral ischemic symptoms.

Emergency carotid thromboendarterectomy for patients with acute ICA occlusion has often been considered contraindicated. This attitude is due to the perceived high incidence of neurologic morbidity and mortality, the fact that it was thought that blood flow must be restored in the first few hours after the occlusion, and because of the previously perceived lack of definite benefit.

As our microsurgical technique, anesthesia methods, and perioperative management through the years have improved, we have improved our ability to reopen these occluded arteries with minimum neurologic morbidity and no operative mortality. We have also been able to achieve a higher patency rate in recent years by developing our current protocol of operating on patients with acute, symptomatic carotid occlusions who have not experienced a decreased level of consciousness, hemiplegia, or aphasia. This approach is viable in appropriately selected patients.

REFERENCES

1. Barnett HJM. Delayed cerebral ischemic episodes distal to occlusion of major cerebral arteries. *Neurology* 1978;28:769–774.
2. Bogousslavsky J, Regli F, Hungerbuhler J-P, Chrzanowski R. Transient ischemic attacks and external carotid artery. A retrospective study of 23 patients with an occlusion of the internal carotid artery. *Stroke* 1981;12:627–630.
3. Cote R, Barnett HJM, Taylor DW. Internal carotid occlusion: a prospective study. *Stroke* 1983;14:898–902.
4. Davie JC, Richardson R. Distal internal carotid thromboembolectomy using a Fogarty catheter in total occlusion. *J Neurosurg* 1967;27:171–177.
5. DeBakey ME, Crawford ES, Morris GC, et al. Surgical considerations of occlusive disease of the innominate, carotid, subclavian, and vertebral arteries. *Ann Surg* 1961;154:698–725.
6. DeWeese JA. Management of acute strokes. *Surg Clin North Am* 1982;62:467–472.
7. Dyken ML, Klatte E, Kolar OJ, et al. Complete occlusion of common or internal carotid arteries. Clinical significance. *Arch Neurol* 1974;30:343–346.
8. Fields WS, Lemak NA. Joint study of extracranial arterial occlusion. X. Internal carotid artery occlusion. *JAMA* 1976;235:2734–2738.

9. Fields WS, Maslenikov V, Meyer JS, et al. Joint study of extracranial arterial occlusion. *JAMA* 1970;211:1993–2003.

10. Fogarty TJ, Crauley JJ, Krause RJ, et al. A method for extraction of arterial emboli and thrombi. *Surg Gynecol Obstet* 1963;116:241–244.

11. Furlan AJ, Whisnant JP, Baker HL. Long-term prognosis after carotid artery occlusion. *Neurology* 1980;30:986–988.

12. Goldberg EM, Goldberg MC, Chowdhury LN, et al. The effects of embolectomy-thrombectomy catheters on vascular architecture. *J Cardiovasc Surg* 1983;24:74–80.

13. Grillo P, Patterson RH. Occlusion of the carotid artery: prognosis (natural history) and the possibilities of surgical revascularization. *Stroke* 1975;6:17–20.

14. Gurdjian FS, Lindner DW, Hardy WG, et al. "Completed stroke" due to occlusive cerebrovascular disease. *Neurology* 1961;11:724–732.

15. Hafner CD, Tew JM. Surgical management of the totally occluded internal carotid artery: a ten-year study. *Surgery* 1981;89:710–717.

16. Hardy WG, Lindner DW, Thomas LM, et al. Anticipated clinical course in carotid artery occlusion. *Arch Neurol* 1962;6:138–150.

17. Hennerici M, Hulsbomer H-B, Rautenberg W, et al. Spontaneous history of asymptomatic internal carotid occlusion. *Stroke* 1986;17:718–722.

18. Hugenholtz H, Elgie RG. Carotid thromboendarterectomy: a reappraisal. Criteria for patient selection. *J Neurosurg* 1980;53:776–783.

19. Hunter JA, Julian OC, Dye WS, et al. Emergency operation for acute cerebral ischemia due to carotid artery obstruction. Review of 26 cases. *Ann Surg* 1965;162:901–904.

20. Kakkasseril JS, Tomsick TA, Arbaugh JA, et al. Carotid cavernous fistula following Fogarty catheter thrombectomy. *Arch Surg* 1984;119:1095–1096.

21. Kusunoki T, Towed DW, Tator CH, et al. Thromboendarterectomy for total occlusion of the internal carotid artery: a reappraisal of risks, success rate and potential benefits. *Stroke* 1978;9:34–38.

22. Kwaan JHM, Connolly JE, Sharefkin JB. Successful management of early stroke after carotid endarterectomy. *Ann Surg* 1979;190:676–678.

23. McCormick PW, Spetzler RF, Bailes JE, et al. Thromboendarterectomy of the symptomatic occluded internal carotid artery. *J Neurosurg* 1992;76:752–758.

24. McCormick PW, Stewart M, Goetting MG, et al. Regional cerebrovascular oxygen saturation measured by optical spectroscopy in humans. *Stroke* 1991;22:596–602.

25. McDowell FH, Potes J, Grock S. The natural history of internal carotid and vertebral-basilar artery occlusion. *Neurology* 1961;11(Pt 2):153–157.

26. Meyer FB, Sundt TM Jr, Piepgras DG, et al. Emergency carotid endarterectomy for patients with acute carotid occlusion and profound neurological deficits. *Ann Surg* 1986;203:82–89.

27. Murphey F, Maccubbin DA. Carotid endarterectomy: a long term follow-up study. *J Neurosurg* 1965;23:156–168.

28. Najafi H, Javid H, Dye WS, et al. Emergency carotid thromboendarterectomy. Surgical indications and results. *Arch Surg* 1971;103:610–614.

29. Nicholls SC, Bergelin R, Strandness DE. Neurologic sequelae of unilateral carotid artery occlusion: immediate and late. *J Vasc Surg* 1989;10:542–548.

30. Ojemann RG, Crowell RM, Roberson GH, et al. Surgical treatment of extracranial carotid occlusive disease. *Clin Neurosurg* 1975;22:214–263.

31. Samson D, Watts C, Clark K. Cerebral revascularization for transient ischemic attacks. *Neurology* 1977;27:767–771.

32. Shaw RS. A method for the removal of the adherent distal thrombus. *Surg Gynecol Obstet* 1960;110:255–256.

33. Shucart WA, Garrido E. Reopening some occluded carotid arteries. Report of four cases. *J Neurosurg* 1976;45:442–446.

34. Spetzler RF, Martin N, Hadley MN, et al. Microsurgical endarterectomy under barbiturate protection: a prospective study. *J Neurosurg* 1986;65:63–73.

35. Thompson JE, Austin DJ, Patman RD. Endarterectomy of the totally occluded carotid artery for stroke. *Arch Surg* 1967;95:791–801.

36. Wade JPH, Wong W, Barnett HJM, et al. Bilateral occlusion of the internal carotid arteries. *Brain* 1987;110:667–682.

37. Walters BB, Ojemann RG, Henos RC. Emergency carotid endarterectomy. *J Neurosurg* 1987;66:817–823.

38. Wilkinson E, Spetzler RF, Carter LP, et al. Intraoperative barbiturate therapy during temporary vessel occlusion in man. In Spetzler RF, Carter LP, Selman WR, et al., eds. *Cerebral revascularization for stroke.* New York: Thieme-Stratton; 1985:397–403.

39. Winslow CM, Solomon DH, Chassin MR, et al. The appropriateness of carotid endarterectomy. *N Engl J Med* 1988;318:721–727.

9

Postoperative Medical Management of the Carotid Endarterectomy Patient

Christopher N. Faber, James K. Lanz, and Antonios Zikos

The major medical complications following carotid endarterectomy include hypertension, intracerebral hemorrhage, myocardial infarction, and thromboembolic disease (16,29,45,73,82,89,92,95,103). Even in experienced centers, the total morbidity and mortality rate approaches 8% (29,89,103). The medical consultant must focus on the prevention of these complications during the preoperative evaluation and, in the postoperative period, be prepared to manage these problems aggressively in the neurosurgical intensive care unit. This chapter reviews approaches to preoperative risk factor assessment and postoperative management of patients undergoing carotid endarterectomy.

CARDIOVASCULAR COMPLICATIONS

Hypertension

No definition of postoperative hypertension has been universally accepted. Several parameters have been used by different centers to define postoperative hypertension including systolic blood pressures exceeding 160

C. N. Faber, J. K. Lanz, and A. Zikos: Department of Medicine, Allegheny General Hospital, Pittsburgh, Pennsylvania 15212.

mmHg (4) to 200 mmHg (104), diastolic pressures exceeding 100 mmHg (27), and postoperative increases of 35 to 40 mmHg over preoperative levels (15,91). Accepting this broad range in definition, hypertension complicates the postoperative course of up to 80% of patients following carotid endarterectomy (27,63,91,104). Risk factors for the development of postoperative hypertension include preoperative hypertension, diabetes, isoflurane anesthesia, high-grade (>75%) carotid stenosis, peripheral vascular disease, and ipsilateral transient ischemic attacks (TIAs) (43,91,92,104).

The hypertensive response occurs approximately 1 to 2 hours postoperatively and persists for an average of 5 to 6 hours with a range of 1 to 24 hours (15). The pathogenesis of postoperative hypertension is not completely understood, but at least one component is intraoperative cerebral ischemia (4). Catecholamines and renin do not mediate this response (43).

Neurologic deficits and death are more frequent in patients with postoperative hypertension (58,104). The combination of postoperative hypertension and hyperperfusion places the patient at increased risk for postoperative hemorrhage. Since postoperative hypertension is much less common in patients who are normotensive preoperatively (27), the best approach to the management of this significant problem is normalization of preoperative blood pressure. In addition, meticulous dissection, sparing the carotid sinus nerves, may mitigate the postoperative hypertensive response (16), although the relative importance compared with preoperative control of blood pressure is debated.

Pharmacotherapy

The management of hypertension in the immediate postoperative period requires rapidly acting agents with short half-lives that can be titrated to achieve the desired range of blood pressure control. Target systolic blood pressure in our patients is less than 160 mmHg, taking into account the preoperative blood pressure. Excessive blood pressure reduction may result in border zone ischemia, especially in patients with poorly controlled preoperative hypertension and in patients with elevated intracranial pressures, and should be avoided. The drugs summarized below represent antihypertensive agents that have been evaluated for postoperative management of hypertension following carotid endarterectomy or other neurosurgical conditions (Table 1).

Sodium Nitroprusside

Sodium nitroprusside is an ultra-short-acting vasodilator that is administered as a continuous intravenous infusion (0.5 to 10 μg/kg/min). It dilates both the arterial and venous capacitance vessels by blocking the action of intracellular calcium. Because of its short half-life, ease of titration, and almost universal effectiveness, nitroprusside has been used as a first-line antihypertensive for immediate control of postoperative hypertension. However, it can decrease cerebral blood flow (CBF) and increase intracranial pressure (ICP) (46,105) and therefore necessitates caution when used in neurosurgical patients. Henriksen and Paulson (46) demonstrated diminished CBF with a 40% reduction in the mean arterial pressure (MAP) in awake patients. This effect was not reproduced in anesthetized patients, suggesting a compensatory activation of sympathetic tone in the awake patient. Turner et al. (105) described a significant rise in ICP during nitroprusside infusions that reduced blood pressure to 70% of baseline. However, once blood pres-

Table 1. *Parenteral antihypertensive therapy for postoperative carotid endarterectomy patients*

Agent	Dosage	Onset (min)	Duration	Side effects
Nitroprusside	IV infusion 0.5–10 μg/kg/min	<1	2–3 min	Hypotension Thiocyanate toxicity Increased ICP
Labetalol	IV bolus 10–60 mg q 10 min IV infusion 0.5–2.0 mg/min	<5	3–6 hr	CHF Heart block Bronchospasm
Enalaprilat	IV bolus 0.625–5 mg IV q 6 h	15	12–24 hr	Cough Angioedema Renal insufficiency
Nitroglycerin	IV infusion 5–200 μg/min	2–5	5–10 min	Headache Increased ICP

CHF, congestive heart failure; ICP, intracranial pressure.

sure is less than 70% of baseline, ICP begins to fall. The potential for nitroprusside to increase ICP is modulated by hypocapnea and hyperoxia (60).

Other potential problems in the use of nitroprusside include hypoxemia due to intrapulmonary shunting (9,86), reflex tachycardia and regional myocardial ischemia (30), tachyphylaxis (20), and abrupt hypotensive episodes that are minimized by the use of the computer-controlled delivery systems (64). Nitroprusside decomposes spontaneously to cyanide, which is then converted to thiocyanate in the liver for subsequent excretion in the urine. Consequently the use of nitroprusside, particularly for long periods of time or in patients with renal failure, can be complicated by thiocyanate or (rarely) cyanide toxicity. Cyanide poisoning induces a lactic acidosis through the inhibition of aerobic metabolism in the cytochrome oxidase system. Thiocyanate toxicity causes blurred vision, tinnitus, confusion, fatigue, nausea, headaches, confusion, psychotic behavior, and seizures (62). Toxicity is rare at infusion rates of 3 μg/kg/min or less for up to 72 hours (21). Thiocyanate levels should be monitored in patients with renal insufficiency or when higher dosages are used. Nitroprusside is photosensitive and must be protected from light. Despite these minor disadvantages, nitroprusside is an excellent antihypertensive for use in the immediate postoperative period.

Labetalol

Labetalol combines both alpha- and beta-receptor blocking activity. By virtue of its beta-blockade, labetalol reduces myocardial oxygen consumption by preventing the reflex tachycardia that may occur after treatment with direct vasodilators. It is an extremely effective antihypertensive agent with a rapid onset of action and low toxicity at conventional dosages. Arterial monitoring is not mandatory because the incidence of precipitous hypotension is rare when it is administered as a bolus (115) or as a continuous intravenous infusion (56). Labetalol is administered in boluses of 20 to 40 mg over 1 minute and as frequently as every 10 minutes thereafter as needed (115). Higher bolus doses of 1 to 2 mg/kg are not recommended due to the possibility of marked hypotensive episodes (108). Continuous intravenous infusion (0.5

to 2.0 mg/min) for as long as 9 days is safe (41). Because it does not undergo renal excretion, labetalol can be used safely in patients with renal insufficiency. As with all beta-receptor blockers, labetalol is relatively contraindicated in patients with significant underlying heart failure, atrioventricular conduction blocks, or bronchospasm.

In neurosurgical patients, labetalol is as effective as nitroprusside in terms of its therapeutic profile and it has fewer side effects (34). Patients treated with labetalol following aneurysm or arteriovenous malformation resection have better blood pressure control and lower ICPs than patients treated with nitroprusside (70). Thus, given the potential adverse effects of nitroprusside (increasing ICP, tachyphylaxis, rebound hypertension, and thiocyanate toxicity), labetalol is an attractive alternative for treatment of hypertension in postendarterectomy patients with no contraindication to beta-adrenergic blockade. Transition to oral antihypertensive therapy is facilitated in the case of labetalol by the availability of both oral and intravenous preparations. The starting oral dose for labetalol is 100 mg twice daily and the usual maximum dose is 200 to 400 mg twice daily.

Nitroglycerin

Intravenous nitroglycerin (5 to 200 μg/min) is an antianginal as well as a weak antihypertensive agent that dilates peripheral capacitance and resistance vessels. Pooling of blood in the capacitance compartment reduces venous return, left ventricular end-diastolic volume (preload), and myocardial wall tension, thus reducing myocardial oxygen demand (114). Nitroglycerin also dilates epicardial coronary vessels and enhances collateral circulation, which improves perfusion to ischemic myocardium (40). Nitroglycerin is only a modestly effective antihypertensive agent that increases ICP and reduces intracranial compliance (23,35). For these reasons, nitroglycerin is not a first-line agent for postoperative hypertension therapy. However, nitroglycerin may be useful in the subset of hypertensive patients with significant coronary artery disease and postoperative myocardial ischemia.

Calcium-Channel Blockers

No experience has been published with calcium-channel blockers in the management of postendarterectomy hypertension. However, nifedipine has been used to treat hypertensive states associated with other neurologic disorders (81,100). Nifedipine (10 to 20 mg), given orally or sublingually, can cause a reflex tachycardia and precipitous hypotension (109). Nifedipine may also increase intracranial pressure and decrease cerebral perfusion pressure (38,100). Finally, reliance on enteral or sublingual absorption limits the usefulness of this agent in the initial management of postoperative hypertension. Nicardipine, an intravenous calcium-channel blocker with antihypertensive properties, may prove more useful in the treatment of postoperative hypertension. The availability of an oral preparation is an additional attractive feature. More experience with this agent, particularly with its effects on CBF and ICP, is required before recommendations can be made regarding its usefulness in the postoperative setting.

Hydralazine

Hydralazine (10 to 20 mg IV) is a potent vasodilator available in intravenous and oral forms. Maximum blood pressure reductions occur within 10 minutes of intravenous administration. Hydralazine can increase intracranial pressure and reduce intracranial compliance (81). Furthermore, the hyperdynamic effects of increased heart rate and cardiac output can exacerbate myocardial ischemia. Due to the frequency of simultaneous coronary artery disease in this patient population, hydralazine should be used judiciously, if at all.

Angiotensin-Converting Enzyme Inhibitors

Angiotensin-converting enzyme (ACE) inhibitors have been used for many years in the treatment of chronic hypertension and congestive heart failure. They do not cause reflex tachycardia, may improve left ventricular performance, and may ameliorate left ventricular ischemia (113). Cerebral blood flow is unchanged in patients with class III and IV heart failure treated with captopril in doses sufficient to reduce blood pressure by 26%. In patients without heart failure, captopril causes a small but insignificant decrease in CBF (75). The availability of intravenous enalaprilat affords ACE inhibitors a potential role in treatment of postoperative hypertension. Enalaprilat (0.625 to 5 mg IV every 6 hours) has a relatively rapid onset of action (15 minutes) and improves cardiac performance (25). Patients with chronic congestive heart failure and a low ejection fraction may benefit the most from these agents, particularly since these patients may not be candidates for beta-blocker therapy. However, given the lack of experience in the neurosurgical patient, ACE inhibitors cannot be recommended as first-line agents in the management of postoperative hypertension. They can be considered as an oral option when switching from nitroprusside, particularly in patients with contraindications to beta-blockers.

Hypotension

Hypotension occurs in 28% to 50% of patients following carotid endarterectomy, with the nadir usually occurring 5 hours postoperatively (15,16,27). This response is frequently associated with a relative bradycardia and is commonly preceded by preoperative hypertension. The most likely cause of this postoperative hypotension is an exaggerated carotid sinus discharge following removal of the atheromatous plaque (15,27,99). Some surgeons believe that this response may be blunted by infiltration of the carotid sinus with lidocaine at the time of surgery (15,16). Postoperative hypotension may be treated with intravenous fluids and vasopressors. Atropine will reverse the bradycardia (27). Postoperative hypotension is best anticipated and prevented, since neurologic complications occur with 7% to 40% of such episodes (15,79).

Myocardial Infarction

Postoperative myocardial infarction, the second most common cause of perioperative morbidity and mortality, complicates about 2% to 3% of carotid endarterectomies (29,80). Bernard et al. (10) reported a cardiac mortality of 20% following endarterectomy. Meticulous patient selection and preparation should circumvent this unusually high mortality rate. Myocardial infarction is also the most frequent late complication, accounting for approximately 50% of late deaths following carotid endarterectomy (57).

Preoperative screening for a recent history of myocardial infarction, the presence of an S_3 gallop or other evidence for heart failure, aortic stenosis, and frequent premature ventricular contractions (PVCs) effectively identifies many patients at risk for perioperative myocardial infarction (39), particularly in the age group over 70 years. Further evaluation may include dipyridamole-thallium imaging (14) and cardiac catheterization. Dipyridamole-thallium imaging allows for noninvasive detection of coronary artery disease in patients who otherwise are unable to exercise.

The coronary syndromes that may follow carotid endarterectomy include exacerbation of stable angina, development of unstable angina, and acute myocardial infarction. Exacerbation of stable angina occurs when myocardial oxygen demand exceeds the impaired myocardial oxygen delivery. Increased oxygen demand may result from postoperative tachycardia or hypertension. Unstable angina and acute myocardial infarction represent a spectrum of disease resulting from various stages of coronary artery plaque disruption, vasoconstriction, and thrombosis (33), which decrease myocardial oxygen supply abruptly. Therefore, if there are symptoms or electrocardiographic (EKG) evidence of postoperative ischemia, unstable angina, or infarction, the goals of therapy are to decrease myocardial oxygen consumption, increase myocardial oxygen supply, and inhibit further coronary artery thrombus formation.

Nitrates, narcotics, and beta-adrenergic blockers all function primarily to decrease myocardial oxygen demand. Nitrates dilate the capacitance vessels and lower preload, thus reducing left ventricular wall stress (114). They also enhance collateral flow to areas of ischemic myocardium (40). Narcotics decrease myocardial oxygen demand by reducing anxiety and by reducing preload (as a result of venodilatation). Beta-adrenergic blockers reduce myocardial oxygen demand by virtue of their negative chronotropic and inotropic effects but are contraindicated in patients with bradycardia, atrioventricular block, or significant heart failure. Finally, diltiazem is cardioprotective in patients who have had a non-Q-wave myocardial infarction, presumably by reducing heart rate (decreasing myocardial oxygen demand) and by preventing coronary vasoconstriction (increasing myocardial oxygen supply) (37).

Intra-aortic balloon counterpulsation is indicated in patients with unstable angina refractory to the medical therapy. Intra-aortic balloon counterpulsation decreases myocardial oxygen demand by reducing afterload. Additionally, by inflating during diastole, diastolic coronary filling is enhanced, thereby increasing myocardial oxygen supply (67).

Systemic heparin or aspirin is used to inhibit further coronary artery thrombus formation, decrease ischemia, and reduce progression to myocardial infarction. Aspirin reduces the incidence of myocardial infarction and death in patients with unstable angina (101,112) and the incidence of reinfarction and death in patients with acute myocardial infarction (53). Heparin also reduces progression to myocardial infarction in patients with unstable angina and may provide additional benefit to patients who have angina that is refractory to aspirin therapy (101).

If evidence exists for continued ischemia or acute myocardial infarction, patients are referred for coronary angiography with angioplasty if possible. Early postoperative patients are not candidates for systemic thrombolytic therapy with its attendant hemorrhagic risks. Coronary angioplasty avoids these hemorrhagic risks, particularly those of intracerebral bleeding (42,69). Angioplasty establishes reperfusion in more than 90% of acute coronary artery occlusions (44,83). The major drawbacks to angioplasty are the requirements for rapid activation of a catheterization team and the potential for early closure of the dilated vessel (102). Coronary artery bypass is considered for patients with persistent symptoms or for those who are not candidates for angioplasty.

VENOUS THROMBOEMBOLISM

Deep venous thrombosis (DVT) and pulmonary embolism (PE) are common complications in the postoperative patient. Depending on the procedure, DVT afflicts as many as 34% of postoperative neurosurgical patients (19) and as many as 60% of patients with hemiparesis secondary to stroke (110). Due to limitations in screening, the true incidence may actually be higher. Risk factors for the development of DVT include age, heart failure, prior DVT, pelvic or lower extremity trauma, and duration of anesthesia (66,97).

The clinical findings in acute DVT include calf pain, swelling, and warmth of the affected extremity. However, the diagnosis of DVT by these clinical features is notoriously imprecise (74,97). Thus, a high index of suspicion must be coupled with more sensitive diagnostic techniques. Several diagnostic options are available. Venography is the gold standard but is invasive and carries the risk of contrast reaction. In addition, the process of performing the study may dislodge clot (12). Radiolabeled fibrinogen detects calf DVT with 83% sensitivity and 93% specificity, but it is insensitive for ileofemoral clots, which have the highest embolic potential (74). Conversely, impedance plethysmography is better for proximal clot detection with approximately a 92% sensitivity and 96% specificity (49). Doppler with real-time ultrasound is a rapidly evolving technology capable of visualizing the venous system of the lower extremity in real time. Incompressibility of the vein is the most useful indicator of thrombosis. Sensitivity of Doppler ultrasound in experienced hands is 98% with a specificity of 96% (111).

Pulmonary embolism occurs in 50% of patients with DVT (74) and most frequently in DVTs that extend above the knee (65). Symptoms of pulmonary embolism include dyspnea, pleurisy, apprehension, and hemptysis. Tachypnea (respiratory rate > 16/min) is present in 90% of patients, with fever, tachycardia, and rales in 40% to 60% (8,50,84,94). Ten percent of patients have a po$_2$ greater than 80 mmHg (8), and the EKG is often abnormal but nonspecific (93). The chest radiograph frequently shows consolidation, elevated hemidiaphragm, or pleural effusion (84).

Definitive diagnosis of pulmonary embolism requires a high probability ventilation-perfusion lung scan or a positive pulmonary arteriogram. A high probability lung scan has a specificity of 97%. Approximately 14% to 30% of patients with acute pulmonary emboli have low or indeterminate probability scans, respectively. Less than 4% of patients with pulmonary emboli have a normal lung scan (78). Therefore high probability and normal lung scans are useful in therapeutic decision-making. Indeterminate and low probability scans require further evaluation with angiography before the diagnosis of pulmonary embolism is secure. However, if DVT is present, angiography is unnecessary since, in the presence of documented venous thrombosis, the decision to treat is not altered by the results of the angiogram.

Since the overwhelming majority of pulmonary emboli originate in the venous system of the lower extremity (87), prevention of deep venous thrombosis will prevent most pulmonary emboli. Four approaches are used for the prevention of DVT: (a) low-dose heparin, (b) coumadin, (c) graduated compression stockings, and (d) pneumatic compression stockings. The National Institutes of Health consensus conference on prevention of venous thrombosis recommends intermittent, sequential pneumatic compression stockings as the preventive measure of choice in neurosurgical patients (68). These devices effectively reduce postoperative DVT by as much as 80% to 90% (51,90,106). The protective mechanism of sequential pneumatic compression is not fully defined. Augmentation of lower extremity blood flow is not the sole mechanism for the protective effect. These devices also enhance the fibrinolytic system, thus promoting clot dissolution (3). The latter mechanism explains the protective effect of arm or single-leg compression device on untreated extremities (55). This modality is cost effective (68) and of proven benefit in the neurosurgical patient (90). Intermittent compression stockings are applied preoperatively or immediately postoperatively and continued for the duration of inactivity.

Subcutaneous heparin is also highly effective in preventing DVT and can be used either alone or with external pneumatic compression stockings in endarterectomy patients (22). Subcutaneous heparin is safe in neurosurgical patients (31) with the possible exception of an increased incidence (approximately 4%) of wound seromas and hematomas (6).

Treatment of DVT and PE in the postoperative setting depends on the proximity to the surgery. In general, anticoagulation is contraindicated for the first 7 to 10 days postoperatively (5). However, since patients with postoperative hypertension may be at increased risk for hemorrhage, the therapeutic decision regarding anticoagulation remains highly individualized. If the patient is not a candidate for anticoagulation, an inferior vena caval filter is placed (54,98). If the patient is anticoagulated, heparin is administered as a bolus of 5,000 U followed by a continuous infusion of 1,000 U/hr, and the infusion is adjusted to maintain the partial thromboplastin time at least 1.5 times control (7). Coumadin therapy is started with heparin, although heparin is continued until the international normalized ratio is 2.0 to 3.0 (corresponding to a prothrombin time of 1.3 to 1.5 times control) with an overlap of 3 to 5 days (48,52). The duration of oral anticoagulation is 3 to 6 months or longer depending on the persistence of clinical risk factors and the speed at which the clot resolves (66).

MISCELLANEOUS COMPLICATIONS

Respiratory Effects

Hypoxic chemoreception may be blunted preoperatively in patients with bilateral carotid occlusive disease. A normal response in such patients may be reactivated after endarterectomy, suggesting that the plaque disrupts blood supply to the carotid body (107). The cerebral blood flow response to carbon dioxide is also blunted preoperatively. Chronic ischemia may cause maximal vasodilatation and preclude further vasodilatation in response to carbon dioxide. This reactivity is restored postoperatively and maintained at 6 months (13).

Short-term mechanical ventilation may be required postoperatively, especially if the patient received intraoperative barbiturates for cerebral protection. Standard ventilator settings are employed: tidal volume 8 to 12 ml/kg, rate 8 to 12/min, Fio_2 50%, positive end-expiratory pressure (PEEP) 0 to 5 cmH$_2$O, and a volume cycled modality (intermittent mandatory or assist-control ventilation). The minute ventilation (rate $\times$ tidal volume) is adjusted to provide normal $paco_2$, and an arterial hemoglobin saturation of >95% is maintained by adjustments in PEEP and Fio_2. PEEP in excess of 3 to 5 cmH$_2$O is rarely necessary in the postoperative endarterectomy patient. PEEP has the potential to decrease MAP with adverse consequences for cerebral perfusion pressure (CPP) and neurologic function (1). However, adverse consequences of PEEP on ICP or CPP were noted infrequently in brain-injured humans (32,88). Patients are ready to wean from the ventilator when their mental status returns to baseline, the gag and cough reflexes return, minute ventilation is less than 10 L/min, pao_2 is ≥60 mmHg on Fio_2 ≤50%, and static lung compliance (tidal volume/peak airway pressure—PEEP) is >30 ml/cmH$_2$O. In most patients, this occurs within the first 12 to 24 hours. High minute ventilation and low lung compliance preclude weaning and should prompt a search for complicating respiratory pathology. Disorders such as emphysema, pulmonary embolism, and sepsis result in high minute ventilation, whereas pulmonary edema, pneumonia, and pneumothorax cause decreases in lung compliance. Weaning proceeds most directly by gradual decrements in the set mandatory respiratory rate.

Renal Effects

Magovern et al. (59) reported a patient with the syndrome of inappropriate antidiuretic hormone secretion (SIADH) following carotid endarterectomy. The diagnosis of SIADH was established by the finding of inappropriately hypertonic urinary osmolality in the setting of hypotonic serum. Significant volume depletion, hypothyroidism, and adrenal insufficiency must be excluded to make the diagnosis of SIADH. This patient developed hyponatremia (S$_{Na}$ = 111 mEq/L) 36 hours postoperatively, in association with a progressive hemiparesis. The patient improved, both neurologically and chemically with fluid restriction. The pathogenesis of the SIADH in this setting was postulated to be focal reperfusion injury since the ipsilateral neurologic deficit was in the same distribution as the preoperative transient ischemic attacks.

Gastrointestinal Considerations

Generally, postoperative endarterectomy patients are not at high risk for stress ulceration. Therefore routine prophylaxis for stress-induced gastric bleeding cannot be supported. If prophylaxis is chosen, antacids should be avoided since they can promote aspiration by increasing gastric volume and are more injurious to the lung than gastric acid if they are aspirated (36). Furthermore, antacids have the highest rate of associated nosocomial pneumonia when compared with H$_2$ blockers or carafate (26). Therefore, if stress gastritis prophylaxis is necessary, carafate or H$_2$ blockers are recommended.

Cranial Nerve Injuries

Injuries to the recurrent laryngeal, superior laryngeal, facial, and hypoglossal nerves have been reported with a combined frequency of 12% to 23% following conventional carotid endarterectomy (47,61) and of 1.7% after microendarterectomy (28). These cranial nerve deficits are frequently mild and usually resolve within the first postoperative year. However, permanent deficits have been reported (61). Bilateral vocal cord paralysis may result in airway obstruction in patients who have bilateral carotid endarterectomy (72). Otolaryngologic examination is recommended for such patients undergoing staged bilateral surgery (47).

Fever

The causes of potential infectious and noninfectious fevers following carotid endarterectomy are many (24). Noninfectious causes of fever include atelectasis, drug reactions, and deep venous thrombosis. Infectious causes include nosocomial pneumonia as well as line, urinary tract, and wound infections. The most common following endarterectomy are wound infections caused by *Staphylococcus aureus* (95). The incidence of wound infection in microendarterectomy is 3.3% (28).

CONCLUSIONS

The major causes of morbidity and mortality following carotid endarterectomy are stroke, intracerebral hemorrhage, myocardial infarction, and thromboembolic disease. All candidates for carotid endarterectomy require a thorough preoperative evaluation including rigorous screening for underlying coronary artery disease and hypertension. Patients with signs or symptoms of poorly controlled coronary artery disease should undergo more detailed preoperative evaluation. Meticulous preoperative control of blood pressure reduces the likelihood of postoperative neurologic and cardiac complications. Postoperative hypertension and hypotension must be anticipated and aggressively treated. Perioperative prophylaxis for deep venous thrombosis is essential for all patients. Close cooperation between the surgeon and consulting medical services ensures optimal preparation and postoperative care for these complex patients.

REFERENCES

1. Aidinis SJ, Lafferty J, Shapiro HM. Intracranial responses to PEEP. *Anesthesiology* 1976; 45:275–286.
2. Akers DL, Brinker MR, Englehardt TC, Kerstein MD. Postoperative somnolence in patients after carotid endarterectomy. *Surgery* 1990;107:684–687.
3. Allenby F, Pflug JJ, Boearman L, Calnan JS. Effects of external intermittent compression on fibrinolysis in man. *Lancet* 1973;1:1412–1414.
4. Archie JP. The relationship of early hypertension following carotid endarterectomy to intraoperative cerebral ischemia. *Ann Vasc Surg* 1988;2:108–113.
5. Bailes, JE. Current treatment of thromboembolic events in neurosurgical patients. *Perspect Neurol Surg* 1990;1:150–164.
6. Barnett HG, Clifford JR, Llewellyn RC. Safety of mini-dose heparin administration for neurosurgical patients. *J Neurosurg* 1977;47:27–30.
7. Basu D, Gallus A, Hirsh J, Cade J. A prospective study of the value of monitoring heparin treatment with the activated partial thromboplastin time. *N Engl J Med* 1972;287:324–327.
8. Bell WR, Simon TL, DeMets DL. The clinical features of submassive and massive pulmonary emboli. *Am J Med* 1977;62:355–360.
9. Benumof JL. Hypoxic pulmonary vasoconstriction and infusion of sodium nitroprusside. *Anesthesiology* 1979;50:451–483.
10. Bernard VM, Johnson WD, Peterson JJ. Carotid artery stenosis: association with surgery for coronary artery disease. *Arch Surg* 1972;105:837–840.
11. Bernstein M, Fleming JF, Deck JH. Cerebral hyperperfusion after carotid endarterectomy: a cause of cerebral hemorrhage. *Neurosurgery* 1984;15:50–56.
12. Bettmann MA, Robbins A, Braun SD, Wetzner S, Dunnick NR, Finkelstein J. Contrast venography of the leg: diagnostic efficacy, tolerance, and complication rates with ionic and nonionic contrast media. *Radiology* 1987;165:113–116.
13. Bishop CC, Butler L, Hunt T, Burnand KG, Browse NL. Effect of carotid endarterectomy on cerebral blood flow and its response to hypercapnia. *Br J Surg* 1987;74:994–996.
14. Boucher CA, Brewster DC, Darling RC, Okada RD, Strauss HW, Pohost GM. Determination of cardiac risk by dipyridamole-thallium imaging before peripheral vascular surgery. *N Engl J Med* 1985;312:389–394.
15. Bove EL, Fry WJ, Gross WS, Stanley JC. Hypotension and hypertension as consequences of baroreceptor dysfunction following carotid endarterectomy. *Surgery* 1979;85:633–637.
16. Cafferata HT, Merchant RF, DePalma RG. Avoidance of postcarotid endarterectomy hypertension. *Ann Surg* 1982;196:465–472.
17. Caplan LR, Pessin MS. Symptomatic carotid artery disease and carotid endarterectomy. *Ann Rev Med* 1988;39:273–299.
18. Caplan LR, Skillman J, Ojemann R, et al. Intracerebral hemorrhage following carotid endarterectomy: a hypertensive complication. *Stroke* 1978;9:457–460.
19. Ceratto D, Adriano C, Fiacchino F. Deep venous thrombosis and low-dose heparin prophylaxis in neurosurgical patients. *J Neurosurg* 1978;49:378–381.
20. Cetnarowski AB, Conti DR. Nitroprusside toxicity and low dose infusion. *Ann Intern Med* 1986;104:895–896.
21. Cohn JN, Burke LP. Nitroprusside. *Ann Intern Med* 1979;91:752–757.
22. Collins R, Scrimgeour A, Yusef S, Peto R. Reduction in fatal pulmonary emboli and venous

thrombosis by perioperative administration of subcutaneous heparin. *N Engl J Med* 1988; 318:1161–1173.

23. Cottrell JE, Gupta B, Rappaport H, et al. Intracranial pressure during nitroglycerin-induced hypotension. *J Neurosurg* 1980;53:309–311.

24. Cunha BA, Tu RP. Fever in the neurosurgical patient. *Heart Lung* 1988;6:608–611.

25. DeMarco T, Daley PA, Lium M, et al. Enalaprilat, a new parenteral angiotensin converting enzyme inhibitor: rapid changes in systemic and coronary hemodynamics and humoral profile in chronic heart failure. *J Am Coll Cardiol* 1987;9:1131–1138.

26. Driks MR, Craven DE, Celli BR, et al. Nosocomial pneumonia in intubated patients given sucralfate as compared with antacids or histamine type 2 blockers. *N Engl J Med* 1987; 317:1376–1382.

27. Englund R, Dean RH. Blood pressure aberrations associated with carotid endarterectomy. *Ann Vasc Surg* 1986;1:304–310.

28. Findlay JM, Lougheed WM. Carotid microendarterectomy. *Neurosurgery* 1993;32: 792–798.

29. Fode NC, Sundt T, Robertson J, et al. Multicenter retrospective review of results and complications of carotid endarterectomy. *Stroke* 1986;17:370–376.

30. Fremes SE, Weisel RD, Mickle DA, et al. A comparison of nitroglycerine and nitroprusside. 1. Treatment of postoperative hypertension. *Ann Thorac Surg* 1985;39:53–60.

31. Frim DM, Barker FG, Poletti CE, Hamilton AJ. Postoperative low-dose heparin decreases thromboembolic complications in neurosurgical patients. *Neurosurgery* 1992;30:830–833.

32. Frost EM. Effects of positive end-expiratory pressure on intracranial pressure and compliance in brain-injured patients. *J Neurosurg* 1977;47:195–200.

33. Fuster V, Badimon L, Badimon JJ, Chesebro JH. The pathogenesis of coronary artery disease and the acute coronary syndromes. *N Engl J Med* 1992;326:310–318.

34. Geniton DJ. A comparison of the hemodynamic effects of labetalol and sodium nitroprusside in patients undergoing carotid endarterectomy. *J Am Assoc Nurse Anesth* 1990;58: 281–287.

35. Ghani GA, Sung YF, Weinstein MS, et al. Effects of intravenous nitroglycerin on the intracranial pressure and volume pressure response. *J Neurosurg* 1983;58:562–565.

36. Gibbs CP, Schwartz DJ, Wynne JW, et al. Antacid pulmonary aspiration in the dog. *Anesthesiology* 1979;51:380–385.

37. Gibson RS, Boden WE, Theroux P, et al. Diltiazem and reinfarction in patients with non-Q-wave myocardial infarction. *N Engl J Med* 1986;315:423–429.

38. Gittin JP, Cottrell JE, Hartung J, Shwiry D. Intracranial pressure during nifedipine-induced hypotension. *Anesth Analg* 1983;62:1078–1080.

39. Goldman L, Caldera DL, Nussbaum SR, et al. Multifactorial index of cardiac risk in noncardiac surgical procedures. *N Engl J Med* 1977;297:845–850.

40. Goldstein RE, Stinson EB, Scherber JL, Seningen RP, Grehl TM, Epstein SE. Intraoperative coronary collateral function in patients with coronary occlusive disease: nitroglycerin responsiveness and angiographic correlations. *Circulation* 1974;49:298–308.

41. Graves JW. Prolonged continuous infusion labetalol. A new alternative for parenteral antihypertensive therapy. *Crit Care Med* 1989;17:759–761.

42. Grines CL, Browne KF, Marco J, et al. A comparison of immediate angioplasty with thrombolytic therapy for acute myocardial infarction. *N Engl J Med* 1993;328:673–679.

43. Hans SS, Prakash S, Hans P. The role of renin and catecholamine production in postcarotid endarterectomy hypertension. *Surg Gynecol Obstet* 1992;174:201–204.

44. Hartzler GO, Rutherford BD, McConahay DR, et al. Percutaneous transluminal coronary angioplasty with and without thrombolytic therapy for treatment of acute myocardial infarction. *Am Heart J* 1983;106:965–973.

45. Healy DA, Clowes AW, Zierler RE, et al. Immediate and long-term results of carotid endarterectomy. *Stroke* 1989;20:1138–1142.

46. Henriksen L, Paulson OB. The effects of sodium nitroprusside on cerebral blood flow and cerebral venous blood gases. *Eur J Clin Invest* 1982;12:389–393.

47. Hertzer NR, Feldman BJ, Beven EG, Tucker HM. A prospective study of the incidence of injury to the cranial nerves during carotid endarterectomy. *Surg Gynecol Obstet* 1981; 151:781–784.

48. Hirsh J. Treatment of pulmonary embolism. *Ann Rev Med* 1987;38:91–105.

49. Hull R, Taylor W, Hirsch J, et al. Impedance plethysmography: the relationship between venous filling and sensitivity and specificity for proximal vein thrombosis. *Circulation* 1978;58:898–902.

50. Hull RD, Hirsh J, Carter CJ, et al. Diagnostic value of ventilation-perfusion lung scanning in patients with suspected pulmonary embolism. *Chest* 1985;88:819–828.

51. Hull RD, Moser KM, Salzman EW. Preventing pulmonary embolism. *Patient Care* 1989; Feb 28:63–81.

52. Hull RD, Raskob GE, Rosenbloom D, et al. Heparin for 5 days as compared to 10 days in the initial treatment of proximal venous thrombosis. *N Engl J Med* 1990;322:1260–1264.

53. ISIS-2 Collaborative Group. Randomised trial of intravenous streptokinase, oral aspirin, both or neither among 17,187 cases of suspected myocardial infarction. *Lancet* 1988;2: 349–360.

54. Jones T, Barnes R, Greenfield L. Greenfield vena cava filter: rationale and current indications. *Ann Thorac Surg* 1986;42:48–55.

55. Knight MT, Dawson R. Effect of intermittent compression of the arms on deep venous thrombosis in the legs. *Lancet* 1976;2:1265–1267.

56. Lebel M, Langlois S, Belleau LJ, et al. Labetalol infusion in hypertensive emergencies. *Clin Pharmacol Ther* 1985;37:615–618.

57. Lee KS, Davis CH. Stroke, myocardial infarction, and survival during long-term follow-up after carotid endarterectomy. *Surg Neurol* 1989;31:113–119.

58. Lehv MS, Salzman EW, Silen W. Hypertension complicating carotid endarterectomy. *Stroke* 1970;1:307–313.

59. Magovern JA, Sieber PR, Thiele BL. The syndrome of inappropriate secretion of antidiuretic hormone following carotid endarterectomy. *J Cardiovasc Surg* 1989;30:544–546.

60. Marsh ML, Aidinis SJ, Naughton BS, Marshall LF, Shapiro HM. The technique of nitroprusside administration modifies the intracranial pressure response. *Anesthesiology* 1979; 51:538–541.

61. Massey EW, Heyman A, Utley C, Haynes C, Fuchs J. Cranial nerve paralysis following carotid endarterectomy. *Stroke* 1984;15:157–159.

62. McDowall DJ, Keaney NP, Turner JM, et al. The toxicity of sodium nitroprusside. *Br J Anaesth* 1974;46:327–332.

63. McKay RD, Newfield P, Reves JG, Brummett C, Morawetz RB. Hypertension and mortality in neuro ICU patients. *Anesthesiology* 1981;55:A101.

64. Meline LJ, Westenkow DR, Pace NL, et al. Computer-controlled regulation of sodium nitroprusside infusion. *Anesth Analg* 1985;64:38–42.

65. Moser KM. Is embolic risk conditioned by location of deep venous thrombosis? *Ann Intern Med* 1981;94:439–444.

66. Moser KM. Venous thromboembolism. *Am Rev Respir Dis* 1990;141:235–249.

67. Mueller HS, Ayers SM, Conklin EF, et al. The effects of intraaortic counterpulsation on cardiac performance and metabolism in shock associated with acute myocardial infarction. *J Clin Invest* 1971;50:1885–1900.

68. National Institutes of Health Consensus Conference. Prevention of venous thrombosis and pulmonary embolism. *JAMA* 1986;256:744–748.

69. O'Keefe JH, Rutherford BD, McConahay DR, et al. Early and late results of coronary angioplasty without antecedent thrombolytic therapy for acute myocardial infarction. *Am J Cardiol* 1989;10:264–272.

70. Orlowski JP, Shiesley D, Vidt DG, et al. Labetalol to control blood pressure after cerebrovascular surgery. *Crit Care Med* 1988;16:765–768.

71. Oster G, Tuden RL, Colditz GA. Prevention of venous thromboembolism after general surgery. *Am J Med* 1987;82:889–899.

72. O'Sullivan JC, Wells GR. Difficult airway management with neck swelling after carotid endarterectomy. *Anaesth Intensive Care* 1986;14:460–464.

73. Owens ML, Wilson SE. Prevention of neurologic complications of carotid endarterectomy. *Arch Surg* 1982;117:551–555.

74. Painter TD. Thrombophlebitis: diagnostic techniques. *Angiology* 1980;31:386–397.

75. Paulson OB, Jarden JO, Godtfredsen J, et al. Cerebral blood flow in patients with congestive heart failure treated with captopril. *Am J Med* 1984;76:91–98.

76. Perdue GD. Management of postendarterectomy neurologic deficits. *Arch Surg* 1982;117: 1079–1081.

77. Piepgras DG, Morgan MK, Sundt TM, Yanagihara T, Mussman LM. Intracerebral hemorrhage after carotid endarterectomy. *J Neurosurg* 1988;68:532–536.

78. PIOPED Investigators. Value of the ventilation/perfusion scan in acute pulmonary embolism. *JAMA* 1990;263:2753–2759.

79. Ransom JH, Imparato AM, Clauss RH, et al. Factors in the mortality and morbidity associated with surgical treatment of cerebrovascular insufficiency. *Circulation* 1969;39: [Suppl I]269–274.

80. Riles TS, Kopelman I, Imparato AM. Myocardial infarction following carotid endarterectomy: a review of 683 operations. *Surgery* 1979;8:249–252.

81. Robertson CS, Clifton GL, Taylor AA, Grossman RG. Treatment of hypertension associated with head injury. *J Neurosurg* 1983;59:455–460.

82. Rosenthal D, Zeichner WD, Lamis PA, Stanton PE. Neurologic deficit after carotid endarterectomy: pathogenesis and management. *Surgery* 1983;94:776–780.

83. Rothbaum DA, Linnemeier TJ, Landin RJ, et al. Emergency percutaneous transluminal coronary angioplasty in acute myocardial infarction: a three year experience. *J Am Coll Cardiol* 1987;10:264–272.

84. Sasahara AA. Current problems in pulmonary embolism: Introduction. *Prog Cardiovasc Dis* 1974;17:161–165.

85. Schroeder T, Sillesen H. Boeson J, Lauresn H, Sorensen PS. Intracerebral haemorrhage after carotid endarterectomy. *Eur J Vasc Surg* 1987;1:51–60.

86. Seltzer JL, Doto JB, Jacoby J. Decreased arterial oxygenation during sodium nitroprusside administration for intra-operative hypertension. *Anesth Analg Curr Res* 1976;55:880–881.

87. Sevitt S, Gallagher N. Venous thrombosis and pulmonary embolism—a clinicopathologic study in injured and burned patients. *Br J Surg* 1961;48:475–482.

88. Shapiro HM, Marshall LF. Intracranial pressure responses to PEEP in head-injured patients. *J Trauma* 1978;18:254–256.

89. Sieber FE, Toung TJ, Diringer MN, Wang H, Long DM. Preoperative risks predict neurological outcome of carotid endarterectomy related stroke. *Neurosurgery* 1992;30:847–854.

90. Skillman JJ, Collins RE, Coe NP, et al. Prevention of deep vein thrombosis in neurosurgical patients: a controlled, randomized trial of external pneumatic compression boots. *Surgery* 1978;83:354–358.

91. Skydell JL, Machleder HI, Baker D, Busuttil DW, Moore WS. Incidence and mechanism of post-carotid endarterectomy hypertension. *Arch Surg* 1987;122:1153–1155.

92. Soloman RA, Loftus CM, Quest DO, Correll JW. Incidence and etiology of intracerebral hemorrhage following carotid endarterectomy. *J Neurosurg* 1986;64:29–34.

93. Stein PD, Dalen JE, McIntyre KM, Sasahara AA, Wenger NK, Willis PW. The electrocardiogram in acute pulmonary embolism. *Prog Cardiovasc Dis* 1975;17:247–257.

94. Stein PD, Willis PW, DeMets DL. History and physical examination in acute pulmonary embolism in patients without preexisting cardiac or pulmonary disease. *Am J Cardiol* 1981; 47:218–223.

95. Sundt TM, Sandok BA, Whisnant JP. Carotid endarterectomy: complications and preoperative assessment of risk. *Mayo Clin Proc* 1975;50:301–306.

96. Sundt TM, Sharbrough FW, Piegras DG, Kearns TP, Messic JM, O'Fallon WM. Correlation of cerebral blood flow and electroencephalographic changes during carotid endarterectomy. *Mayo Clin Proc* 1981;56:533–543.

97. Swann KW, Black PM. Deep venous thrombosis and pulmonary emboli in neurosurgical patients: a review. *J Neurosurg* 1984;61:1055–1062.

98. Swann KW, Black PM, Baker MF. Management of symptomatic deep venous thrombosis and pulmonary embolism on a neurosurgical service. *J Neurosurg* 1986;64:563–567.

99. Tarlov E, Schmidek H, Scott R, Wepsic J, Ojemann R. Reflex hypotension following carotid endarterectomy: mechanism and management. *J Neurosurg* 1973;39:323–327.

100. Tateishi A, Takanobu S, Takeshita H, Suzuki T, Tokuno H. Effects of nifedipine on intracranial pressure in neurosurgical patients with arterial hypertension. *J Neurosurg* 1988;69:213–215.

101. Theroux P, Ouimet M, McCans J, et al. Aspirin, heparin, or both to treat acute unstable angina. *N Engl J Med* 1988;319:1105–1111.

102. Topol EJ, Califf RM, George BS, et al. A randomized trial of immediate versus delayed elective angioplasty after intravenous tissue plasminogen activator in acute myocardial infarction. *N Engl J Med* 1987;317:581–588.

103. Toronto Cerebrovascular Study Group. Risks of carotid endarterectomy. *Stroke* 1986;17: 848–852.

104. Towne JB, Bernhard VM. The relationship of postoperative hypertension to complications following carotid endarterectomy. *Surgery* 1980;88:575–580.

105. Turner JM, Powell D, Gibson RM, et al. Intracranial pressure changes in neurological patients during hypotension induced with sodium nitroprusside or trimethophan. *Br J Anaesth* 1977;49:419–425.

106. Turpie AG, Gallus AS, Beatie WS, Hirsch J. Prevention of venous thrombosis in patients with intracranial disease by intermittent pneumatic compression of the calf. *Neurology* 1977;27:435–438.

107. Vanmaele RG, DeBacker WA, Willemen MJ, et al. Hypoxic ventilatory response and carotid endarterectomy. *Eur J Vasc Surg* 1992;6:241–244.

108. Vlachkis ND, Maronde RF, Maly JW, et al. Pharmacodynamics of intravenous labetalol and follow-up therapy with oral labetalol. *Clin Pharmacol Ther* 1985;38:503–508.

109. Wachter RM. Symptomatic hypotension induced by nifedipine in the acute treatment of severe hypotension. *Arch Intern Med* 1987;147:556–558.

110. Warlow C, Ogston D, Douglas AS. Venous thrombosis following strokes. *Lancet* 1972; 1:1305–1306.

111. White RH, McGahan JP, Daschbach MM, Hartling RP. Diagnosis of deep-vein thrombosis using duplex ultrasound. *Ann Intern Med* 1989;111:297–304.

112. Willard JE, Lange RA, Hillis LD. The use of aspirin in ischemic heart disease. *N Engl J Med* 1992;327:175–181.

113. Williams GH. Converting-enzyme inhibitors in the treatment of hypertension. *N Engl J Med* 1988;319:1517–1525.

114. Williams JF, Glick G, Braunwald E. Studies on cardiac dimensions in intact unanesthetized man. V. Effects of nitroglycerin. *Circulation* 1965;32:767–771.

115. Wilson DJ, Wallin JD, Vlachachis N, et al. Intravenous labetalol in the treatment of severe hypertensive emergencies. *Am J Med* 1983;75(S):94–102.

10

Advances in Intervention for Carotid Disease

Julian E. Bailes, Arvind Ahuja, and
Donalee A. Davis

Advances in the medical and surgical care of patients with carotid atherosclerotic disease have been remarkable in recent years. Improvements in anesthetic technique and perioperative critical care have allowed us to successfully intervene in sicker patients and to affect positively their outcome from the atherosclerotic process and cerebral ischemia. In most cases, carefully selected patients undergoing carotid endarterectomy are prevented from suffering cerebrovascular accidents and the attendant neurologic morbidity.

As we look to the future of treatment for patients with carotid atherosclerotic processes, we will benefit from past experience and present knowledge. Several research areas appear to be likely to contribute to our understanding, to careful selection of appropriate patients, and to surgical techniques. Improvements in cerebral protective mechanisms will be forthcoming, both technically and pharmacologically. The immediate impact will be on our ability to choose the appropriate patient in terms of medical illnesses, neurologic condition, and determination of the patients for whom surgical intervention will improve on the natural history of the arterial disease.

The patient with asymptomatic carotid artery stenosis has traditionally posed a complex management problem in attempting to decide whether intervention is warranted and efficacious. The recent release of the Asymptomatic

J. E. Bailes and A. Ahuja: Department of Neurological Surgery, Allegheny General Hospital, Pittsburgh, Pennsylvania 15212.
D. Davis: Department of Neurovascular Diagnostic Ultrasound, Allegheny General Hospital, Pittsburgh, Pennsylvania 15212.

Carotid Atherosclerosis Study (ACAS) results has markedly advanced our understanding and helps to clarify this previously unclear clinical picture. This chapter discusses some historical thought concerning asymptomatic carotid atherosclerotic disease and attempts to summarize the state of our present knowledge, particularly in light of the recent ACAS results. Along these lines, the use of noninvasive carotid examination, particularly Doppler ultrasound testing, has become increasingly important in screening patients for possible surgery. All too often, surgeons have overlooked the impact as well as the technical aspects of this noninvasive, cost-effective, reliable, and increasingly important examination. The basics of Doppler ultrasound including newer color Doppler analysis are presented. This overview may serve to interest some surgeons who have previously been unfamiliar with this imaging modality.

As has often been said, one of the aims of surgical research is to reduce or eliminate invasive procedures. Advances will be made in medical treatment, providing reduction or elimination of severe atherosclerotic processes. In addition, less invasive procedures will be brought to the forefront in the treatment of atherosclerosis. Carotid angioplasty is currently in its infancy but should continue to grow and, in all likelihood, endovascular techniques will provide increasing capabilities to treat patients in a safer, cost-effective, and less invasive manner.

ASYMPTOMATIC CAROTID STENOSIS

The future risk of cerebral ischemic events in asymptomatic patients has been the source of debate for many years. There has been uncertainty and ongoing debate concerning the implications of asymptomatic carotid stenosis and especially the efficacy of prophylactic carotid endarterectomy. The presence of cervical carotid bruits has been noted as a marker for extracranial carotid artery disease. Asymptomatic cervical bruits are present in approximately 4% of people older than 40 and in about 8% of normal persons older than 75 (62).

Occasionally bruits are caused by innocuous arterial pattern variations such as large-vessel tortuosity, anemia, or other hyperkinetic circulatory disorders secondary to systemic illnesses. It is believed that as the degree of stenosis increases, so does the presence and harshness of the bruit, up until the time that a marked reduction of blood flow past the lesion or total arterial occlusion occurs. Cervical bruits do not always reliably determine the location of the stenotic lesion, and up to one-third of patients with carotid stenotic lesions will not have bruits (17). Ocular bruits originate from a variety of causes including arteriovenous malformations, vascular tumors, hyperdynamic circulatory conditions, periorbital lesions, and Paget's disease, among others (62). Carotid siphon stenosis and contralateral carotid occlusion may also give rise to ocular bruits (30,66).

In patients age 40 or older and especially in those with concomitant peripheral and/or coronary atherosclerosis, carotid bruits always deserve consideration and may serve as a guide for further investigation. The degree of atherosclerotic change and characteristics and the location of the stenotic lesion are inadequately determined by the clinical examination. Further diagnostic evaluation (beginning with noninvasive techniques such as Doppler ultrasound, magnetic resonance angiography, or digital subtraction angiography) is required before a definitive diagnosis is made and treatment plan formulated.

While some authors have recommended surgical intervention for any patient with carotid narrowing, defining the population at risk and deciding in which patients endarterectomy improved on the natural history has been a difficult task. Historically, it has been felt that the natural history of asymptomatic carotid artery stenoses could likely vary between patient populations. For instance, patients with severe (greater than 90%) stenosis, complex ulcer formation, or severe ulcerative lesion are at greater risk than patients without these features. Progressive carotid stenosis, as documented by serial examinations, has also been considered a harbinger of an advanced and dynamic atherosclerotic process, which placed the asymptomatic patient at higher risk. Concomitant coronary artery disease likewise implies a more extensive atherosclerotic process and may indicate a more aggressive approach to previously asymptomatic carotid disease in selected patients. Clinicians have felt that men may experience more subsequent cerebral ischemic events and previously asymptomatic carotid artery stenosis, a finding supported by the ACAS data.

Studies with serial arteriograms performed over several years have shown a significant increase in the size of the atheromatous lesions. Javid et al. (47) found that 52% of atheromas progressed in size, with an increase greater than 25% annually and 34% of lesions with recurrent stenosis or thrombosis occurring in 7.4% of patients.

Several studies have attempted to determine a natural history of occlusive carotid artery disease in patients with asymptomatic carotid bruits. In 1980 Heyman et al. (42) reported the results of a population-based study in Evans County, Georgia in which 1,620 persons, aged 45 years or older, were surveyed. These patients had been previously asymptomatic for cerebral or cardiac ischemic disease and had asymptomatic cervical bruits noted on physical examination. On a 6-year follow-up analysis a significantly greater risk of stroke in men than in women was noted (odds ratio, 7.5 and 1.6, respectively). However, the laterality and the location of the carotid bruits often did not correlate with the type of subsequent cerebrovascular accident. In only three persons did cerebral infarction occur ipsilateral to the cervical carotid bruit. In two people in this study, massive intracranial hemorrhage resulted in their deaths. During the 6-year evaluation period, this study confirmed 90 deaths, 36 of which resulted from cerebrovascular accident and 54 from ischemic coronary disease. Therefore cervical carotid bruits, especially in men, proved to be more of a risk factor for death from ischemic heart disease than from cerebrovascular accidents (42).

In the Framingham study, Wolfe et al. (80) analyzed 171 persons for 8 years who had asymptomatic cervical carotid bruits. They found an increased incidence of bruit varying from 3.5% of the population aged 44 to 54 years to 7.0% for those 65 to 79 years old. An increased incidence was seen in patients who had hypertension and diabetes mellitus. They found an increased incidence of cerebral ischemic events: transient ischemic attacks (TIAs) in 8 persons and cerebrovascular accidents in 21. This represented a stroke rate more than twice that expected for the age and sex of this population. However, the location of the stroke was often different from the territory supplied by the ipsilateral turbulent carotid artery. The type of stroke varied and was more frequently seen as aneurysmal subarachnoid hemorrhage, lacunar cerebral infarction, and cardiac-origin embolization. In addition, a 2.5 times increased risk of myocardial infarction and subsequent mortality in patients with carotid bruit was found. They concluded that the presence of a carotid bruit was a marker for generalized atherosclerotic disease and in particular for cardiovascular morbidity and mortality.

In a prospective study, Wiebers et al. (79) analyzed a referral population of 566 patients with asymptomatic carotid bruit, comparing them with 428 patients in a population-based cohort without carotid bruit, who were free of cerebrovascular symptoms. They followed each person until death or for a 5-year period and found that of patients with asymptomatic carotid bruit, the annual stroke rate was 1.5% a year or 7.5% at 5 years. By contrast, in patients without the presence of carotid bruit, they found a stroke rate of 0.5% a year or 2.4% at 5 years. They also found that patients with localized carotid bruit were not significantly different (in terms of future cerebrovascular ischemia) from those whose physical examination disclosed diffuse carotid bruits. They concluded that patients with asymptomatic, diffuse, or localized carotid bruit have three times the incidence of ischemic stroke than patients without such bruits (79). Hennerichi et al. (41) prospectively studied 339 patients with asymptomatic carotid stenosis who were admitted for serial Doppler ultrasound examination. Of these patients, 199 had slight or moderate stenoses, 36 had severe stenoses, and 49 had documented internal carotid artery occlusion. They found an annual mortality rate of 7% and a stroke mortality of 0.6% at 7-year follow-up. Ten patients died secondary to cerebrovascular accidents and 41 died from cardiac causes. They also found that the risk of cerebrovascular accident without premonitory cerebral TIAs was low, 0.4%, a rate not favoring prophylactic endarterectomy for neurologically asymptomatic patients (41).

A prospective 23-month study of 500 patients with asymptomatic cervical carotid bruits was reported by Chambers and Norris (17). They found a 6% incidence of cerebral ischemic events, both TIAs and strokes, at 1 year and a 4% mortality rate. Only 1% of patients suffered a stroke without warning TIAs, with a 1-year stroke risk rate of 1.7%. An increased incidence (up to 5.5%) of cerebrovascular accident was found in patients with greater than 75% stenosis. Norris et al. (63) reported on 696 patients with asymptomatic carotid stenosis who were followed prospectively for a mean of 41 months. They found that TIAs occurred in 75 patients, and 29 suffered from stroke. During this time, 132 patients had ischemic coronary events, with 59 dying from myocardial infarction and only 5 from stroke. The annual stroke rate in patients with carotid stenosis of 75% or less was 1.3%, increasing to 3.3% in patients with greater than 75% carotid stenosis. With this severe degree of stenosis, the combined TIA and stroke rate was 10.5% annually, with three-fourths of the cerebral events ipsilateral to the narrowed vessel. Taking into account other etiologies of ipsilateral stroke such as hemorrhage and lacunar infarction, they estimated that the spontaneous ipsilateral annual stroke rate was below 2% in the highest risk group.

The Carotid Artery Stenosis and Narrowing Operation versus Aspirin (CASANOVA) study group was a multicenter trial of 410 patients with asymptomatic carotid disease angiographically defined as 50% to 90% stenosis. The efficacy of carotid endarterectomy in combination with antiplatelet therapy was compared with medical treatment using antiplatelet therapy alone. The patients were similar in regard to degree of stenosis, age, sex, and medical conditions. They considered only stroke and not TIAs the primary end point of the study. The total major/minor complication rate of surgery was 11.4%, with a total stroke rate of 3.0% and mortality rate of 1.2%. Their results showed no difference between carotid endarterectomy and medical treatment compared with medical treatment alone. They excluded patients in the high-risk group of greater than 90% stenosis, however (15).

Libman et al. (51) reported a retrospective study of 215 patients with asymptomatic carotid stenosis; 107 had carotid endarterectomy and 108 medical treatment alone. The mean follow-up period was 44 months. A 4.7% incidence of postoperative ipsilateral stroke was seen in carotid endarterectomy patients. Comparing carotid endarterectomy with medical management, this study showed no significant difference in the 5-year risk of ipsilateral stroke, stroke in any distribution, or survival free of any stroke.

Endarterectomy appeared to be of benefit for diabetic patients, those with a smoking history, those without myocardial infarction, and those with prior contralateral carotid distribution cerebral ischemic symptoms. Among carotid endarterectomy patients, independent predictors with the worst long-term outcome were history of myocardial infarction, age greater than 65 years, and systolic blood pressure on admission greater than 160 mmHg (51).

Several surgical studies have reported a benefit of carotid endarterectomy for patients with asymptomatic carotid bruit. Thompson et al. (76) reported their series of 132 patients who underwent 167 carotid endarterectomies for asymptomatic cervical carotid bruits, with a 15-year follow-up examination. They compared this surgical series with a control group of 138 patients with asymptomatic carotid bruits who were managed conservatively. Their operative results showed two transient and two permanent cerebral ischemic events and no operative mortality. During the follow-up period, 91% of the surgical patients remained asymptomatic and three (2.3%) developed nonfatal stroke at 11, 26, and 67 months postoperatively. Among the control group, 21 (15.2%) patients suffered cerebrovascular accidents at a mean interval of 20 months following discovery of the bruit. During this long period of follow-up, 43 of 132 (32.6%) patients in the carotid endarterectomy group died and 50 of 138 (36.2%) patients in the control group died. Cardiac events were the cause of death in 72% of the carotid endarterectomy patients and 48% of the control group patients. They concluded, with their respectable surgical complication rate, that patients with an asymptomatic carotid bruit may be improved upon by endarterectomy if selected appropriately. Meissner et al. (53) reported a retrospective study of 640 neurologically asymptomatic patients, 292 of whom had carotid artery stenotic lesions that were analyzed by ocular pneumoplethysmography to be pressure-significant. In 348 patients, a carotid bruit without a pressure-significant lesion was noted. The annual stroke rate for the first 3 years was 3.4% and 1.5% in the abnormal and normal ocular pneumoplethysmography groups, respectively, with a 0.5% rate in an all age- and sex-matched population. Considering both TIA and stroke, the annual total neurologic event rate was 5.2% compared with 2.3% in the normal group, with 50% of all neurologic ischemic events occurring ipsilateral to the ocular pneumoplethysmography abnormality. They concluded that patients with asymptomatic carotid occlusive disease deemed pressure-significant are at a twofold greater risk for cerebrovascular accident than those patients with normal ocular pneumoplethysmography and at a sevenfold greater risk than the general population (53). In a smaller study of 82 patients with TIAs and pressure-significant carotid lesions, Wiebers et al. (78) found a higher rate of ipsilateral cerebral ischemic symptoms than in patients without pressure-significant lesions.

Many clinicians have felt that high-grade carotid stenosis (greater than 90%) represents a higher risk and more ominous natural history than a lesser degree of narrowing. Indeed, several studies of asymptomatic carotid stenosis have excluded patients with a high degree of stenosis (15). Roederer et al. (67) studied a group of 167 asymptomatic patients who were followed with serial Doppler ultrasound studies. For the entire population, the yearly incidence of neurologic ischemic symptoms was 4%. However, in patients with an 80% to 99% diameter-reducing stenosis, 47% developed an ipsilateral TIA, stroke, or carotid occlusion within the 3-year follow-up. Bogousslavsky et al. (9) likewise found that high-grade stenosis of the carotid artery is associated with an increased neurologic risk. Moneta et al. (58) studied 129 asymptomatic high-grade (80% to 99%) internal carotid artery stenoses in 115 patients. Seventy-three carotid lesions were managed conservatively, and 56 carotid endarterectomies were performed in patients with a similar medical and cardiac risk profile. At 2-year follow-up, a dramatic reduction was seen in both cerebral ischemic events and carotid occlusion demonstrated for the surgically treated group. Their operative neurologic morbidity was 1.8% with no mortality. In the conservative medically managed group, a 28% incidence of TIAs and a 19% incidence of stroke were seen versus 5% and 4% in the endarterectomy group, respectively. In the medically managed population, eight of the nine strokes occurred within 9 months of diagnosis of a high-grade lesion, and none of the eight was preceded by TIA symptoms. These authors concluded that carotid endarterectomy, provided a low surgical complication rate exists, is indicated for patients with asymptomatic high-grade internal carotid artery stenosis (9).

The ACAS Report

A more definitive answer to the question of operative benefit in patients with asymptomatic carotid stenosis rested upon the results of planned large, randomized, clinical trials (3). The ACAS was commissioned to be such a study and to examine results in patients with asymptomatic carotid stenosis of greater than 60% reduction in diameter. The National Institute of Neurological Disorders and Stroke announced interim results of the ACAS trial in a Clinical Advisory in the fall of 1994. The objective of this study was to ascertain whether patients with severe but asymptomatic carotid artery stenosis benefit from carotid endarterectomy. The study was to consider perioperative risk of any stroke or death regardless of etiology and to explore a possible reduction in the overall 5-year risk of fatal and nonfatal ipsilateral carotid distribution cerebrovascular accidents. A total of 1,662 patients from 39 centers in the United States and Canada were entered during a 5-year period between December 1987 and December 1993. Randomization was done in patients between 40 and 79 years of age who had at least 60% carotid artery stenosis at the cervical origin of the internal carotid artery, as measured by angiography or Doppler ultrasonography. Life expectancy of at least 5 years was a criterion. Patients were excluded if they had symptoms associated with TIA or stroke or previous carotid endarterectomy of the randomized artery. In addition, medical conditions precluding adequate follow-up or that made 5-year survival unlikely were cause for exclusion.

Two groups were formulated, consisting of 828 patients who received carotid endarterectomy and 834 patients who had medical management only. All patients received 325 mg/day of aspirin and counseling to reduce atherosclerotic risk factors such as hypertension, obesity, and tobacco use. The male/female ratio was 2:1 and approximately half of the patients were between the ages of 60 and 69 years old. Thirty-seven percent of patients were 70 years of age or older and 95% were Caucasian.

The interim results of the randomized trial (terminated early in July 1994) demonstrated a marked beneficial effect in the surgical cohort. At the time of the report, the median follow-up was 2.7 years, consisting of 4,465 patient years of end-point observation. The aggregate risk of any stroke or fatality in the perioperative period for the carotid endarterectomy cohort was 2.3%. Using a Kaplan-Meier method in an intention-to-treat analysis, aggregate risk data over the 5-year follow-up period showed that the primary outcome (stroke) occurred in 4.8% of the surgical patients and in 10.6% of the medical management only patients. This means that the relative risk reduction conferred by carotid endarterectomy was 55% (23% to 73%, 95% confidence interval, $p = 0.004$).

As other studies have suggested, carotid endarterectomy for asymptomatic carotid stenosis was also shown to carry a greater risk reduction in men (69% relative risk reduction in men; 16% in women). The study showed that carotid endarterectomy was beneficial, with a statistically significant absolute reduction of stroke of 5.8% within 5 years and a relative risk reduction of 55%. Because the trial reached statistical significance in favor of surgery, on the recommendation of the study data monitoring committee participating physicians were notified immediately and advised to reevaluate patients who did not receive surgery (61).

As is the case for any intervention, perioperative neurologic morbidity and mortality as well as coronary and medical complications must be kept at an absolute minimum to improve on the natural history of carotid atherosclerotic disease. In the ACAS study, the aggregate risk of any stroke or death in the perioperative period of the endarterectomy cohort was 2.3%. The authors of the interim result study emphasized that the success of carotid endarterectomy in patients with asymptomatic internal carotid artery stenosis depends on performance by surgeons and medical centers to reach a perioperative morbidity and mortality rate of less than 3%. Such performance includes careful selection of patients and postoperative management of risk factors, both medical and neurologic.

In summary, the ACAS preliminary study reported on the first large, prospective multicenter clinical trial that demonstrated unequivocal results and favored carotid endarterectomy for patients with asymptomatic narrowing between 60% and 99%. We await formal publication to explore this population in greater detail with additional statistical analysis and in-depth study to explain the clinical results, including the apparent difference between the sexes.

NONINVASIVE CAROTID DOPPLER IMAGING

Background

The techniques for real-time ultrasound evaluation of the carotid artery have been made possible over the last two decades by technologic advances. Olinger (64) was one of the earliest researchers to obtain pictures of the carotid artery and its plaques using B-mode ultrasound techniques. Essentially the technique involved enough energy and frequency levels in the transducer to emit sound in the 1 to 10 million cycles/s range with adequate energy levels to permit resolution of 1 mm or less at depths of up to 4 cm.

B-mode scanning is a brightness mode scanning with each point on a display representing the reflection from some structure and the brightness point representing the energy level of the reflected sound. Real time was introduced by displaying many images per second on a monitor in such a way that the eye could detect movement of the wall and structures within the wall of a moving vessel (82).

Two major techniques have been used to produce this elusion of movement. The first involved the linear array, by which large numbers of sound-emitting transducers would emit their sound and receive back the reflections. Alternating detectors would rapidly proceed down a line of similar detectors and emitters thus producing the elusion of motion. This technique allows plaque formation to be visualized but offers no information other than its presence.

A second technique utilizes a mirror that reflects the sound between 30 and 120 times/s. Using a single transducer or a circular array of transducers, this reflection resulted in a higher level of resolution and elimination of artifacts. Resolution of the wall of a carotid vessel has been dependent on the frequency of the emitted sound. Higher frequencies have the capability of deeper penetration. Carotid ultrasound examinations usually require a 7.5- to

10-MHz transducer. The square of the diameter of the transducer is directly proportional to the resolution capacity.

Duplex ultrasound, developed in the last decade, combines high-resolution B-mode imaging with Doppler analysis (Fig. 1). Traditional B-mode instruments designed for the abdomen are ineffective for the carotid examination because they do not possess adequate spatial or gray-scale resolution. Carotid examinations require specially designed instruments for near-field work (high-resolution, superficial-structure scanners). The Doppler components of the duplex instrument may be pulsed or continuous wave. All Doppler systems are designed to allow the operator to select the precise location of Doppler sampling within the B-mode display (72). This is accomplished by varying both the Doppler angle and the depth of the range gate from which the Doppler signals are accepted (Fig. 2).

Through advancements in computer technology and transducer design, duplex systems today have a two-dimensional color-coded flow image superimposed on a two-dimensional B-mode image (Fig. 2). All modern duplex devices utilize fast-Fourier-transform frequency spectrum analysis for processing Doppler shift information. Many systems are equipped with computer capabilities for measuring blood velocity ratios, spectral broadening, and blood flow (36). Flow characteristics can be displayed at certain points within a vessel while producing real-time images of the walls. Figure 3 demonstrates an abnormal spectral analysis that corresponds to luminal narrowing from atheromatous plaque. The addition of color flow helps to identify the presence of carotid lesions that are hemodynamic or contain ulcerations. An array of color intensities reflects eddying currents and blood flow turbulence not visualized on the traditional duplex instruments (Fig. 4).

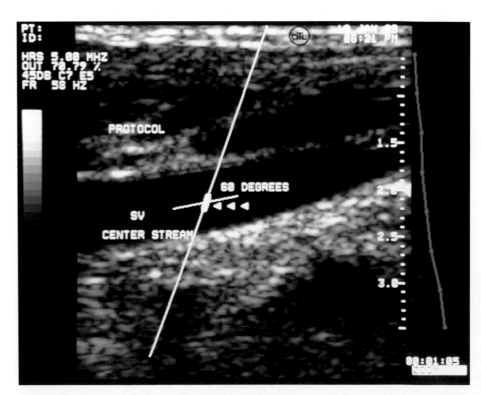

Figure 1. Carotid protocol. The sample volume is located in the center stream of the vessel with the angle 60° to the vessel axis.

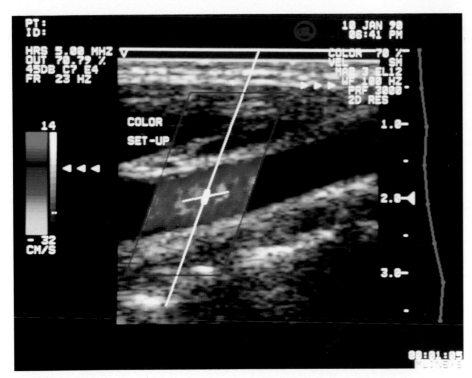

Figure 2. Color set-up. The arrows to the left define a recommended color map and the color scale. The zero baseline, demonstrated by blue, is one-third of the scale. Flow toward the brain is red and occupies two-thirds of the scale.

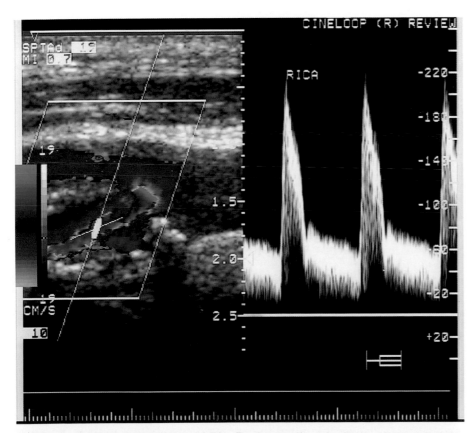

Figure 3. Abnormal spectral analysis. Peak systolic velocity is measured at the point of maximum stenosis. Greater than 250 cm/s corresponds to a critical stenosis of 80% to 90%.

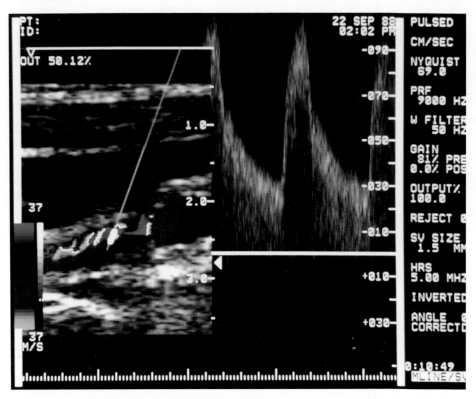

Figure 4. Hemodynamic lesion. Increased velocity is seen as a bright orange or white color jet. Turbulence is typically mottled in color flow imaging. Spectral analysis confirms hemodynamic state.

Sonic Anatomy of the Carotid Artery

The routine technique of demonstrating carotid vessels employs analysis of both cross sections and longitudinal sections (7). Longitudinal sections are taken in multiple planes so the internal carotid artery can be readily distinguished from the external carotid artery by virtue of the anatomic branching. The vessel wall demonstrates a fine distinct line that is an apparent intimal equivalent. While the reflection itself is not strictly the intima, it represents an intact internal lining structure for the vessel. This real-time image not only shows vessel anatomy but also demonstrates the presence of plaque formation that may extrude into the lumen. Cross-sectional analysis will give a more accurate picture of the exact degree of involvement. Real-time ultrasound gives information about vessel walls and plaque, and an angiogram evaluates the lumen alone with only indirect evidence on plaque (84).

Plaque Morphology

Plaques may be detected down to 1 mm in size and may display numerous sonic physiologic characteristics. Their location varies from anterior to posterior and from medial to lateral, but most are seen on the posterior medial wall. Their shape often has a stalagtite-like feature, with varying degrees of involvement. Plaques are noted to have marked variation in their presentation and are characterized as hard or soft depending on the intensity with which they reflect sound. The surface may be smooth or irregular, suggesting ulcerations. Ulcers are readily detected on longitudinal section and are easily identified with color-flow Doppler. Echogenicity refers to the echoes produced when sound waves are reflected from different tissue densities (46). Anechoic describes an echo-free region appearing the same as the flowing blood. Lipid deposits and intraplaque hemorrhage have a hypoechoic or low-level echogenicity. Hyperechoic plaques are bright (high-level) echoes associated with increased collagen content. These plaques demonstrate a phenomenon termed *shadowing*. One of the major difficulties encountered can be caused by the presence of a highly calcific plaque formation and its shadowing, which obscures visualization of the vessel lumen (Fig. 5). Plaque texture is characterized as homogenous or heterogenous. Uniform echo patterns over a smooth intimal surface are homogenous, whereas more complex echo patterns over irregularly shaped areas are referred to as heterogenic. Thrombus formations are weakly echogenic and considered to be homogenous (Fig. 6). Heterogenic plaque formations often contain ulcers and associated intraplaque hemorrhage (Fig. 7). Such ulcers are missed on angiograms because the contrast is kept out of the crater by the clot (8).

Role of Ultrasound in Screening

Real-time ultrasound is an extremely accurate and valuable test and is enhanced by the application of Doppler. Imaging alone can often detect the presence of a total occlusion (Fig. 8). In certain areas real-time analysis alone can be inaccurate (83). A totally occluded vessel leaving no stump may well be overlooked, or an external carotid artery that branches early may well be mistaken for a common carotid artery with its internal and external

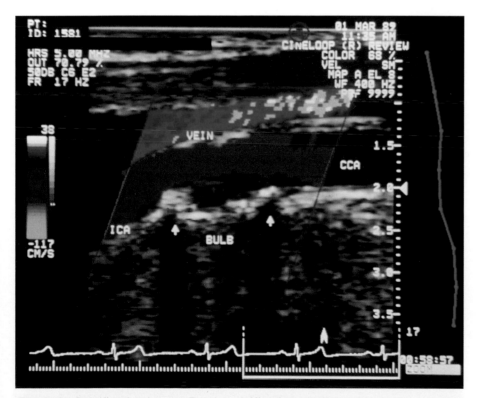

Figure 5. Calcification image. Dense calcification produces an acoustic shadow that obscures adequate visualization. Spectral analysis is needed to document flow velocity changes.

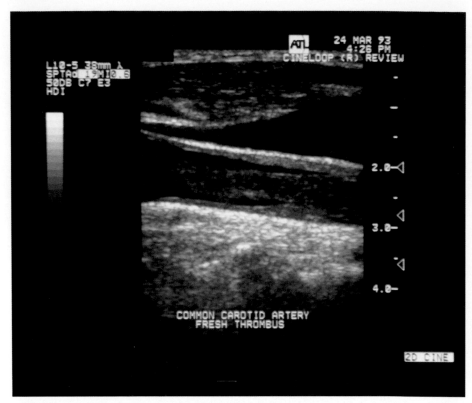

Figure 6. Carotid thrombus. Thrombus formations are demonstrated as speckled, weakly echogenic material filling the arterial lumen.

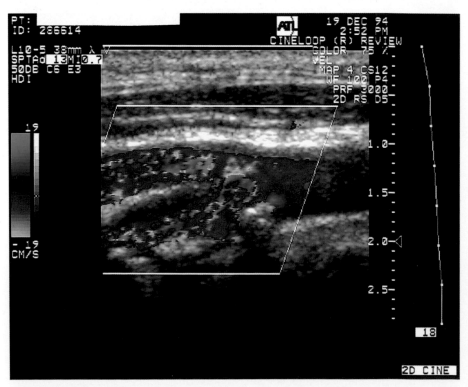

Figure 7. Heterogenic plaque formations. This type of plaque is complex and has a greater incidence of intraplaque hemorrhage and ulceration as seen here.

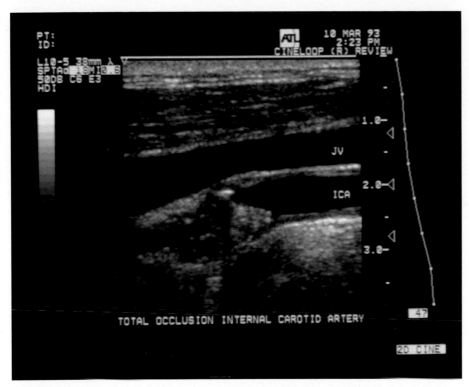

Figure 8. Total occlusion. This occlusive plaque has a complex echo pattern extending from the bifurcation into the internal carotid.

branches. A "normal" result could be obtained when in actuality the internal artery is occluded. Doppler analysis will prevent common mishaps. Furthermore, an extremely dense plaque may well preclude real-time analysis of softer plaque material and may cause the plaque to be underestimated. Doppler analysis within the hyperechoic shadowing can demonstrate much higher frequency shifts, alerting the technician to the fact that a higher degree of obstructive disease may actually be present.

Unique Principles and Concepts of Ultrasound

The major implication of hypertension as a risk factor in the production of stroke is well understood. Ultrasound has contributed an interesting and frightening addition to this story. We have observed many cases in which the plaque is quite large and the vessel is totally occluded during diastole and open at the 20% to 30% range during systole. This is frequently not appreciated during angiography, although we will often see a zone where no dye is appreciated between the common carotid and somewhere up the internal carotid artery and then a good column of dye beyond. This motion is clearly dependent on adequate pressure to continue the physiologic motions of the vessel and may well require a relatively hypertensive state to continue the adequate vascular motion in order to open the vessel for adequate flow during the cardiac cycle. It may well provide a good explanation for numerous strokes during orthostatic hypotensive episodes and during the relative orthostatic period of sleep. It certainly will also add to the concern of the clinician presented with a patient who is hypertensive and who has evidence of vascular disease, including bruits or previous TIAs. Knowledge of the anatomy of an extracranial vessel prior to antihypertensive therapy may well help us to prevent iatrogenic stroke.

The problems of showers of emboli or of multiple small infarcts and repeated small TIAs have been evaluated to a certain extent in the past by pathologic and angiographic studies and are now further studied by routine ultrasound investigation. Small emboli can come from very small apparently innocuous plaques, and we have routinely found small superficial ulcerations in what would appear to be otherwise smooth plaques. Correlation of this data needs to be obtained and tagged radioplatelet studies that are currently in progress may provide the evidence we are seeking. Furthermore, understanding the efficacy of antiplatelet and anticoagulant-type therapeutic regimens can be markedly enhanced with a noninvasive study allowing analysis of the wall of the extracranial vessels. The progression of plaques can be demonstrated in longitudinal form since ultrasound studies have been demonstrated to be highly replicable, and variations in a plaque over time are easily recognized. One need no longer look blindly for the result of a particular program, in terms of the final stroke result; we can now watch the pathologic process and intervene should there be signs of marked progression. Numerous studies need to be undertaken in a way superior to the previously blind statistical analyses, which required a much longer period and allowed a large number of tragedies to occur. Predicting who will be helped by aspirin may even allow certain numbers of women to use this therapy, even though statistical studies show no efficacy.

Follow-up studies in the postendarterectomy period have also been extremely valuable and have shown numerous cases in which large pieces of plaque material were left behind when the plaque was removed. These stalagtites have provided a source of emboli from clot formation and have often also acted as flap valves producing extremely tight blockade of flow. Repeat surgical procedures have been undertaken based on this noninvasive detection of remnant plaque and further angiographic analysis. Often, however, the symptomatology and the stalagtite have been unaccompanied by any angiographic evidence and surgery has been based on ultrasound evidence. Intraoperative ultrasound is now commercially available as a check on the completeness of plaque removal at surgery.

Summary

Duplex Doppler examination of extracranial carotid vessels has proved to be a valuable tool in the detection of atheromatous lesions. This technology incorporates both anatomic as well as physiologic information and has been a major reason for reduction in stroke over the last two decades. Numerous research studies are underway that will illuminate the efficacy of therapeutic and surgical interventions and provide us with an understanding of the nature of this progressive plaque disease.

INTRACRANIAL THROMBOLYSIS

Stroke is the third leading cause of death in North America and affects approximately 500,000 people each year in the United States alone (19,81). Among the patients who survive a stroke, significant functional deficit occurs. Of all the different etiologies, thromboembolic occlusion remains the most common cause of ischemic stroke. The primary step in preventing strokes is to identify patients with risk factors such as hypertension or diabetes mellitus and try to modify them. A secondary preventive measure would be to recognize patients at significant risk of stroke such as those with TIAs. Treatment of these patients is the subject of review in this book.

The tertiary preventive method is to implement treatment that would reduce the area of infarction and decrease the sequelae of ischemic stroke. This generally involves acute intervention with medications such as calcium-channel blockers (60), glutamate-receptor antagonists (12), or opiate-receptor antagonists (6). The aim is to reduce the "penumbra" area around the infarct, thus hopefully decreasing the actual area of infarct and minimizing the extent of resulting neurologic deficit.

Another method being studied involves the use of thrombolytic agents to recanalize the thrombosed vessel. One way of doing this is to give thrombolytic drugs intravenously. Brott et al. (11) reported on 74 patients who received intravenous recombinant tissue plasminogen activator at 0.35 to 1.08 mg/kg for acute stroke. Thirty-percent of patients had measured neurologic improvement by 2 hours after initiation of treatment, and 46% had improvement at 24 to 48 hours. A major risk of therapy remains conversion of a bland stroke to a hemorrhagic one. However, none of the patients who received recombinant tissue plasminogen tissue activator less than 0.58 mg/kg had a hemorrhagic stroke. This is currently being studied further in a randomized trial (10).

Using a rabbit model, Mohr et al. (57) demonstrated that intra-arterial administration of thrombolytic agents can produce a more rapid and a more effective thrombolysis with a smaller amount of the thrombolytic agent. Cardiac studies have also shown that a lower rate of systemic hemorrhagic complications may be seen with intra-arterial delivery of thrombolytic agents in patients with coronary occlusion (22).

With the recent development of microcatheter and guidewire technology, it is now possible to catheterize intracranial vessels subselectively with minimal morbidity and mortality. Microcatheter technology and the positive results from experimental and clinical cardiac trials have prompted efforts to apply this technique in acute treatment of stroke. Initial studies have been limited to patients presenting within 6 hours of onset of symptoms, similar to the intravenous thrombolytic therapy protocol. Many randomized trials are currently in progress utilizing different agents such as urokinase (Fig. 9), prourokinase (which is a precursor of urokinase), and recombinant tissue plasminogen activator.

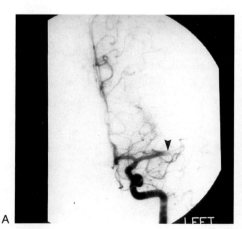 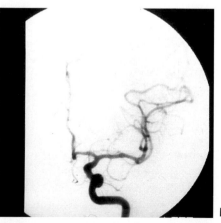

Figure 9. A 49-year-old man presented with a left hemisphere stroke secondary to a cardiac emboli. An anterior posterior angiogram demonstrated occlusion of the middle cerebral artery (*arrows,* **A**). A microcatheter was placed in the clot and 750,000 U of urokinase was delivered over 1 hour with complete recanalization and dramatic clinical improvement **(B)**.

Barnwell et al. (5) reported ten patients who had successful vessel recanalization with significant clinical improvement following intra-arterial thrombolytic treatment. The key to this thrombolytic treatment is early intervention, for which it is crucial that the general population recognize early signs and symptoms of stroke and seek help in a expeditious fashion.

CAROTID ANGIOPLASTY

Dotter and Judkins (24) introduced flexible dilators for angioplasty of femoral and iliac arteries. In 1974, Gruntzig and Hopff (37) made a major contribution by introducing a double-lumen balloon catheter. Since then, percutaneous transluminal angioplasty (PTA) has played a significant role in treatment of occlusive disease of renal, coronary, and extremity arteries. Angioplasty of supra-aortic arteries has been slower to gain acceptance. Kerber et al. (49) and Mullen et al. (59) in 1980 first reported angioplasty of carotid arteries. Since then, many cases of successful carotid angioplasties have been reported (32,43,75,77).

Tsai et al. (77) in 1986 reported a series of 27 patients who had 29 PTAs; of these, 78% had atherosclerotic lesions. The average age of patients was 72 (range, 34 to 84 years). In this series, a dramatic reduction in stenosis was seen, but all lesions were not quantified. All patients were doing well 3 to 4 months after the procedure. Limited long-term follow-up is available, but 8 patients demonstrated evidence of no restenosis 4 months to 4 years after PTA. Theron (74) reported on his experience with 32 cases of atherosclerotic lesion of the common carotid artery bifurcation. In this study, 12% of patients had permanent neurologic deficits secondary to embolism (9%), or vessel dissection (3%). Theron further modified the PTA method by introducing a distal balloon for protection from embolism. He reported on 51 patients with carotid atherosclerotic lesions. Using cerebral protection, only 2% of the patients had permanent neurologic deficits from vessel dissection, and no case of embolism was observed. In spite of this series with very good results, a potential risk of distal embolism, rupture of the vessel wall, and carotid thrombosis remains (74). Embolization and stroke have not proved to be as great a risk as predicted from atherosclerotic stenosis of the carotid artery (1,75,77).

Patients with intracranial atherosclerotic lesions are difficult to treat surgically, but they can be offered an alternative with PTA. Many small series report a beneficial effect for PTA. Ferguson et al. (29) established the North American Cerebral Percutaneous Transluminal Angioplasty Register (NAC-PTAR) to evaluate a multicenter study of clinical and angiographic outcome following PTA in patients with intracranial atherosclerosis who were not candidates for surgical treatment. They reported 102 patients who had 113 angioplastic procedures. The average stenosis before angioplasty was 80% and was reduced to 30% after PTA, a statistical difference ($p < 0.0001$). Complications that were seen in 13.7% of the patients included death (two patients), stroke, and TIA. However, the natural history of intracranial atherosclerotic lesions should be kept in mind while interpreting these results. These carry a high morbidity and mortality. Occlusion of the middle cerebral artery with atherosclerosis carries an immediate mortality of about 30% and poor outcome in over 50% of cases (1). Occlusion of an atherosclerotic basilar artery resulted in death in 86% of the cases (38). Clearly intracranial angioplasty offers a good treatment modality. It is being modified continuously to decrease the morbidity and mortality.

At this point in time, PTA is not a total substitute for surgical management—which achieves good results. Angioplasty has a role in patients who are not good surgical candidates due to risk of anesthesia, coronary artery disease, age, or location of atherosclerotic plaque.

Technique

A 6-F Cordis Envoy catheter (Cordis, Miami, FL) is inserted through the femoral artery and positioned in the appropriate vessel, e.g., common carotid or vertebral artery proximal to the lesion (1) (Fig. 10). We commonly use a Stealth balloon (Target, Freemont, CA) for atherosclerotic lesions. Initial diagnostic angiography is performed using "washers" to measure the parent vessel size and the degree of stenosis. Based on this, appropriate-sized balloons are selected. The balloons are bench tested with nonionic, full-strength Isovue 260 contrast media. A Stealth has only a single lumen through which a guidewire is placed and protrudes through the distal balloon lumen. Using the real-time digital subtraction angiography technique, the balloon is placed through the guide catheter and across the stenosis. Next, the steerable guidewire is removed from the Stealth balloon, and a special occlusion wire that allows closure of the distal part of the balloon for inflation is placed. The occluding valve wire is locked in place with a torque device and inflation of the Stealth balloon is then performed up to 8 to 10 atmospheres of pressure for up to 5 to 10 seconds for each inflation. After the angioplasty, postprocedure angiography is performed through the guide catheter. If a good result is seen, the balloon is removed. The patient is monitored in the intensive care unit, remains on heparin for 24 to 48 hours, and is maintained on aspirin postoperatively (Fig. 11).

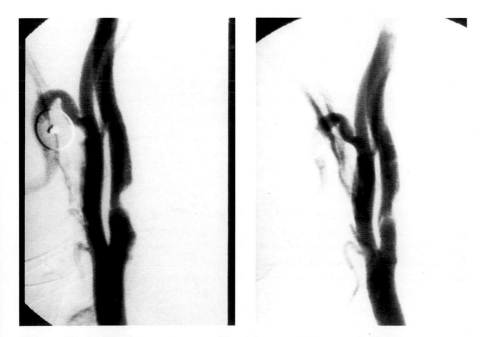

Figure 10. A lateral common carotid angiogram demonstrating proximal internal carotid atherosclerosis preangioplasty **(A)** and postangioplasty **(B)**.

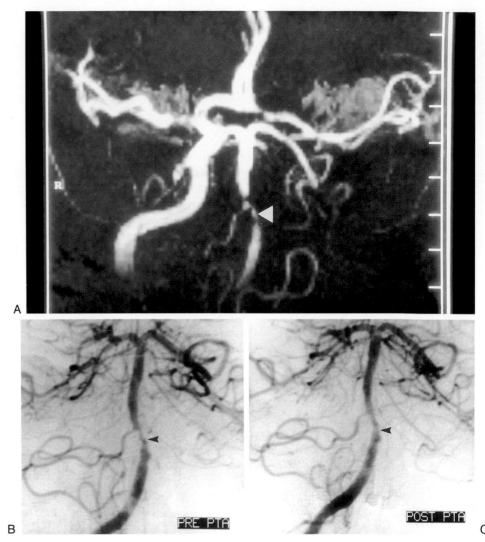

Figure 11. A: A magnetic resonance angiography of a 65-year-old demonstrating a midbasilar stenosis (*arrow*) in a patient with posterior circulation transient ischemic attacks that were unresponsive to medical treatment. **B:** An anterior posterior vertebral angiography demonstrated atherosclerotic stenosis (*arrow*) of the basilar artery. **C:** An angioplasty with a Stealth balloon was performed with good angiographic and clinical results (*arrow*).

FIBROMUSCULAR DYSPLASIA

Fibromuscular dysplasia (FMD) is uncommon and of unknown etiology (21,71). It usually involves primary aortic branches in a nonatheromatous segmental pattern. Cerebral FMD is most often seen in middle-aged women. The diagnosis is usually made when the patients are being evaluated for ischemic, hemorrhagic, or nonspecific neurologic symptoms. The most common angiographic pattern is a "string of beads" (Fig. 12), thought to be secondary to ridges of fibroproliferative tissue. The most common location of FMD is the distal internal carotid artery (65), but it can also affect vertebral and intracranial arteries. In approximately 15% of cases, the patients also have renal FMD, which usually occurs in younger patients and can present with hypertension. In 60% to 86% of patients, FMD affects the bilateral

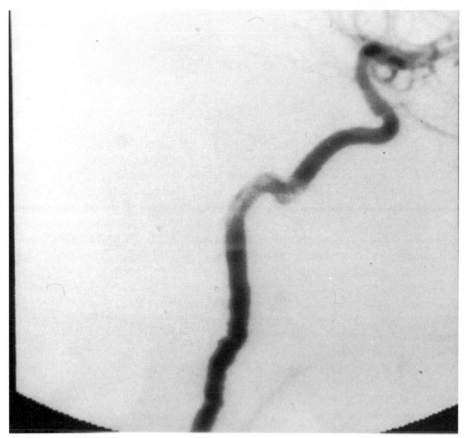

Figure 12. A 55-year-old woman had angiography for subarachnoid hemorrhage. Cervical angiography demonstrated irregular zones of widening and narrowing of vessel lumen consistent with fibromuscular dysplasia.

internal carotid artery. A higher incidence of cerebral aneurysms is seen in patients with FMD.

The relationship between cerebral FMD and ischemic symptoms is not very clear. Patients with FMD clearly present with ischemic symptoms in selective cases. Two mechanisms may be responsible for the ischemic symptoms. The "string of beads" pattern can produce a hemodynamically significant stenosis secondary to each ring of fibrous muscular proliferation, causing stenosis, which is additive and can produce significant stenosis. Another etiology may be the formation of thrombosis due to rheology change in blood in the vicinity of a web, which can be seen as a source of emboli (25,55,56,71). However, all these factors may not be of major significance clinically. Corrin et al. (21) observed only three ischemic events occurring in 79 patients followed for an average of 5 years. In this series, up to one-half of the patients had atherosclerotic lesions appropriate to their symptoms (21,71). In view of these findings, the angiographic finding should be interpreted cautiously and the angiographic and clinical findings need to be correlated. Patients should have medical management initially and surgical or endovascular therapy considered in case of medical management failure. Surgical approach is limited due to the high location of FMD (in the carotid vessel near the skull base), which is associated with greater surgical morbidity and mortality (26).

Earlier, transluminal dilatation was done by biliary duct dilators (26,71,73). These are rigid dilators introduced via a carotid arteriotomy. Better results have been obtained with PTA through a transfemoral approach. The technique of transluminal angioplasty is similar to the angioplastic technique described earlier.

RADIATION-INDUCED ANGIOPLASTY

The long-term side effects of radiation are gaining clinical significance as the life expectancy of cancer patients increases. Radiation can affect normal tissue and can lead to vasculopathy. After cervical radiation, patients may have symptomatic radiation-induced carotid angiopathy (20). Physicians have recognized this as the cause of TIA as patients survive longer after radiation therapy (4,13). Radiation-induced large-vessel atheromatous disease has become a well-recognized condition since the first experimental and clinical observations in the 1940s and 1950s (20). Symptomatic radiation-induced carotid artery stenosis was first described by Glick (35) in 1972, and additional case reports have followed (13,20,27). Attempts have been made to determine the incidence and risk factors of this disease; however, the incidence, natural history, associated predisposing risk factors, and relationship to site and dose of radiation are still unknown (27,32,35).

Elerding et al. (27) found a 6.3% incidence of stroke in 910 patients who had had previous radiation for Hodgkin's lymphoma, non-Hodgkin's lymphoma, and head and neck cancer. They also prospectively evaluated 118 patients with carotid artery stenosis for a 9-year period (27). Carotid duplex imaging was abnormal in 25% of patients who had received previous radiation and abnormal in 6.4% of nonirradiated patients. Moritz et al. reported a 30% incidence of moderate-to-severe stenosis with carotid duplex imaging in 53 irradiated patients followed for an average of 28 months; this was a fivefold higher incidence of stenosis than observed in a nonirradiated group. Clearly, atherosclerotic process is accelerated in irradiated lesions. The etiology is presumed to be a premature and progressive atherosclerosis (43). Time between irradiation and onset of symptoms has ranged from 3 months to 30 years. Completed strokes carry a high morbidity and mortality (43,48).

Atkinson et al. (4) reported seven patients with radiation-associated atheromatous disease of the cervical carotid artery and reviewed the literature. The authors identified a certain group of patients who exhibited less evidence of coronary and peripheral vascular disease and demonstrated a tendency for unusual distribution of atheromatous disease compared with a control group. These patients also had extensive postradiation skin atrophy and fibrosis of tissues overlying the radiation-induced stenotic lesions. Others have found these lesions to be extensive and circumferential on angiography (27,69). Extensive scarring in the cervical region and the extreme adherence of plaque to the vessel wall make surgical resection difficult, sometimes necessitating resection of arterial segments (4). Radiation-induced angiopathic lesions in the cervical segment of the carotid artery are usually long and adhere to the vessel wall, posing a higher risk during surgical resection than shorter atherosclerotic lesions of the carotid bifurcation (70). Surgical intervention is discouraging due to the extent of the lesion as well as the high chance of causing cranial nerve palsies from dissection in radiation-induced scar tissue. A less invasive transfemoral PTA technique has been recommended for high-risk surgical candidates or for patients with lesions that encompass a long segment of carotid or that are surgically inaccessible (4) (Fig. 13).

Angioplasty of the cerebral vessels is not without risk. Since radiation-induced plaques are extremely adherent, transluminal angioplasty may offer a theoretical advantage by affording less likelihood of distal embolization. The risk of vessel rupture may be reduced by choosing a balloon with a

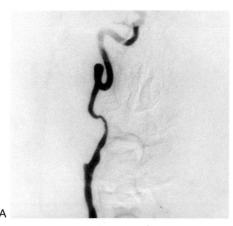
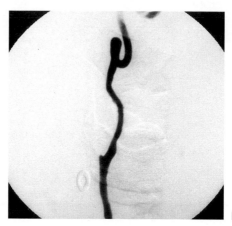

A   B

Figure 13. A 62-year-old woman who presented with right hemispheric transient ischemic attacks. Her history is significant for a laryngeal carcinoma that had been previously operated on and received radiation. An anteroposterior common carotid angiography demonstrated long stenosis of the right internal carotid artery **(A)**. Patient had carotid angioplasty with good angiographic results **(B)** and no neurologic deficits. Patient continues to remain asymptomatic 6 months after angioplasty.

maximal inflation diameter that does not exceed the vessel's original luminal diameter. Vessel wall fibrosis in radiation-induced carotid artery stenosis may also afford an additional measure of safety. Ahuja et al. (2) reported an example of radiation-induced bilateral carotid atherosclerosis successfully treated with PTA. Percutaneous angioplasty in an awake patient offers the advantage that the neurologic examination may be performed during this procedure. In addition, avoiding the risk of general anesthesia in a patient population that frequently has serious medical contraindications to anesthesia reduces morbidity and mortality. The hospital stay and recuperation time are greatly diminished when compared with routine surgical intervention.

Considerable experience is accumulating with angioplasty for cervical carotid bifurcation and internal carotid artery atherosclerotic narrowing. Potential risks are considerable, and methods for protecting the cranial circulation against distal embolization during angioplasty are being developed. Initial results are promising, and in some cases angioplasty may eventually replace carotid endarterectomy.

REFERENCES

1. Ahuja A, Gutenman LR, Hopkins LN. Angioplasty for basilar artery atherosclerosis. Case report. *J Neurosurg* 1992;77:941–944.
2. Ahuja A, Blatt GL, Gutenman LR, Hopkins LN. Angioplasty for symptomatic radiation-induced extracranial carotid artery stenosis: core report. *Neurosurgery* 1995;36 (*in press*).
3. The Asymptomatic Carotid Atherosclerosis Study Group. Study design for randomized prospective trial of carotid endarterectomy for asymptomatic atherosclerosis. *Stroke* 1989; 20:844–849.
4. Atkinson JLD, Sundt TM Jr, Dale AJD, Cascino TL, Nichols DA. Radiation-associated atheromatous disease of the cervical carotid artery: report of seven cases and review of the literature. *Neurosurgery* 1989;24:171–178.
5. Barnwell SL, Clark WM, Nguyen TT, et al. Safety and efficacy of delayed intraarterial urokinase therapy with mechanical clot disruption for thromboembolic stroke. *AJNR* 1994; 15:1817–1822.
6. Biller J. Medical management of acute cerebral ischemia. In: Barnett HJM, Hachinski V, eds. *Cerebral ischemia: treatment and prevention. Neurol Clin* 1992;10:67.
7. Blasberg DJ. Duplex sonography for carotid artery disease: an accurate technique. *AJNR* 1982;3:609–614.

8. Bluth EL, McVay LV, Merritt CR, Sullivan MA. Identification of ulcerative plaque with high resolution duplex carotid scanning. *J Ultrasound Med* 1988;7:73–76.

9. Bogousslavsky J, Despland P-A, Regli F. Asymptomatic tight stenosis of the internal carotid artery: long term prognosis. *Neurology* 1986;36:861–863.

10. Bozzao L, Fantozzi LM, Bastianello S, Bossao A, Fieschl C. Early collateral blood supply and late parenchymal brain damage in patients with middle cerebral artery occlusion. *Stroke* 1989;20:735–740.

11. Brott TG, Haley EC Jr, Levy DE, et al. Urgent therapy for stroke: part I. Pilot study of tissue plasminogen activator administered within 90 minutes. *Stroke* 1992;23:632–640.

12. Buchan AM, Xue D, Huang Z-G, et al. Delayed AMPA receptor blockade reduces cerebral infarction induced by focal ischemia. *Neuroreport* 1992;2:473–476.

13. Byhardt RW, Moss WT. The heart and blood vessels. In: Moss WT, Cox JD, eds. *Radiation oncology. Rationale, technique, results*. St. Louis: CV Mosby;1989:277–284.

14. Caracci BF, Zukowski AJ, Hurley JJ, Neunheim KS, Auet AI. Asymptomatic severe carotid stenosis. *J Vasc Surg* 1989;9:361–366.

15. The CASANOVA Study Group. Carotid surgery versus medical therapy in asymptomatic carotid stenosis. *Stroke* 1991;22:1229–1235.

16. Caserella WJ. Noncoronary angioplasty. Results and complications of percutaneous transluminal angioplasty. *Curr Probl Cardiol* 1986;11:155–165.

17. Chambers BR, Norris JW. Clinical significance of asymptomatic neck bruits. *Neurology (NY)* 1985;35:742.

18. Chambers BR, Norris JW. Outcome in patients with asymptomatic neck bruits. *N Engl J Med* 1986;315:860–865.

19. Chambers BR, Norris JW, Shurvell BL, et al. Prognosis of acute stroke. *Neurology* 1987; 37:221–225.

20. Conomy JP, Kellermeyer RW. Delayed cerebrovascular consequences of therapeutic radiation. A clinicopathologic study of a stroke associated with radiation-related carotid arteriopathy. *Cancer* 1975;36:1702–1708.

21. Corrin LS, Sandok BA, Houser OW. Cerebral ischemic events in patients with carotid artery fibromuscular dysplasia. *Arch Neurol* 1981;38:616–618.

22. Del Zoppo GJ, Ferbert A, Otis S, et al. Local intra-arterial fibrinolytic therapy in acute carotid territory stroke. *Stroke* 1988;19:307–313.

23. DeMonte F, Peerless SJ, Rankin RN. Carotid transluminal angioplasty with evidence of distal embolization. Case report. *J Neurosurg* 1989;70:138–141.

24. Dotter CT, Judkins MP. Transluminal treatment of arteriosclerotic obstruction. Description of a new technic and a preliminary report of its application. *Circulation* 1964;30: 654–670.

25. Effeney DJ, Ehrenfeld WK, Stoney RJ, Wylie EJ. Fibromuscular dysplasia of the internal carotid artery. *World J Surg* 1979;3:179–186.

26. Ehrenfeld WK, Wylie EJ. Fibromuscular dysplasia of the internal carotid artery. Surgical management. *Arch Surg* 1974;109:676–681.

27. Elerding SC, Fernandez RN, Grotta JC, Lindberg RD, Causay LC, McMurtrey MJ. Carotid artery disease following external cervical irradiation. *Ann Surg* 1981;194:609–615.

28. Ferguson R. Getting it right the first time. *AJNR* 1990;11:875–877.

29. Ferguson RDG, Ferguson JG, Lee LI. Endovascular revascularization therapy in cerebral athero-occlusive disease. In: Hopkins LN, ed. *Neurosurgery clinics of North America*. Philadelphia: WB Saunders; 1994;511–527.

30. Fisher CM. Cranial bruit associated with occlusion of the internal carotid artery. *Neurology (NY)* 1957;7:299.

31. Freischlag JA, Hanna D, Moore WS. Improved prognosis for asymptomatic carotid stenosis with prophylactic carotid endarterectomy. *Stroke* 1992;23:479–482.

32. Freitag G, Freitag J, Koch RD, Wagemann W. Percutaneous angioplasty of carotid artery stenoses. *Neuroradiology* 1986;28:126–127.

33. Furlan AJ. Natural history of atherothromboembolic occlusion of cerebral arteries: carotid vs vertebrobasilar territories. In: Macke, et al., eds. *Thrombolytic therapy in acute ischemic stroke*. Berlin: Springer-Verlag:1991.

34. Garrido E, Montoya J. Transluminal dilatation of internal carotid artery in fibromuscular dysplasia: a preliminary report. *Surg Neurol* 1981;16:469–471.

35. Glick B. Bilateral carotid occlusive disease following irradiation for carcinoma of the vocal cords. *Arch Pathol* 1972;93:352–355.

36. Grant EG, Tessler FN, Perrella RR. Clinical Doppler imaging. *AJR* 1989;152:707–717.

37. Gruntzig A, Hopff H. Perkutane Rekanalisation chronischer arterieller verschlusse mit einem neuen Dilatationskatheter. Modifikation der Dotter-technik. *Dtsch Med Wochenschr* 1974;99:2502–2505.

38. Hacke W, Zeumer H, Ferbett A. Intra-arterial thrombolytic therapy improves outcome in patients with acute vertebrobasilar occlusive disease. *Stroke* 1988;19:1216.

39. Hasso AN, Bird CR, Zinke DE, Thompson JR. Fibromuscular dysplasia of the internal carotid artery: percutaneous transluminal angioplasty. *AJR* 1981;136:955–960.

40. Hayward RH. Arteriosclerosis induced by radiation. *Surg Clin North Am* 1972;52:359–366.

41. Hennerichi M, Hulsbomer H-B, Hefter H, Lammerts D, Rautenberg W. Natural history of asymptomatic arterial disease. Results of a long-term prospective study. *Brain* 1987;110: 777–791.

42. Heyman A, Wilkinson WE, Heyden S, et al. Risk of stroke in asymptomatic persons with cervical bruits. *N Engl J Med* 1980;302:838–841.

43. Higashida RT, Tsai FY, Halbach VV, et al. Transluminal angioplasty for atherosclerotic disease of the vertebral and basilar arteries. *J Neurosurg* 1993;78:192–198.
44. Hobson RW II, Weiss DG, Fields WS, et al. Efficacy of carotid endarterectomy for asymptomatic carotid stenosis. *N Engl J Med* 1993;328:221–227.
45. Howard VJ, Howard G, Harpold GJ, et al. Correlation of carotid bruits and carotid atherosclerosis detected by B-mode real-time ultrasonography. *Stroke* 1989;20:1331.
46. Imparato AM, Riles TS, Gorstein F. The carotid bifurcation plaque: pathologic findings associated with cerebral ischemia. *Stroke* 1979;10:238–245.
47. Javid H, Ostermiller WE, Hengesh JW, et al. Natural history of carotid bifurcation atheroma. *Surgery* 1970;67:80–83.
48. Kadir S, White RI Jr, Kaufman SL. Prevention of thromboembolic complications of angioplasty by critical patient selection. Presented at the 82nd Annual Meeting of the American Roentgen Ray Society, New Orleans, Louisiana, May 10–14, 1982.
49. Kerber CW, Cromwell LD, Loehden OL. Catheter dilatation of proximal carotid stenosis during distal bifurcation endarterectomy. *AJNR Am J Neuroradiol* 1980;1:348–349.
50. Lamberts HB, DeBoer WGRM. Contributions to the study of immediate and early x-ray reactions with regard to chemoprotection. VII. X-ray-induced atheromatous lesions in the arterial wall of hypercholesterolaemic rabbits. *Int J Radiat Biol* 1963;6:343–350.
51. Libman RB, Sacco RL, Shih T, et al. Outcome after carotid endarterectomy for asymptomatic carotid stenosis. *Surg Neurol* 1994;41:443–449.
52. Mayo Asymptomatic Carotid Endarterectomy Study Group. Results of a randomized controlled trial of carotid endarterectomy for asymptomatic carotid stenosis. *Mayo Clin Proc* 1992;67:513–518.
53. Meissner I, Wiebers DO, Whisnant JP, O'Fallon WM. The natural history of carotid artery occlusive lesions. *JAMA* 1987;258:2704–2707.
54. Messert B, Marra TR, Zerofsky RA. Supraclavicular and carotid bruits in hemodialysis patients. *Ann Neurol* 1977;2:535–536.
55. Mettinger KL. Fibromuscular dysplasia and the brain: II. Current concept of the disease. *Stroke* 1982;13:53–58.
56. Mettinger KL, Ericson K. Fibromuscular dysplasia and the brain: observations on angiographic, clinical and genetic characteristics. *Stroke* 1982;13:46–52.
57. Mohr JP, Gautier JC, Hier DB, Stein RW. Middle cerebral artery. In: Barnett HJM, Stein BM, Mohr JP, Yatsu FM, eds. *Stroke*. New York: Churchill Livingstone ;1986:377–450.
58. Moneta GL, Taylor DC, Nicholls SC, et al. Operative versus non-operative management of asymptomatic high-grade internal carotid artery stenosis: improved results with endarterectomy. *Stroke* 1987;18:1005–1010.
59. Mullen S, Duda EE, Patronas NJ. Some examples of balloon technology in neurosurgery. *J Neurosurg* 1980;52:321–329.
60. Murphy J. UK-calcium antagonist trial (TRUST). *J Neurol* 1990;237:130.
61. National Institute of Neurological Disorders and Stroke. Clinical advisory: carotid endarterectomy for patients with asymptomatic internal carotid artery stenosis. NIH, September 28, 1994.
62. Norris JW. Head and neck bruits in stroke prevention. In: Norris JW, Hachinski VC, eds. *Prevention of stroke*. New York: Springer-Verlag;1991:103.
63. Norris JW, Zhu CZ, Bornstein NM, Chambers BR. Vascular risks of asymptomatic carotid stenosis. *Stroke* 1991;22:1485–1490.
64. Olinger CP. Ultrasonic carotid echoarteriography. *AJR Radium Ther Nucl Med* 1969,106. 282–295.
65. Osborn AG, Anderson RE. Angiographic spectrum of cervical and intracranial fibromuscular dysplasia. *Stroke* 1977;8:617–626.
66. Pessin MS, Paris W, Prager RJ, et al. Ausculation of cervical and ocular bruits in extracranial occlusive carotid disease. *Stroke* 1983;14:246.
67. Roederer GO, Langlois YE, Jager KA, et al. The natural history of carotid arterial disease in asymptomatic patients with cervical bruits. *Stroke* 1984;15:605–613.
68. Sams A. Histological changes in the larger blood vessels of the hind limb of the mouse after x-irradiation. *Int J Radiat Biol* 1965;9:165–174.
69. Silverberg GD, Britt RH, Goffinet DR. Radiation-induced carotid artery disease. *Cancer* 1978;41:130–137.
70. Smith RR. Radiation-associated atheromatous disease of the cervical carotid artery: report of seven cases and review of the literature [Comment]. *Neurosurgery* 1989;24:178.
71. So EL, Toole JF, Dalal P, Moody DM. Cephalic fibromuscular dysplasia in 32 patients: clinical findings and radiologic features. *Arch Neurol* 1981;38:619–622.
72. Spencer MP. Frequency spectrum analysis in Doppler diagnosis. In: Zeiebel WJ, ed. *Introduction to vascular ultrasonography*. Florida: Grune & Stratton;1986:53–81.
73. Starr DS, Lawrie GM, Morris GC Jr. Fibromuscular disease of carotid arteries: long term results of graduated internal dilatation. *Stroke* 1981;12:196–199.
74. Theron J. Angioplasty of brachiocephalic vessels. In: Vinnela F, et al., eds. *Interventional neuroradiology: endovascular therapy of the central nervous system*. New York: Raven Press;167–181.
75. Theron J, Raymond J, Casasco A, Courtheoux F. Percutaneous angioplasty of atherosclerotic and postsurgical stenosis of carotid arteries. *AJNR Am J Neuroradiol* 1987;8:495–500.
76. Thompson JE, Patman RD, Talkington CM. Asymptomatic carotid bruit: long-term outcome of patients having endarterectomy compared with unoperated controls. *Ann Surg* 1978;188:308–316.

77. Tsai FY, Matovich V, Hieshima G, et al. Percutaneous transluminal angioplasty of the carotid artery. *AJNR Am J Neuroradiol* 1986;7:349–358.

78. Wiebers DO, Folger WN, Forbes GS, et al. Ophthalmodynamometry and ocular pneumoplethysmography for detection of carotid occlusive disease. *Arch Neurol* 1982;39: 690–691.

79. Wiebers DO, Whisnant JP, Sandok BA, O'Fallon WM. Prospective comparison of a cohort with asymptomatic carotid bruit and a population-based cohort without carotid bruit. *Stroke* 1990;21:984–988.

80. Wolfe PA, Kannel WB, Sorlie P, McNamara P. Asymptomatic carotid bruit and risk of stroke. The Framingham study. *JAMA* 1981;245:1442–1445.

81. Wolf PA, Kannel WB, McGee DL. Epidemiology of strokes in North America. In: Barnett HJM, Stein BM, Mohr JP, et al. eds. *Stroke: pathophysiology, diagnosis, and management.* New York: Churchill Livingstone;1986:19–29.

82. Zagzebski JA. Physics and instrumentation in Doppler and B-mode ultrasonography. In: Zwiebel WJ, ed. *Introduction to vascular ultrasonography.* Florida: Grune & Stratton; 1986:53–81.

83. Zwiebel WJ, Crummy AB. Sources of error in Doppler diagnosis of carotid occlusive disease. *AJNR* 1981;2:231–242.

84. Zwiebel WJ, Austin CW, Sackett JF, et al. Correlation of high resolution B-mode and continuous wave Doppler sonography with arteriography in the diagnosis of carotid stenosis. *Radiology* 1983;149:523–532.

Subject Index

Subject Index